We
Are
Deageable

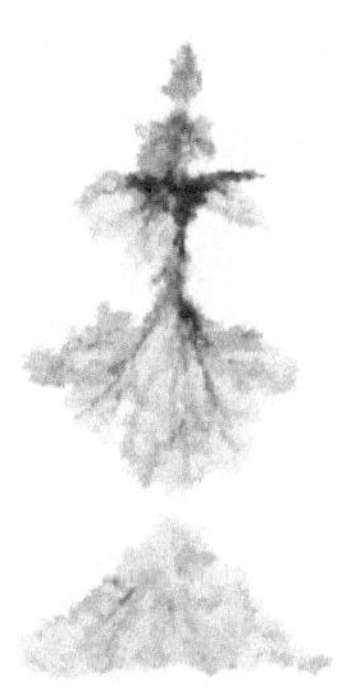

We can nutritionally slow down aging

and stay truly youthful

Anti-aging foods together with

lifestyle changes can help you live a longer

and disease-free life

Preface

Have you ever wondered why you couldn't open a stuck jar lid when you're 40? Or why you seem destined to get illnesses as you grow older? These are consequences of the waves of aging that first struck you at the age of 34, as well as lifestyle choices you made yesterday that lead you down the path of illness in later life.

These days, the most important thing in the world is not wealth, but health. As the old saying goes, health is something that can't be bought with money. If you're suffering from a serious illness like type 2 diabetes, heart disease and cancer, modern medicine is not a reliable path to a cure, but to palliative relief.

When I went to the rich house, I saw the rich ate boring expensive foods like fish maw, shark fin, abalone and sea cucumber. He said that these foods provide therapeutic benefits and boost his health. What he may not know is that there is a whole lot more healthful foods in nature than just these pricey bites.

As you age, you move to the stage of decline. But, in nature, there are anti-aging foods you can use to ward off the harm of aging and to arrest aging itself. Today, what harm your body the most are the accumulated insults of your aging cells and lifestyle choices you made yesterday. There are ways to nutritionally intervene in the aging process, protect you from chronic ailments of old age and prolong your vitality for as long as possible, which many people don't know how to do.

Throughout "We Are Deageable," I will show you how we can slow down or even reverse the aging process. You will see another corner of the power of natural, anti-aging foods and lifestyle changes that can strengthen cells in the body to slow down aging, fight diseases, and extend lifespan.

The mission of this book is to tell you the story of nasty diseases that afflict people. It also aims to explain a little about how the foods we eat can lead to health problems that often baffle us. Moreover, I exemplify some interruptions in my health that are the path less traveled. At the end it reveals how to obtain an ability to bounce back from ill health based on science that is important to extend lifespan, since your longevity depends on it.

I am not a medical-care provider. Although I, as a biochemist, have been studying and battling diseases for more than 20 years; some 80% of what I know has been learned through literature reviews, of which I would like to share with you. Hope that knowledge and techniques from this book can be applied to the fight against the chronic ailments of old age and can improve your health or even to extend your lifespan, because life beyond 90 or even 100 is a bonus.

However, this book does not provide treatment or medical advice, nor does it prescribe medication to the public. Before implementing any information from this book, it's important to carefully weigh the pros and cons. If you are currently taking medications or have existing health issues, it's advised to consult your physician or healthcare professional before beginning any dietary program suggested in this book. Still, I strongly believe that by committing to the natural and preventive practices outlined in this book, you can expect to enjoy a long life filled with health and prosperity.

Finally, if this book can assist you in achieving good health and help you avoid medication at the age of 60 and beyond, there is nothing that would bring me greater happiness. I can't imagine anything that would bring me more joy than that.

N. Tongyoo
tongyoo@uclmail.net

Choose what to read

Part 4

Part 1

CHAPTER 1

Your health is your wealth

"Life is like a box of chocolates. You never know what you're gonna get." This well-known quote is from the 1994 film Forrest Gump, in which Tom Hanks played the lead role. Like Forest Gump, I was once in the military too. But I felt I wasn't on the right career path. Then I started on my own career-change journey. I exposed to different career fields and I met people from diverse professions including farmers, teachers, doctors, nurses, soldiers, merchants and laborers. Though each of those people has a different occupation and social status, one thing that they have in common is a health problem.

Personally, I've never had to sit on a bench at a bus stop and listen to someone talking about his life for 3 hours until my ear off. But, by chance, I found myself listening to people sharing their stories of pain, despair, and the relentless struggles they and their loved ones faced due to illness. Oddly enough, I have heard people with health problems make statements such as.

"Having money or gold is unequal to good health" or
"Having millions of dollars isn't worth as much as having good health" or "If there is a pile of gold in front of me, while I am very sick, I don't care."
I heard those words a lot, but at that time I didn't feel anything. Until one day, I heard a word like those from my close friend who has $10 million in his net worth said something similar, "Millions of dollars aren't better than good health."

A different view of health and well-being

At a young age, it's common to feel as though you don't need to actively participate in taking care of your health. Typical thoughts might include, "My body is already healthy," or "I don't have any illnesses, so there's no need to exercise or look after myself." Often, people believe that medical professionals are solely responsible for their health. Many of us live for the moment, with no plans for tomorrow, and engage in unhealthy habits like drinking alcohol, smoking, and eating junk food, without taking proper care of themselves. One day, they may wake up in their 40s or 50s with a serious health issue, like diabetes and heart diseases, and find themselves regretting their past choices that can't be undone.

Take my friend, for example. She works tirelessly and, upon returning home, only wants to rest on her comfortable sofa. On weekends, she prefers to remain sedentary, reading Chinese novels on her phone while sipping iced coffee and consuming sweets. When I suggested she take time to exercise and avoid unhealthy foods, she ignored my advice. Like many others, she believes her body is in great shape and doesn't need exercise or dietary restrictions. She thinks she can eat whatever she wants. My friend is an example of someone who works hard towards financial security, aiming to enjoy life in retirement. While she strives for success in her career, she neglects her health.

Now, reflect on your own situation and ask yourself: can you be sure that future wealth will guarantee good health? What would success be without it? People often forget that money can't buy health, and without it, life can be miserable. If you value your health as much as a box of chocolates, be cautious not to consume them all at once, saving some for a rainy day.

As we've reached this point, many people may agree that a successful life is one with good health, not a life plagued by health problems. We can't reach our full potential if our souls are trapped in a physically ill body. Just as an injured athlete can't complete a race, a person with health issues may not be able to live their life to the fullest. From a broader perspective, health is a fundamental aspect of happiness as is one of our basic needs, alongside food, shelter, and clothing.

Test your perspective and understanding of health

People from diverse backgrounds might hold differing views on health, shaped by factors like age, education, and socio-economic status. Let's assess your understanding of health facts. Take a look at the next three simple questions—their answers might surprise you. Choose the response you believe is the most accurate.

Question 1. From the figures below, which sequence accurately represents the aging of skin?

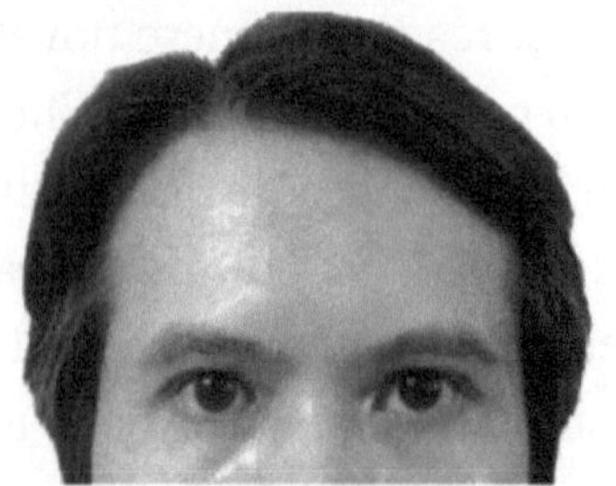

Figure (a)

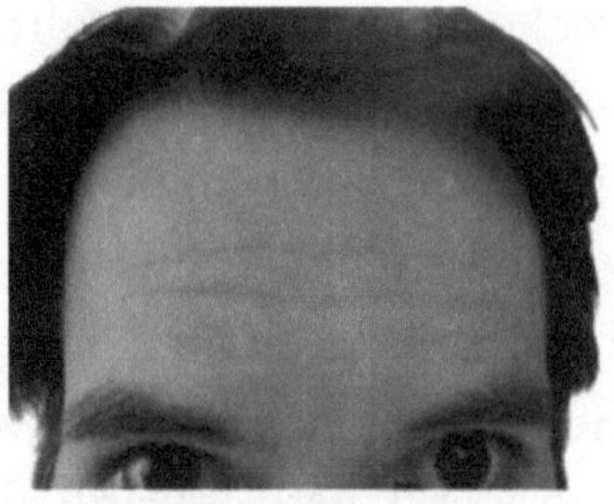

Figure (b)

☐ The sequence of aging skin is Figure (a) ➔ Figure (b)
☐ The sequence of aging skin is Figure (b) ➔ Figure (a)

Question 2. How long can humans potentially live?
☐ 120 years
☐ More than 120 years

Question 3. Can people reverse type 2 diabetes without medication?
☐ Yes
☐ No

***

Answers

Question 1. From the figures below, which sequence accurately represents the aging of skin?

Answer: The sequence of aging skin is Figure (a) ➔ Figure (b)

Question 2. How long can humans potentially live?

Answer: More than 120 years

Question 3. Can people reverse type 2 diabetes without medication?

Answer: Yes

Explained answer; how skin changes with age

Question 1. The natural aging process and the impact of various environmental factors contribute to skin changes over time, as depicted in Figure (a) and Figure (b). UV light, air pollution, and exposure to smoke are factors that can cause the breakdown of vital skin components like elastin, collagen, and hyaluronic acid. This leads to reduced skin elasticity, resulting in wrinkles, sagging, and thinning skin—particularly on the face. If you see more wrinkles, it might mean your body is aging quickly.

Let's talk about what wrinkles can tell us about your inner health. Cells in your body are continually dividing, but when cells become damaged or die, your body replaces them with new ones. Cell damage occurs not only in skin cells but also in all body tissues and organs, such as the heart, muscles, liver, and kidneys. As a result, the telltale signs of age-related cell degeneration within your body's tissues and organs may vividly emerge on your face. Wrinkles symbolize your body's message that the tissues and organs inside you are damaged.

But if you are still relatively young and just beginning to notice wrinkles on your face, there is a window of opportunity to rejuvenate your skin cells and minimize the appearance of these wrinkles. However, if it's too late, repairing damaged skin and removing wrinkles becomes difficult. If left untreated, over time, wrinkles can deepen, become more noticeable, and eventually permanent and irreversible.

In fact, Figure (a) is a photo I took recently in March 2020, while Figure (b) was captured five years ago. At the age of 45, I had the chance to rejuvenate my skin cells and eliminate my forehead wrinkles, allowing my skin cells to recover when it was still possible. Note that the following images have not been altered by any app or digital technique used to de-age a person or an actor in a photo or film.

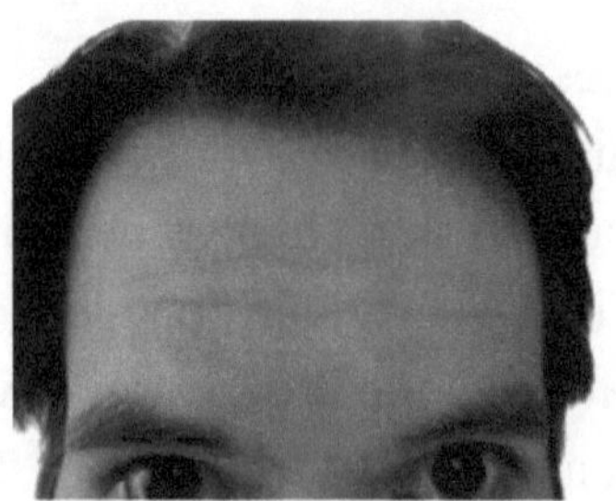

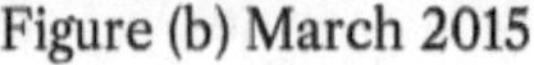

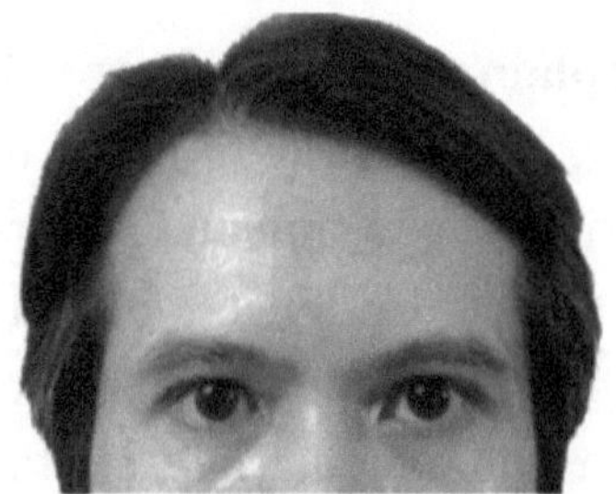

Figure (b) March 2015   ➜   Figure (a) April 2020

Forehead wrinkles that appear at a young age can be erased. The two photographs provided were captured using a digital camera (Sony Digital Camera, Model No. DSC-W310) and have not been altered or edited.

I believe there are others who have managed to achieve a more youthful appearance naturally. One such example is the famous movie actor Will Smith, who has maintained a youthful face over the years. Another notable example is singer-actor Jennifer Lopez, who, despite being over 50 years old, has managed to keep her face looking youthful. There is surely something special in their routines that bolsters their physical health and slows down, or even reverses, the aging process. The secret of de-aging could be within your grasp too!

The notion that certain lifestyle habits can slow down or even reverse the aging process is not a new concept. In recent years, there has been a growing interest in understanding the science of aging and the impact of specific lifestyle choices on how we age. It's true that lifestyle choices can significantly influence the way we age. However, it's crucial to recognize that genetics also play a significant role in the aging process. Actually, genes are vital when we're young, but as we age, how we live and our surroundings matter most, making up 70% of our chances of staying healthy. Genetics become less important, just 30%, as we get older. While we can't change our genetic makeup, we can make informed choices to support our bodies and minds as we grow older. By making better lifestyle choices, you can reduce aging's impact and enhance your life's quality over time, potentially extending your years. That's why I propose the idea of "We Are Deageable," suggesting we can counteract aging's effects, which is the essence of this book.

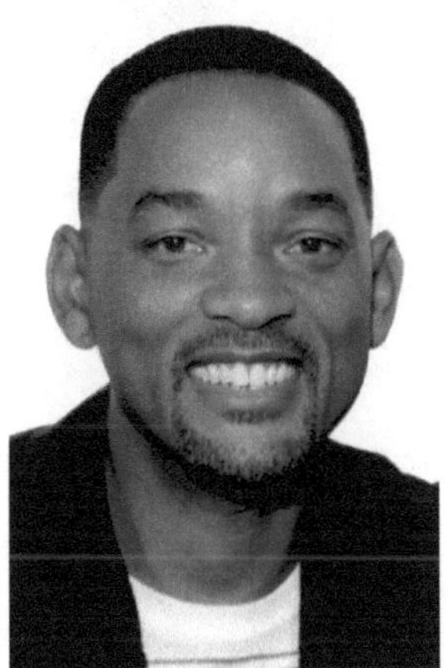

At the age of 51, Will Smith appears youthful, and he is able to run every morning.[1]

There is scientific proof that a person can really rejuvenate his or her body, defy aging or even reduce wrinkles on the skin by eating a healthy diet, getting enough sleep, exercising regularly and more,[2] in addition to the dark pigment that slows Will Smith's aging, However, neglecting self-care and health can have opposite effects.

Explained answer; humans can live beyond 120 years

Question 2. People can live longer than 120 years. The oldest human ever recorded is Jeanne Calment (1875-1997), who lived to be 122 years and 164 days old. Even at 100 years old, she could still ride a bike and walk around like most people. Her secret to longevity included a healthy diet consisting of extra virgin olive oil, 2 pounds of chocolate per week (an average of 100 g per day), and wine. Her record age remains unsurpassed to this day.

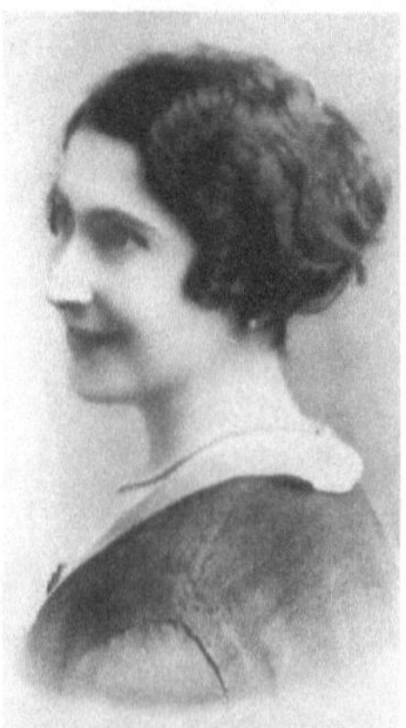

Jeanne Calment, pictured in 1915 at age 40, lived a record-setting 122 years.[3]

Did you know that even cells with the same genetic makeup and environment can age differently? In yeast, for example, half of the cells may experience aging due to a decline in DNA stability, while the other half ages as a result of mitochondrial dysfunction. As for human cells, they don't immediately die when damaged; instead, they become old cells first. However, there are only 4 ways human cells can die: cell death from stress, injury, self-destruction, and aging. In fact, around 60 billion cells, or 60 g of cells, die daily in your body. Don't be concerned, though. It's just the body's regular way of recycling cellular stuff.

Fascinatingly, yeast cells can live and reproduce indefinitely under the right conditions, unlike us humans. As we age, our cells accumulate damage, and our bodies' ability to repair this damage declines. This leads to declining health and, eventually, the end of life. This is the course of life's transitions.

Aging increases our likelihood of facing chronic health problems, such as heart disease, diabetes, and arthritis. Cognitive decline and increased susceptibility to infections are also the ill effects of aging. In essence, before we die, almost everyone of us must confront a series of illnesses along the way.

But what if we could fix the wear and tear in our cells and delay aging like Jeanne Calment did and live longer? Under the right conditions, it might help us enjoy more years of good health. This could be achieved through a combination of various approaches, such as: eating foods that can promote the abilities of cells and tissues to enhance aging tolerance, regular exercise, reducing stress, ensuring adequate sleep and pursuing scientific advancements in the area of anti-aging. On the other hand, neglecting to address the aging process can make you aging faster and sensitive to nasty diseases.

Explained answer; how people can reverse type 2 diabetes without medication.

Question 3. This may be good news for people with type 2 diabetes, as studies showed that type 2 diabetes can be reversed without drugs or injecting insulin even for patients who have had type 2 diabetes for over 10 years.[4,5] The interventions that help people achieve remission do not require hospitalization or medication, but rather lifestyle changes and healthy diets.

In summary, it's a fact that no one wants to grow old, become sick and make frequent visits to the hospital. Good physical and mental health is what we all need. Yet to live a healthy and happy life, one must work towards it like work for wealth. There's no denying that good health is a person's most valuable asset. This is a secret that all wealthy people know.

CHAPTER 2

Vicious cycle in the treatment of chronic disease

Once I graduated from university, I lived without much thought. When I had a job, salary, and, of course, purchasing power, the very first things I did were shopping, traveling, drinking and eating a lot. Fast food was one of my early bad eating habits. At one point, I ate fried chicken on almost a daily basis. Later, at the age of 30, I transitioned to eating Korean-style barbecue grill, which is a paid self-serve meal where customers can eat everything in the restaurant for a set price, similar to a western-style all-you-can-eat buffet. Perhaps many of you may have been fans of fast food and all-you-can-eat buffets, but I have since given them up.

I reflect on those years and what inspired me to consume junk food, blackened pork chops, and starchy or fatty foods. Then I began to realize that there are wrinkles appearing on my forehead at the age of 40. "Hey, hey, hey, what's going with my face?" "Why does this happen to my body, but not to someone who is my age?" Once again, what happened to me is a common trend where people neglect their health, and it shows on their faces, often realizing it too late. Young people often prioritize other aspects of their lives and don't pay much attention to their health and wellness until they get older or reach middle age. Not many people know that health in their 20-40s is as important as in later in life. In fact, the choices a person makes in terms of diet, exercise, and lifestyle during these formative years have a significant impact on their overall well-being and quality of life as they age.

The health decline in your late 20s

Did you know that there are more and more working-age people spend more years being unhealthy? There is evidence that people's health begins to decline more or less at age 27. In 2017, Blue Cross-Blue Shield, a prominent health insurer, conducted an eye-opening analysis of its 55 million American policyholders aged 21-36. They discovered that the health of young Americans took a nosedive starting at age 27, with conditions like depression, diabetes, obesity, and heart disease on the rise. This is unfortunate for the United States, the world leader in medical technology. While the 55 million Americans in the study may not represent the global population, it's still disconcerting to consider that individuals in other nations could face similar health challenges. Should this be the case, significant economic and social consequences could arise for countries worldwide. In my opinion, a man in his late 20s should be in good health to pursue his dream career and to live a disease-free life. He shouldn't have to worry about his illness at all.

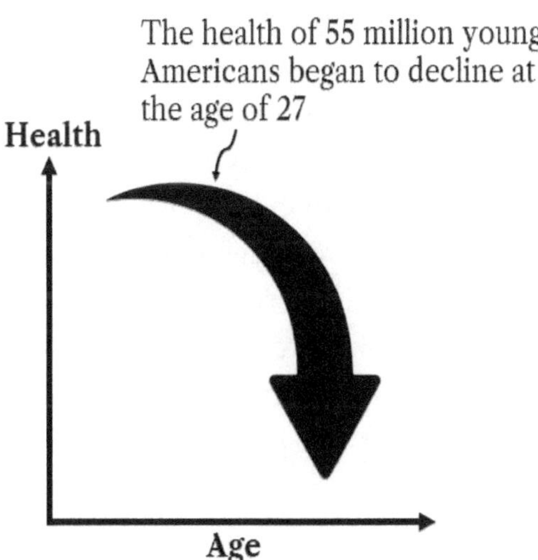

The data from the leading health insurer, Blue Cross-Blue Shield revealed that the young Americans' health began to decline at the age 27.[1]

Health is extremely important in your life, but the reality is that in today's society, there are many people with poor health. This is the reason for the emergence of a new condition in society called the "deteriorating health society." A society with a situation where many people have poor health and a chronic illness may have an impact on the quality of life and development of society and the population in the long run.

The root causes of illness

We're all aware that health issues can originate from 1) germs, 2) genetic errors, and 3) other causal factors such as excessive weight, fat build up in our bodies, low levels of hormones and more.

However, nowadays, the leading cause of death worldwide is not due to germs or genetic anomalies, but rather an anomaly within the body itself. Bugs that have entered our body are defeated within no time, but if inside one's body is abnormal, the body will take a longer time to fight. Eventually in the end, the body often fails and loses the fight. It appears that the body is better equipped to defend against external attacks, rather than internal ones. Also, biological aging and what you eat every day can greatly influence or even worsen existing illnesses and overall health.

Your life is essentially a reflection of your choices. However, many fail to realize the profound implications of poor decisions. While we can't choose to evade aging, we certainly can opt for a healthier lifestyle. The twin perils of biological aging and poor lifestyle choices can wreak havoc on our bodies over time. After years of unhealthy aging and detrimental lifestyle decisions, you may have caused harm to your body's cells. This prolonged unhealthy existence can pave the way for chronic diseases like type 2 diabetes, obesity, high blood pressure, atherosclerosis, heart disease, osteoarthritis, and cancer. Some individuals, unfortunately, undergo a more rapid aging process, resulting in early onset of chronic health conditions and physical frailty. This accelerated aging shortens their lifespan and compromises the quality of their lives.

Despite the progress made in medicine over recent decades, chronic diseases can't be cured by any medication. They usually don't occur randomly but are the consequences of actions that will inevitably bear results.

When you make poor lifestyle choices, your body reflect it by being more broken. The more poor lifestyle choices you make, the more your body will reflect it by becoming more unhealthy. And it's you that have to repay karma until the end of life. During a payback period, you might have to live your life between home and hospital and spend years in pain and treatment. These outcomes are the result of unhealthy lifestyle decisions that you must come to terms with.

Treatment for one health problem may cause the worse health problem

People think that medical treatment is the best way to make symptoms of the disease go away and get back to good health quickly. But here is the real situation of a person with underlying medical conditions. He wants his symptoms to go away and his illness to be cured as soon as possible. He goes to see a medical doctor; he receives the medicine and hopes that it will lead to a cure. But what if a person is not infected with a germ, but has a condition that medication can't eliminate the root cause of? What if the medicine a doctor prescribed could only ease disease symptoms and allow him to lead a palliative life for the remainder of his days?

Giving patients a medicine is a practice of modern medicine that has been taught continually in medical schools. It's a job of a good doctor to prescribe an appropriate medication to treat the disease. In my view this kind of approach is like a high-speed treatment because it serves its purpose of making the symptoms disappear and restoring good health quickly. Of course, patients also like this kind of treatment because it's a quick fix. But they forget that this modern medical treatment doesn't apply well to chronic diseases that have no effective treatment or cure. This rapid-acting medication is only an effective way to treat infections and fighting the spread of infectious diseases.

Doctors also know that medical treatments may have carryover effects in other areas of the body. Although some medicines may have a lower carryover effect than the other, some may have certain side effects that are almost unavoidable. Actually, any over-the-counter or prescription medicine is of an amount of a chemical greater than normally found inside our bodies. After swallowed, it can give an immediate effect to cellular function of the trillions of cells in the body. Possibly, the use of one drug is doomed to create for more problems than it would solve. For several diseases, when trying to treat one health problem, it may cause the worse problem. This is always a problem.

Vicious cycle in the treatment of chronic disease

Using medications to handle a chronic condition is reminiscent of the storyline in the movie "Groundhog Day." It may turn into an ongoing loop of pill-taking, symptom observation, and dosage adjustments. The use of synthetic drugs, which are medications that are chemically synthesized in a laboratory, is often the primary mode of treatment for chronic diseases. The treatment is a cycle that is impossible to escape until the end, as there is no cure for chronic diseases and medications must be taken for the rest of the patient's life. This cycle can be frustrating and exhausting for patients, who may feel like they are not making any progress in their treatment.

Allow me to explain the origin of this cyclical issue. It all starts when an individual suffers from a long-term illness and seeks medical help at a hospital. The doctor prescribes medication to alleviate the disease's symptoms. However, after taking the medicine for some time, it often has adverse effects on other cells, tissues, and organs in the person's body, leading to new symptoms. The patient then returns to the doctor, who now must treat the new symptoms with another drug, while the initial symptoms persist. More medications can only help the person maintain a normal life until his death. If a person is living with a chronic condition, he has to accept that his chronic condition can't be cured by any drug. This is the "vicious cycle in the treatment of chronic disease." This vicious cycle has also subjected doctors and nurses, particularly in places with limited healthcare infrastructure, to endless hardship.

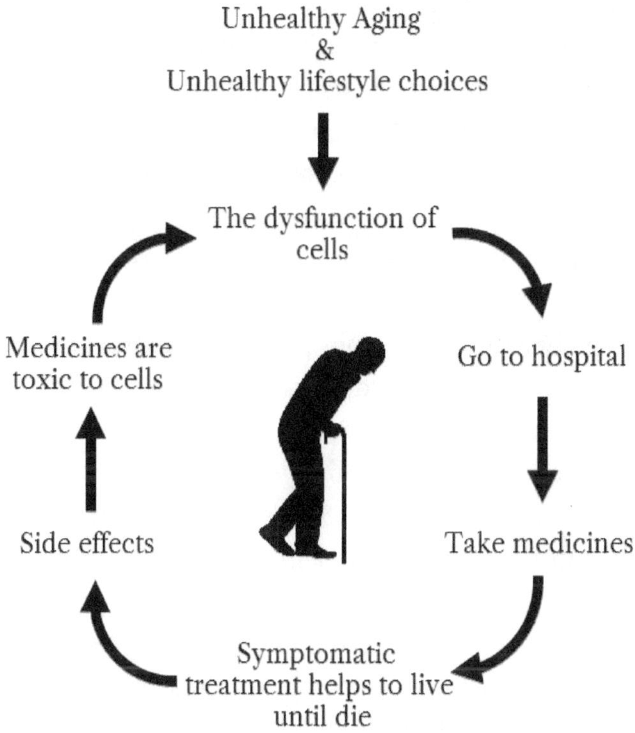

Vicious cycle in the treatment of chronic disease.

For those who have health conditions and regularly take medicines to manage their illnesses, I don't mean that they should stop taking them. You are already in the vicious cycle, stop taking your medicines could do harm to your health. But I didn't mean it's too late. There are ways to reverse your health conditions without drugs. However, if you are in a healthy condition, you should take care of yourself now and postpone the period of time that you have to take medications as further as possible.

These days we all see elderly patients taking a medicine as if it's a food. Many people think that looks normal for the present day. In the vicious cycle, patients want to get rid of their pain and suffering fast. This is an invisible force. If everyone believes that the fastest way to fix a broken body is to continuously take the medicine and take more when it runs out, this will only perpetuate the vicious cycle in the treatment of chronic disease. Taking medicine continuously is a situation of which it will go on forever. Patients who take their medicines regularly may become overused. For older people, long-term use of medications has more serious adverse effects on vital organs such as the liver and kidneys, which deteriorate with age, than benefits.

Likewise, more medicines prescribed to treat the side effects of previously prescribed medicines will create endless problems. Currently, for instance, there the data showed that 1 in 3 Americans uses lot of awful medicines on a regular basis and 40% of Australian people aged 50 and older take 5 or more medicines.[2,3] The use of multi medicines is also common in people with multiple chronic conditions.

In older people, there is evidence that there is no proven benefit of multi medicines, but rather increase the risk of adverse reactions.[4] Evidence suggested that the use of multiple medications by older adults strongly increases the risk of adverse effects and even leading to hospitalizations.

Taking 2 medicines raises one's chance of having an adverse reaction by 13%.

Taking 5 medicines raises one's chance of having an adverse reaction by 58%.

And the risk of having an adverse reaction increases to 82% if taking 7 medicines or more.

As we age, there is also a loss of elasticity of the heart and a shrinking liver and kidneys.[5] Imagine, if multiple side effects of the use of lot of awful medicines were combined with multiple chronic conditions, how could an old man's body with shrinking organs be able to endure this? There are also a few facts that you need to know. Clinical trials often perform in younger subjects (18-55 years old), for this reason, the benefits of medicines in older people in their 60s and beyond is unclear.[6] More importantly, prescription drugs are the third leading cause of death behind cancer and heart disease.[7]

The worst war by death toll

The question of how to end the never-ending war on nasty diseases like type 2 diabetes, obesity, high blood pressure, atherosclerosis, heart disease, osteoarthritis, and cancer is a difficult one. I personally believe that the war won't be succeeded in ending war, but by stopping the war before it happens.

Preventive healthcare is the most effective and least resource-intensive strategy in the fight against chronic diseases. It also offers economic benefits by reducing the financial burden on healthcare systems and society as a whole. By adopting healthy behaviors and lifestyle habits, one can take care of oneself and delaying the effects of aging, which can prevent chronic diseases from occurring, making it more effective than waiting for treatment from a doctor.

In our body, infection, inflammation, stress and aging are alike—they cause cell damage. But cell damage is reversible. If a cell is damaged, the body will first try to repair by itself. If the underlying cause is resolved, then the damaged cell can be transformed back into a normal cell. If not, the body can clear away damaged cells and replace with newer, healthier ones. With this body's way of compensatory cellular changes, the body can recover without the need for medication.

Moreover, medications cost money, while preventive care services could save millions upon millions. Implementing disease prevention and health promotion programs can lead to significant cost savings. As Benjamin Franklin once said, "An ounce of prevention is worth a pound of cure." In my view, investing in early prevention is the best way to safeguard your health. Imagine how fantastic it would be if an older adult hadn't visited a hospital for the past 30 years.

Furthermore, when an older adult falls ill, it becomes a burden on their children or those around them, as well as the hospital, public health system, and government. Today, the world has become a place where many people get sick, making it the only planet in the universe full of intelligent beings struggling with illness.

How can we escape from the vicious cycle?

Every cycle has a driving force. One of the ways to escape the vicious cycle in the treatment of chronic disease is to eliminate that force. It's time to fight aging and chronic diseases without medicines. It's time for everyone to extend his/her lifespan and seek medications later on in life.

As science advances, now we can learn to live healthier lives. Good health can be fostered. Chronic diseases can be prevented by eliminating the risk factors. In order to do that, we need to make healthy lifestyle choices, change our habits, slow down aging and create a longer period of good health.

A famous quote by Hippocrates, spoken over 2,400 years ago, states, "Let food be thy medicine, and medicine be thy food." This suggests that doctors can use food as a means to cure diseases. In line with this, Harvard health experts also believe that we can ward off harmful diseases by consuming healthy foods such as vegetables, fruits, whole grains, legumes, and nuts while reducing our intake of unhealthy foods like red meat, sugar, and refined grains.

They suggest people switch up their diets. For instance, in every kilogram of food you eat, aim for 300 grams of vegetables, 300 grams of fruit, 232 grams of whole grains (like rice, wheat, and corn), and 125 grams of legumes or beans. Additionally, you should limit your consumption of meat products like beef, pork, and chicken to about 40 g a day and restrict your sugar and fat intake to just 25 g a day. Harvard health experts believe that if humans can adopt this suggested plant-based diet, reduce meat-based products, and avoid unhealthy foods such as processed foods and those containing added sugar, it could prevent 11 million deaths a year and keep millions of people away from the doctor. This is truly a remarkable idea.

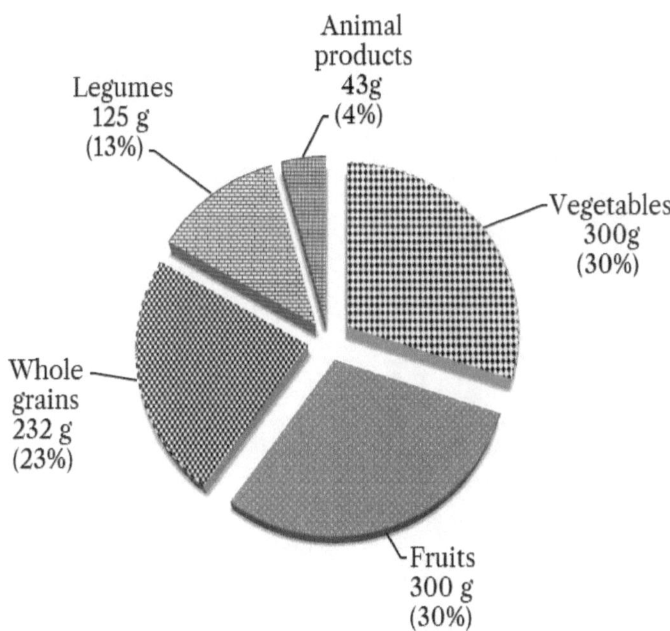

The amount of a plant based-diet recommended by Harvard health experts.[8] Fill one third of your plate with vegetables, another third with fruits, a quarter with whole grains, and the rest with beans or legumes.

The Canadian government's dream diet

Some say government is soulless. But that's not always true. For example, Canada's government has been working hard to prevent long-term illnesses among its citizens. They've been promoting healthy eating habits for a long time. And their most recent dietary guide from 2019 is bold. It encourages Canadians to fill half of their plate with fruits and vegetables, a quarter with whole grains, and the remaining quarter with proteins. This diet is thought to mirror the stone-age diet. The Canadian food guide also recommends making water your drink of choice, which goes against the way many people have been eating and drinking their whole lives. However, this is a healthy and wise choice.

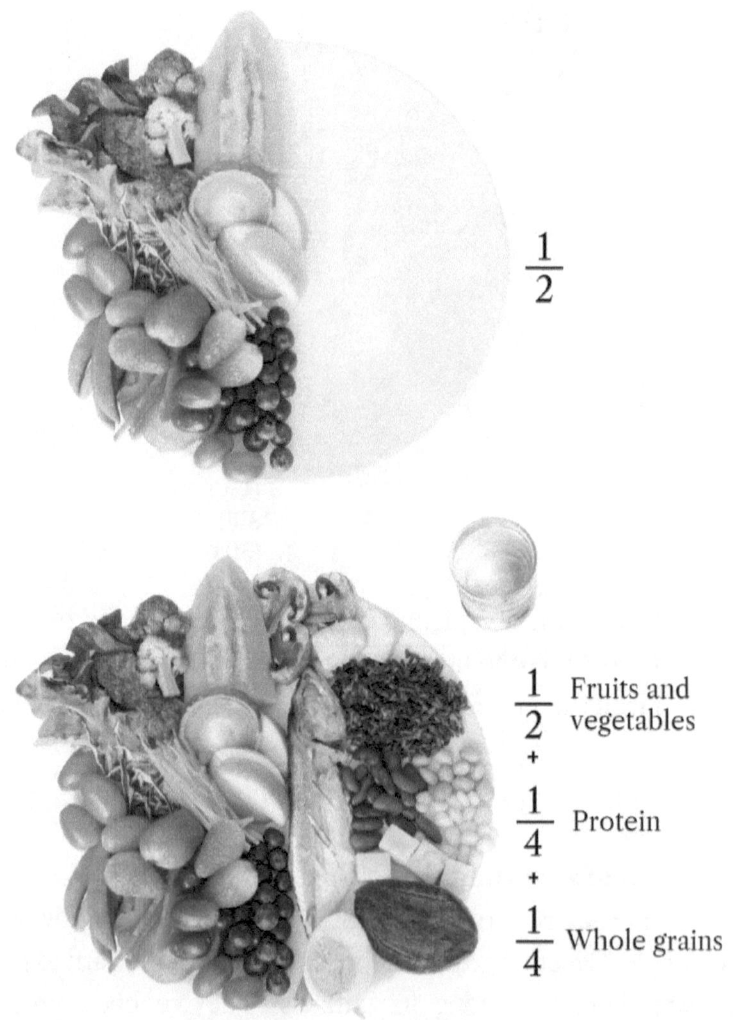

An example of the Canadian government's dream diet

Let's go back to Will Smith once more. At the age of 50, Will Smith treats himself with a daily dose of running. But most of the people in 50s run to hospital for more medicines, hoping that once they take medicines, they will get well soon. Not many people think that, by the age of 50, they should exercise regularly and make healthy lifestyle choices in order to prevent or fight off diseases.

For chronic conditions, medicines do not resolve the root causes of disease, but used as symptomatic treatment that extends a misery life to the end. In fact, the real healing power lies in your body's defenses that can deal with a disease that has not fully developed and including your determination to change the way you live and use of foods as a tool to prevent and reverse diseases.

Natural foods that can be found in nature and accessible to everyone are the keys to slow down aging and fight off chronic diseases sustainably. By eating a healthy diet that makes up 80% of your overall food intake, it may result in a positive impact on 80% of your body's functioning. Though millions of people receive the Canadian government's message, only a few can adhere to the advice. However, I believe that if every individual taps into the true healing power of real foods, we can fill the gap that even modern medicine could not bridge. In the near future, there may be a minimal need for doctors.

Part 2

Macrocosm of Aging

CHAPTER 3

Growing old, old cells and old-cell-destroying substances

Have you ever wondered why the queen bee, which is genetically similar to worker bees, lives 20 times longer than the workers? If you believe that the world was created according to the Bible, there is a record that humans once lived for hundreds of years. The Bible says that Adam lived 930 years and Noah lived 950 years.[1] But, later something changed and God set a limit on human lifespan, stating "I won't let my life-giving breath remain in anyone forever. No one will live for more than 120 years." It was a command from God that human lifespan will not exceed 120 years. Then after the biblical flood, the life expectancy for humans becomes gradually shorter. At the present day, a maximum human lifespan is about 120 years.[2] Is it possible that humans were ever perfect and lived past 900 years? Is this just a record written by the eyewitnesses? If it's true, why did everything change after the Flood?

In the 13th–16th Centuries, during the Little Ice Age, the Basque people in northern Spain faced food shortages and natural selection subsequently occurred. Those who survived tend to have mitochondria—the powerhouses of the cell—that work more efficiently. However, "you can't make an omelet without breaking eggs." The drawback to more efficient mitochondria is: it produces a lot of free radicals, which can lead to cartilage degeneration and development of rheumatoid arthritis. Though natural selection has strongly favored Basque people with the energy-efficient mitochondrial trait, there are negative consequences. Today, rheumatoid arthritis is the most common condition in European population descended from Basque people.[3]

Actually, humanity has faced generations of famines. These periods of scarcity have shaped genetic changes in humans, which were passed down from one generation to the next. For the Basque people, this included errors in their mitochondria. Struggling for the survival of human race in the past brings more free radicals, which can cause damage to DNAs and cells throughout the body, not only damage a joint.

Basically, free radicals in our bodies occur all the time as long as we eat and metabolize nutrients for energy. The more food you eat, the more free radicals are produced. This keeps your body continuously busy dealing with the constant threat of free radicals.

People aren't afraid of chronic diseases

There was a time when people were spread out and not too many of us around. Back then, outbreaks of diseases didn't happen that often, so people weren't too scared of them. But as time went on and more people started living close together, around the Middle Ages, things changed. People became really scared of catching diseases like smallpox, measles, and cholera. Diseases like these could spread quickly and made a lot of people sick. For years, these terrible diseases clung on and claimed lives. Sometimes a deadly outbreak killed most of the population, leading to a breakdown of civilization. For example, typhoid fever, that is thought to be a reason of the fall of the Aztec Empire. Or, the Black Death that arrived at the port of Sicily in Italy in 1347 before spreading across Europe, killing as many as 200 million people—a third of the world population at that time.

But, now with medical advances, we have vaccines, antibiotics and the know-how to beat infectious diseases; the world in which we are today has no fear of those nasty contagious diseases anymore. Those diseases, these days, fade and many of them are gone.

However, the human race's struggle with maladies is not over yet. In recent history, westernized populations have become plagued by civilization diseases like type 2 diabetes, obesity, hypertension, heart disease, cancer, osteoporosis, Parkinson's and Alzheimer's. These chronic diseases are rare or virtually absent in hunting and gathering society and other non-westernized populations. Despite current medical advances, we have yet to be able to defeat these nasty diseases.

Chronic diseases differ significantly from infectious diseases. Unlike an infectious disease that the threat can be seen when someone near you has signs and symptoms, chronic diseases are difficult to recognize and aren't immediate threat. We can't say exactly when diabetes, high blood pressure, heart disease, cancer, osteoporosis, Parkinson's or Alzheimer's will occur inside us. That why people don't fear chronic diseases. Today, chronic diseases are the main causes of death worldwide. The incidence of chronic diseases exponentially increases with age and commonly found in elderly population. Such as the incidence of cancer that increase in exponential fashion with age.

As you know that suffering from a chronic disease can feel like being stuck in an endless cycle, where efforts to address one health problem before it worsens can result in new health issues that ultimately bring you back to the initial problem. If there is no intervention or break, this cycle will continue until the last minute of life. It's estimated that two-thirds of all death each year caused by age-related maladies.

Diseases associated with aging are complex and multifaceted, as numerous processes contribute to their onset and progression. Yet, it's key to remember that changes in our hormones and the aging process itself are two primary factors that considerably impact the emergence of these ailments.

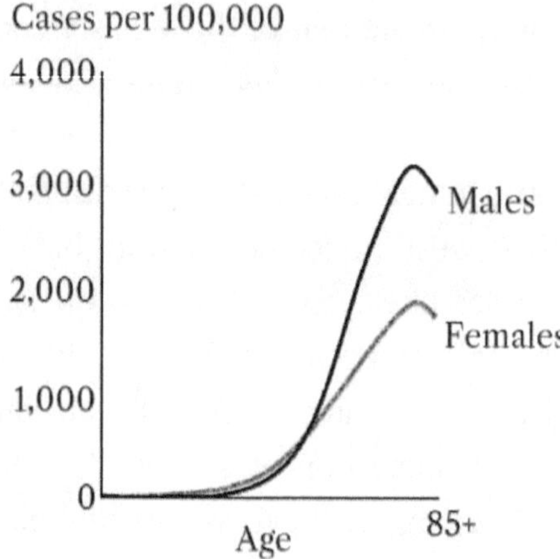

Rates of new found cancer cases in the United States increase in exponentially fashion with age.[4]

Reproduction and hormones have a built-in timeline

Scientists believe that the human body is genetically programmed to age in a certain way. Aging is connected to sexual reproduction, which involves the transmission of genetic material to produce new life and pass on our genes to the next generation. According to this hypothesis, after reaching reproductive age (around 20 years old), we spend another 20 years raising our children. Therefore, the natural lifespan of humans should not exceed 40 years.

In humans, the extended post-reproductive lifespan may have evolved to provide support to younger generations. Following our reproductive years, nature starts a new phase in life, shifting from growth to decline. This occurs as hormone production decreases, with cells reallocating resources towards conservation. Normally, all human cells function according to a biological clock, but after reproductive age, cells divert resources to savings, results in reduced hormone production and a subsequent decline in biological functions. In other words, when we stop growing, we start aging. Aging can be recognized by physical signs like wrinkles, poor eyesight, slow walking or memory loss. It can even lead to heart, bone, and muscle deterioration. At any given moment, some of the cells in your body may already be retired, starting the body's full aging process.

Our hormone levels start to decline as early as our late 20s and continue to diminish with age. The gradual decline of growth hormone, for instance, plunges to only 50% of its youthful levels. What's more, by the time we hit 30, our melatonin production takes a hit, potentially impacting your sleep quality. Between the ages of 45-55, our DHEA levels—responsible for producing sex hormones— also drop, leading to menopause in women and andropause in men. Meanwhile, by 60, our thyroid hormones, which regulate metabolism, growth, and development, start to wane as well. These decreasing hormone levels play a significant role in aging and the development of age-related illnesses.

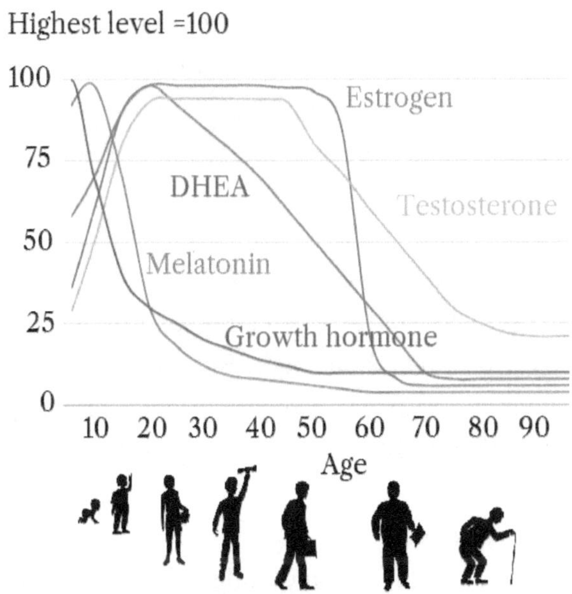

The levels of important hormones in human body at different points of life.[6]

The decline of hormones, also known as the loss of "hormonal magic," is believed to be a contributing factor to the decline of young people's health. As hormones decrease, our bodies age faster, and even a slight hormonal shift can affect our well-being in significant ways. In men, for instance, a slight decrease in testosterone levels can result in fatigue, reduced muscle mass, decreased libido, and erectile dysfunction. Take menopause, for another example, which usually occurs around 50. Lower estrogen levels before time put women at a higher risk of heart disease and osteoporosis. However, for women in their reproductive years, they can still conceive and carry a pregnancy to term, thanks to the continuous ovulation. So, despite aging, the hormonal magic in women is not completely lost until they reach their 50s, when ovulation stops. This is a built-in timeline of hormonal changes in our bodies that define our health.

There is a clear sequence of steps in your body that can be exploited to make small tweaks to hormone levels, much like altering a computer program. Humans can naturally increase their reduced hormones, as exemplified by the story of elderly Okinawans who have managed to delay the decline in DHEA levels as they age, which will be discussed later. However, it's important to first understand the cellular causes of aging.

What are the cellular causes of aging?

People age differently. You can be an immune ager, a kidney ager, a liver ager or a metabolic ager. But when it comes to aging at the cellular level, apart from changing in gene expression patterns that can occur with age, there are more factors that cause aging at the cellular level:

Genome decay

Chemicals, UV rays from sunlight, germs, viruses, cigarette smoke, unhealthy food as well as overeating, all of these can damage DNA, cause genome decays, cell aging and lead to more complex biological changes in cells and tissues in other negative ways. When genome decays, it can cause genes in a cell to mutate or change and then cause the cell to grow out of control and become cancerous.

Telomere shortening and senescence

Telomere shortening is one of the reasons why we age. Every time a cell divides, the ends of a chromosome called telomeres get shorter about 50 bases. And the division of each cell is limited to about 70 times before cell death or senescence. If the cells don't die after this, they will become senescent cells. Telomere shortening may be the body's way of checking mutations in cells and eliminating cancer-prone cells.

Additionally, senescent cells can be created when cells are exposed to harmful substances or toxins. Senescent cells, also referred to as old cells, can remain in the body and aren't yet eliminated or die. In this zombie-like state, a senescent cell will lose its power of division and growth. But they possess the ability to communicate with other cells, enabling them to influence neighboring cells and the surrounding tissue environment. These zombie cells accumulate as we get older. These cells are also resistant to self-destruction; even when prompted to die, they don't, allowing them to accumulate further in tissues over time.

Regarding its benefits, senescent cells can be found in your body as early as the age of 5, helping to stimulate stem cells to grow and initiate repairs. Plus, senescence may be part of an evolutionary process designed to prevent the damaged cells become cancerous. The mechanism by which aging cells stop dividing is also the body's way of making sure that abnormalities or damages won't pass on to future offspring. So, if there are damaged cells in your body, your body won't be encouraging cells to grow and multiply, but rather age or die.

Nonetheless, senescent cells contain DNA damages that can't be repaired. When cells become senescence, they are enlarged. Inside these cells is full of waste products that can't be removed. Our bodies then have to send immune cells to destroy senescent cells. However, the efficiency of this process declines with age. So, in which parts of the body, if there are a lot of senescent cells, it's as if a battlefield between senescent and immune cells. This battlefield is also a source of inflammation.

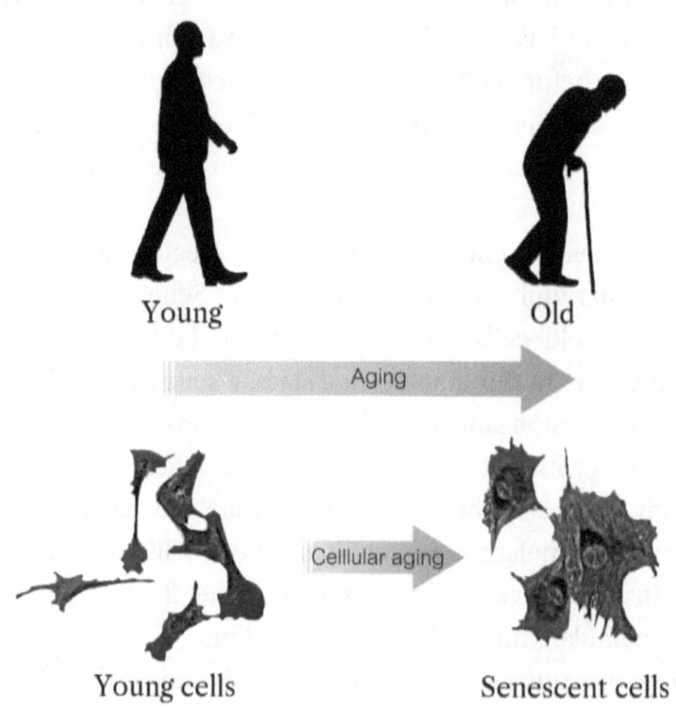

Senescent cells or old cells accumulate as we get older.

Senescent cells damage vital organs

When senescent cells accumulate in large quantities within vital organs, such as the brain, liver tissues, joints, cataracts in the eyes, and arterial walls, it results in the development of various diseases. The greater the number of senescent cells in your body, the more susceptible you become to illness. Especially in older people, their whole bodies contain up to 0.1% of senescent cells, which is more than the number of immune cells.[7] Hoping for the immune system to get rid of senescent cells is very unlikely. The older you are, the more difficult it's to eliminate senescent cells. Senescent cells also release a range of inflammatory molecules, which contributes to tissues dysfunction and aging itself. In addition, senescent cells induce nearby cells to become senescence, and make the situation worse. Too many senescent cells in the body could be a ticking time bomb for chronic diseases. The more they pile up, the more your body systems get affected, leading to malfunctioning organs and ultimately, death.

There are also other causative factors of aging such as mitochondrial dysfunction, decreased autophagy, epigenetic changes and stem cell exhaustion. It's important to provide this information for you. All of these are fundamental knowledge that you can use to fight against age-related diseases and aging itself.

Stem cells can divide indefinitely

Although nature programs all human beings to die, it also offers wonders. While aging cells stop dividing and enter senescence at one point in time, stem cells can develop into diverse types of cells in the body and divide indefinitely to produce themselves. Stem cells divide to replace damage cells and repair tissues or organs. Stem cells are present in almost all parts of the body; they are in adipose tissue, spine, bloodstream, liver, pancreas, brain, heart, kidneys, skin, teeth, gut and other organs. It's not known exactly how many stem cells are in the human body. However, most stem cells are in: adipose tissue contains about 1 in 100 to 1 in 1,000 mesenchymal stem cells that can differentiate into bone, cartilage, and fat cells; and the digestive system contains around 1 in 1,000 to 1 in 10,000 intestinal stem cells that help regenerate the gut lining. Where there are stem cells, there is the site of the "Fountain of Youth" that damaged, old or dying cells are repaired, replaced or renewed.

The ability of stem cells is remarkable, as in the case of human liver regeneration, even if three-quarters of the liver is lost, the remaining one will unbelievably regrow on its own to its normal size within a few months. This is a fountain of youth in you, but you are unaware of it. Instead, you are doing things that destroy or deteriorate your stem cells. What leads to stem cell deterioration and decline is, for example, cigarette smoke, alcoholic beverages, sugar, and even aging itself.

As soon as you inhale cigarette smoke, whether from first-hand smoking or second-hand smoke, the stem cells will stop working for 24 hours. In this 24-hour period, it can be an important moment to repair damaged cells or restore wear and tear in your body. Alcohol consumption reduces the activity of stem cells in the brain. Diabetes also disrupts the function of stem cells. When the body can't regulate the levels of sugar in your blood, stem cells become exposed to elevated blood sugar levels, which can decrease their activity and capability to divide. Sugar also slows down the movement of stem cells to other parts of the body. Moreover, as we age, the number of older stem cells increases while the overall count of stem cells decreases. Biological aging is a cause of stem cell exhaustion and deterioration. Plus, wherever senescent cells are found, they induce surrounding cells to also undergo senescence or aging. Ultimately, tissue repair in your body will be compromised or fail because it's too many senescent cells. This is why the mend of damaged tissues or organs in the elderly is slower than in younger and healthier adults, or even irreparable.

So as not to make senescent cells the cause a deteriorating body, aging and chronic diseases, can we get rid of senescent cells? Or is there any way to rejuvenate less active and older stem cells?

In fact, the removal of senescent cells and enhancing the regeneration of stem cells can be achievable. There are various approaches to remove senescent cells and enhance the regeneration of stem cells. Getting rid of senescent cells could restore the body's strength, help to eliminate inflammation in vital organs, treat chronic diseases and revive your body.[8,9] Enhancing the regeneration of stem cells would also be highly beneficial.

***

Old-cell-destroying substances

Getting rid of senescent cells lurking in heart, liver, kidneys or brain can help restore their functions and increase the lifespan. This can be exemplified by scientific evidence. For instance, killing senescent cells resulted in treated mice living 25% longer than those in control groups, along with a reduction in age-related diseases such as kidney dysfunction, heart dysfunction, and cancer.[8,10] This is the proof of principle. If mice were humans, this could mean an increase in lifespan from 80 years to 100 years. In humans, a small clinical trial published in the journal EBioMedicine in 2018 found that removing senescent cells from patients with a rare genetic disorder improved their physical function and quality of life.

Substances that can selectively destroy old cells in the body are called "senolytics." Most of senolytics are natural and man-made compounds, and one of the well-known natural senolytics is quercetin. In humans, quercetin along with dasatinib could eliminate senescent cells from fat tissues, and increased the patient's healthspan.[8] Importantly, scientists believe that getting rid of only 30% of the senescent cells is enough to help lessen the symptoms of a disease. Moreover, the use of senolytics doesn't need to be used continuously as with conventional drugs, since taking senolytics periodically is sufficiently effective.

Quercetin is light yellow, and a chemical of plant origin. It's a colored flavonoid that can be found in a variety of fruits and vegetables. Quercetin is soluble in fat and, in human body, has a half-life of 1-2 hours.

Actually, the quercetin can be found in red onions ranging from 32 to 2,405 mg/100 g depending on its source.[11] Quercetin is also found in red kidney beans, 300 mg/100 g, neem flowers and leaves, 200 mg/100 g, caper, 146 mg/100 g and onion leaves, 140 mg/100 g.[12] To prevent the loss of quercetin, foods rich in quercetin should be cooked at less than 120°C for no more than 30 minutes.

In fact, in nature, quercetin is normally present as quercetin glycosides, quercetin bound to glucose, that are more stable and better absorbed. Quercetin glucosides are found in cowpea, 69 mg/100 g.[13] In human, 3-17% of quercetin is well absorbed by the small intestine.[14] Eating foods containing quercetin with the main meals can reduce the breaking down of quercetin by stomach acid. In a promising study, 5 participants received 225 g of fried onion—equivalent to 50 mg of quercetin. A blood test 2 hours later showed that the participants had 0.248 mcg/ml of quercetin in their plasma. And after 10 hours, quercetin was still found in the plasma at 0.01 mcg/ml.[14,15] It indicated that the digestive system of human can absorb quercetin from natural foods very well.

Fisetin is another senolytic found in natural foods. In laboratory experiments, fisetin was the most effective senolytic for clearing off senescent cells, followed by curcumin, luteolin and resveratrol. Fisetin could effectively kill off 50% of the aging cells in lab dish. When tested in older mice—equivalent to 75 years old humans—that received 60 mg/kg of fisetin (human dose will be 5 mg/kg) for 10 weeks, it was found that fisetin could extend lifespan in older mice by 10%. Fisetin was also found to enhance the liver and pancreas function in aged mice, and a single treatment can have long-lasting effects over time.[16] Experts believed that the healthspan improvement in tested animals didn't depend on continued presence of circulating fisetin in the blood because the half-life of fisetin is about an hour. But it's likely due to its ability to getting rid of senescent cells. Based on a clinical trial conducted with U.S. volunteers, there have been no reports of adverse side effects of fisetin.[17] But for some reason medical professionals recommend taking moderate amounts of fisetin. In a clinical trial conducted by Mayo Clinic researchers, participants were given only 20 mg/kg of fisetin for 2 days in a row, and only once a month. In the future, when this first clinical trial in humans is done, we will see how effective fisetin as senolytic actually is.

Curcumin, a part of turmeric with up to 9,000 mg per 100 g, can activate certain enzymes that cause programmed cell death or apoptosis in senescent cells. Curcumin has been shown to effectively eliminate 30% of aging cells in laboratory experiments.[16]

Luteolin, a compound in many fruits and veggies, can block the pathways that cause senescence, preventing the buildup of senescent cells in the body. This helps the immune system target and remove these cells. Research has shown that luteolin can remove up to 15% of senescent cells in laboratory studies.[16] Luteolin can be found in onion leaves at 39 mg/100g and celery leaves at 17 mg/100g.

Senolytics	Natural food sources and senolytic content (mg/100g)* [11,13,14,18,19,20]	Senescent cells that killed off in test tubes[16]
Fisetin	Strawberries, 16 Apple, 2.6	25-50%
Curcumin	Turmeric, 9,000	20-30%
Luteolin	Onion leaves, 39 Celery leaves, 17	10-15%
Resveratrol	Merlot grapes, 0.125 Red wine, 1.0 Apple, 0.04	5-10%
Quercetin	Red onion, 2,405 Red kidney beans, 300 Neem leaves, 200 Caper, 146 Cowpea, 69 Pak choy, 39	<5%

Senolytics are also effective for restoring stemness of stem cells

As we age, stem cell activity declines. Although stem cells are able to produce themselves, they lose their regeneration capacity and efficiency over time. When stem cells get exhausted, they become senescent cells, and if these aging cells aren't eliminated, they will cause serious illnesses. Just like, as people say, a few rotten apples can spoil the whole barrel.

In addition to being a senolytic, fisetin, curcumin, and resveratrol can also be, I refer to, "stemness rejuvenator" that can reverse stem cell aging and restore their stemness.

However, in older people, it's likely to take longer time than in younger people to rejuvenate aging cells with stemness rejuvenators because older people may have a greater number of senescent cells. Additionally, if you wish to remove old cells, they don't readily die because they possess mechanisms to resist it. This makes their elimination from the body more challenging. By scientific methods, it has been revealed that, in older mice, it took 2-5 times longer time to rejuvenate older stem cells to become younger ones. This rejuvenation process can range from 30 to 50 days for stem cells to regain their youthful characteristics.

Typically, scientists use a method called "reprogramming" to revitalize aged stem cells in laboratories. In fact, in a mouse model, natural compounds like fisetin, curcumin, and resveratrol supercharge the process, turning normal cells into stem cells up to 6 times faster.[16,21] In addition, age doesn't matter—whether the cells are from adolescents or centenarians, they can be transformed into youthful stem cells in a lab dish.[22]

As a mouse is a stand-in for human, it's plausible that stem cell rejuvenation observed in mice could also apply to humans. And natural compounds such as fisetin, curcumin, and resveratrol may be just as effective in enhancing cell reprogramming and give rise to stem cells. In the experiments, the success rate of reviving cells using fisetin, curcumin, or resveratrol is around 0.1-1.5%.[8] This implies that out of every 1,000 human cells, one cell can be rejuvenated, and this small percentage may give rise to stem cells. There are over 1,000,000,000,000 cells in the human body, of which 0.1% of them are senescent cells, and around 100,000 senescent cells are in the circulation.[23,24] If stem cell rejuvenation is achieved for every 1,000 cells, fisetin, curcumin and resveratrol may be able to revert millions of aging cells to youthful ones.[25,26] These revivified cells may bring about the revivification to your tissues and organs. Consequently, eating foods rich in stemness rejuvenators could help delay health issues that come with aging and extend a person's lifespan. It's one of the methods to avoid succumbing to illness and conquer the aging process.

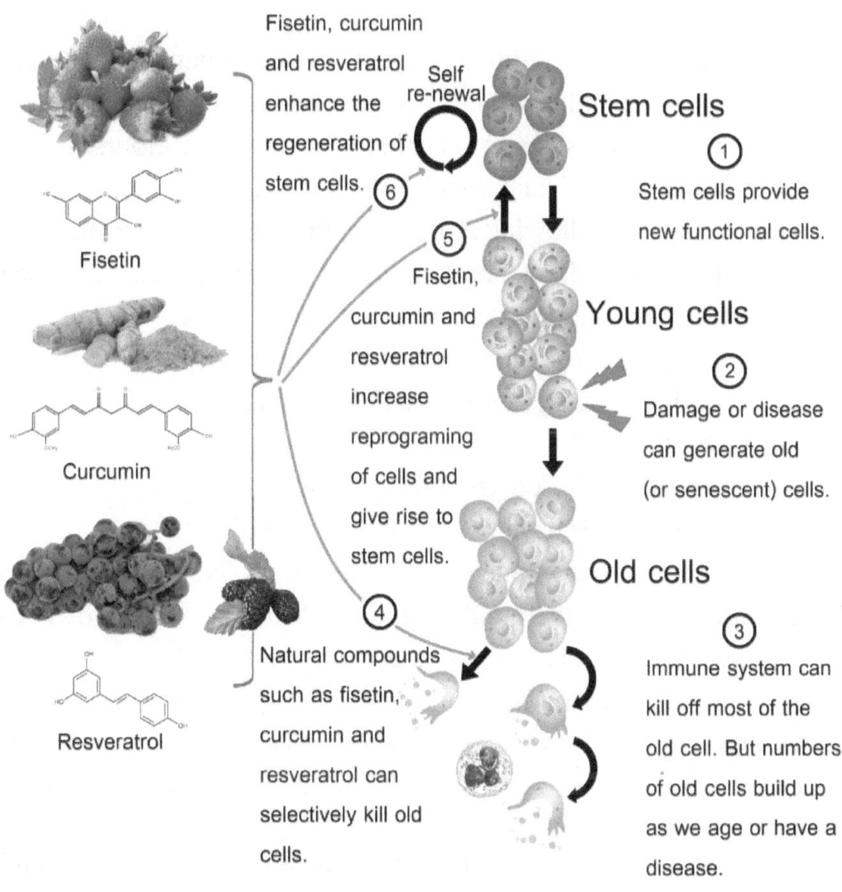

The image illustrates the importance of using senolytics to clear senescent cells–old and damaged cells–periodically in order to rejuvenate cells, delay aging, and prevent maladies. Rejuvenating aged stem cells can also enhance the regeneration of aging bodies, further delaying aging and warding off diseases. Natural compounds like fisetin, curcumin, and resveratrol, found in certain foods, can help counteract the decline in cellular and stem cell function.[16,24,25]

Bioenhancer needs for senolytics and stemness rejuvenators

Getting the most out of senolytics and stemness rejuvenators can be tricky. They are often not absorbed well and break down quickly in our stomach and gut. That is where a bioenhancer comes in.

Piperine is a naturally occurring bioenhancer that can maximize bioavailability of other active ingredients and improves absorption. Piperine stays in our blood for about 1-2 hours. It also reduces stomach acid and blocks the liver from breaking down certain compounds, allowing more to get into our bloodstream.

For the best effect, about 20 mg of piperine is needed. Given that a single black peppercorn holds about 3 mg of piperine, you would need about 5-7 peppercorns to get this effect.[26]

Piperine increased curcumin absorption by 2,000%, in a study in human volunteers.[27]

Piperine increased resveratrol absorption up to 1,544% in mice, but human trials have not shown clear results.[28]

For quercetin, taking it with substances like vitamin C and bromelain (an enzyme found in pineapples) has been shown to increase the body's ability to use quercetin effectively.

Another way to get the most out of curcumin is to eat it with fats. Curcumin dissolves in fats, not water, so eating it with good fats like olive oil, coconut oil, or fish oil can help our bodies absorb it better.

In the end, eating natural foods packed with nutrients and beneficial compounds is usually the healthiest approach. Plus, our bodies are designed to absorb and use these ingredients from natural foods most effectively.

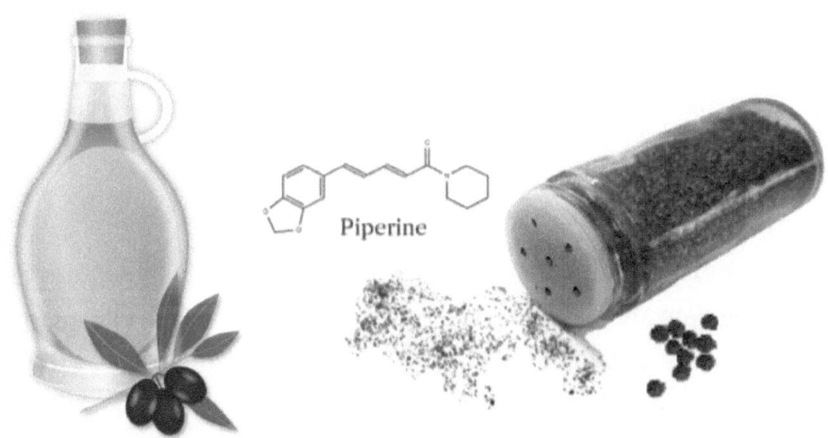

About 5-7 black peppercorns, equivalent to 20 mg of piperine, are able to enhance the absorption of curcumin and resveratrol in the body. Olive oil can also increase curcumin bioavailability.

In brief, it's like a queen bee that doesn't live long because of its genetics—both the queen bee and worker bees share similar genes. The difference is that worker bees feed on nectar, but the queen bee is fed only royal jelly. This rich royal jelly diet changes a queen bee genetically and allows her to achieve longer lifespan. The idea is that aging can be nutritionally controlled and manipulated. Certain nutrients can alter gene expression and cellular function within an organism. You can delay aging and extend healthspan too by eating food rich in senolytics and stemness rejuvenators and allow yourself to live longer and healthier life.

CHAPTER 4

Sugar: the real enemy of your body

"หวานลิ้นกินตาย" is a Thai expression that has been around for a long time means "fine words but no parsnips." But if Thai people listen to this metaphor and infer the meaning literally without translation, this expression is also true. Its meaning without translation for Thai people is similar to "for those with a sweet tooth shall lick the dust." Why? It's because consumption of added sugars ruins your health and increases the risk of dying from chronic diseases.

In fact, the sweet dangers of sugar on your health have been known since 1972, when a British physician at the University of London, John Yudkin, published his book, entitled, Pure, White and Deadly.[1] He revealed that sugar is the main cause of overweight, obesity and subsequent diseases, including diabetes, atherosclerosis, heart disease, digestive disease, liver disease, metabolic syndrome and many other chronic diseases. But the whole world was skeptical until 30 years later, in 2002, the World Health Organization (WHO) finally realized the dangers of sugar and declared to limit sugar intake to less than 10% of total daily calories.[2] Later, John Yudkin's home country, United Kingdom, suggested that its citizens should limit sugar intake to 5% of total daily calories due to cavities and tooth decay reasons. Since consuming 10% of sugar, or 50 g of sugar per day, still a problem causing people to suffer from dental caries, which have a profound effect on their health. Only limiting sugar intake to less than 5% of total daily calories can reduce tooth decay. Believe it or not, 80% of the world's population has tooth decay.[3] That was the WHO agreed and recommended limiting added sugars to less than 5% of total daily calories or no more than 25 g per day in 2014.[4] This recommended practice is supposed to be used around the world.

Statistical figures in Thailand, an upper middle-income country, in 2011 revealed that an average Thai consumed about 29 kg of sugar a year. Of course, this exceeds the recommended limit of 10% and 5% of daily calorie needs. You may not surprise that what has happened next. There are more than 5 million Thai people suffering from diabetes and the number is rising.[5] Don't Thai people believe their idiom "for those with a sweet tooth shall lick the dust"?

Sugar sells: the truth behind the bestselling drinks

Thailand is the largest consumers of soft drinks in Southeast Asian nations; the average Thai person consumes 41 liters of soft drinks a year. If soft drinks contain 10% sugar, it means that an average Thai consumes more than 4 kg of sugar from soft drinks a year. Thais have a sweet tooth, about a third of Thai working-age people also consume soft drinks or sugar-sweetened beverages on a daily basis.[6] And for Thai children, they consume 25-50 g of sugar a day.[7] Let's do the math, and you will find that Thai children eat about 9-18 kg of sugar a year.

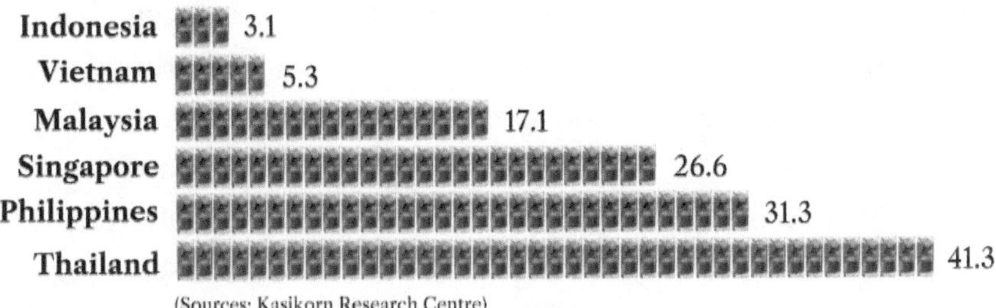

Thailand's soft drink consumption in 2011 (liters/person/year).

Children may not know how much sugar they consume because sugar can be disguised as sucrose, glucose, fructose or syrup in snacks, soft drinks, fruit juices and processed foods. They have also more chance to expose to sugar bouts through festivals, celebrations on various occasions or when visiting relatives or friends who offer them sugary treats. Indeed, children are more prone to consumption of added sugar because they have a natural preference for sweet tastes.

Let's take a further look at how 5 million Thai people with type 2 diabetes consume sugar. In 2018, a survey of 304 sugar consumption behaviors among Thai people with type 2 diabetes aged 52-57 years old revealed that these patients consumed an average of 43 g of sugar daily, or almost twice as much as the WHO's recently recommended sugar intake per day.[8] It's alarming to note that some Thai children take in more sugar (50 g daily) than Thai adults with type 2 diabetes. It's uncertain if Thais truly heed the WHO's advice. It's indeed an unfortunate reality.

Although there may be some Americans who have read Pure, White and Deadly, the fact remains that 10% of the poorest Americans consume sugar-sweetened beverages or carbonated drinks twice as often as 10% of the richest Americans.[9] This suggests that socio-economic status plays a significant role in the consumption of added sugar, with those in lower income brackets having a higher likelihood of consuming sugar-sweetened beverages. Also, kids from poorer families often have fewer choices for healthy food. Many of the areas where they live lack big food stores or markets that sell fresh, good-for-you foods. More often, these neighborhoods have more small shops or fast-food spots, which usually offer less healthy choices.

Moreover, in particular, for those with children who frequently consume sugary beverages, it's also crucial to recognize how sugar can affect your children's brains. Evidence shows that sugar consumption can result in poor school performance. Higher consumption of sugary beverages has been linked to lower test scores in spelling, grammar, reading, writing, and numeracy.[10]

This could be due to inflammation of the blood vessels in the brain caused by sugar consumption, which impairs cognitive function and language abilities. What's more, studies have found that individuals who consume high amounts of sugar during childhood may experience poor learning and memory as they grow older.[11] Furthermore, continued high sugar intake into adulthood has been linked to the shrinkage of the hippocampus, the area of the brain responsible for long-term memory processing.

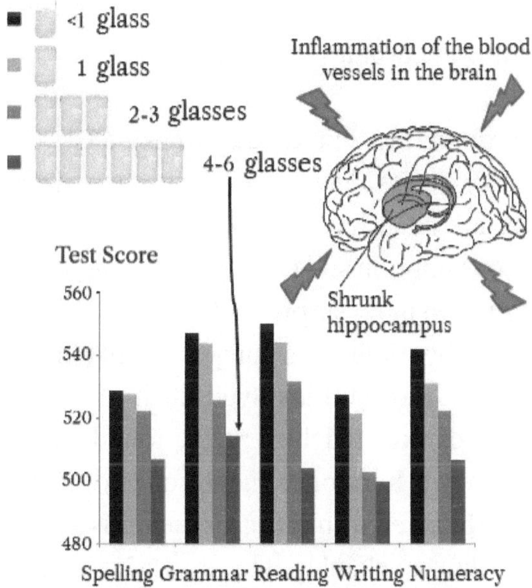

Higher consumption of sugary beverages was associated with lower test scores in spelling, grammar, reading, writing and numeracy in children aged 8-15 years.[10] Continued high sugar intake into adulthood has been linked to the shrinkage of the brain.

Because sugar sweetened beverages are bad for children, so I hasten to add the best strategy for limiting sugary beverage intake for your kids. According to research,[11] the best tactic is "to keep sugary beverages, even juice or sports drink, out of the house and don't buy them at all." The study suggested that "we should educate our children and tell them what these drinks are made of, and why they aren't healthy, and cause diseases like obesity and diabetes."

But, if you consume it, your children are going to consume it too. Children often imitate what they see other people, especially family members, doing. For the people you love, you must abstain from sugary beverages, and drink water instead. Did you know? If you drink 500 ml or 2 cups of water before your meals every day for 8 weeks, you could lose as much as a kilogram of your weight.[12] If you aren't sure giving up sugary drinks is reasonable, you should see Mexico—the world's leader in the obesity epidemic. That now Mexico has banned the sale of sugary drinks to children—an important setting in curbing obesity and diabetes.

The carbonated drinks make you hungry

Nowadays, it's widely known that sugary drinks are not good for our health, as studies have indicated a clear relationship between sugary drink consumption and obesity. However, a study by scientists has revealed an even more surprising fact: drinking carbonated drinks can cause obesity by stimulating hunger and making us feel hungry all the time. The study, which involved 20 healthy male participants who consumed carbonated beverages, found that their levels of ghrelin, the hunger hormone, increased by about 500%.[13] This suggests that carbonated drinks trigger feelings of hunger, which may be the missing link explaining why excessive consumption of soft drinks leads to obesity.

However, in real life, people who consume soft drinks or carbonated drinks may also tend to eat other unhealthy foods and have low levels of physical activity. It's worth noting that this study involved a small sample size of male volunteers, and studies involving larger populations may yield more convincing results. Nevertheless, the evidence really suggests that carbonated drinks trigger feelings of hunger and may lead to weight gain in men. This could be why large beverage companies like Coca-Cola fund research to convince us that lack of exercise, not diet, is the primary cause of obesity in the United States.[14]

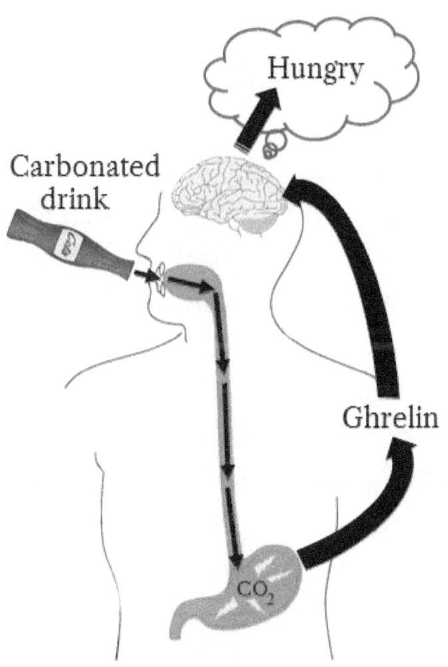

Carbon dioxide in carbonated drink stimulates the production of ghrelin, a hunger hormone, which in turn triggers felling of hungry, increases food intake and may lead to weight gain in men.[13]

Shock cells with sugar

Humans didn't evolve to eat sugar. Human ancestors had to walk for miles and miles to find sweet fruits. When eating fruits, it doesn't mean that sugars in fruits will enter the bloodstream immediately; instead, our digestive system slowly digests and absorbs them. Today's sugary drinks contain ready-to-take in sugars for the body to absorb all at once—our bodies don't have to waste time and energy spending on digestion anymore. Sugar-sweetened beverages also contain more readily absorbed sugars such as fructose and glucose that can be absorbed more easily than the table sugar, sucrose. When they enter into the body, our cells become startled and shocked due to the sudden high sugar content. This is similar to placing cells instantaneously in sugar syrup, which could result in gene expression that differs from the usual.

The forgotten findings

In addition to the book that has been overlooked in many countries, research conducted in 1973[15] that warned us of the dangers of sugar has also been forgotten. This research revealed that sugar is an enemy of our immune system, causing us to lose control of it almost instantly. When an individual consumes 100 g of glucose, fructose, sucrose, honey, or orange juice, the immune response, especially the white blood cells that defend the body against pathogens and infections, is immediately reduced by 40% and shut down for 5 hours. It's worth reiterating that "sugar can suppress the white blood cells of the immune response for up to 5 hours." Sugar doesn't decrease the number of defensive white blood cells, but rather hinders their function. Imagine if this window of time coincides with the body's need to fight off cancer, it could result in missed opportunities to combat the disease and allow it to progress.

Do you think that consuming 100 g of sugar is too much? As a reference, that amount is equal to consuming 25 teaspoons of sugar. And to give you an idea, here are some examples of foods and their sugar content per 100g: drinking a 1-liter bottle of soda, a 1-liter bottle of fruit juice or 4 cans of 250 ml energy drink. It's concerning that these types of drinks are often readily available in schools, vending machines, and convenience stores.

After sugar shuts down the immune system for 5 hours, it lowers your defense by 20%

After more than 40 years of being forgotten, the findings were finally proved that people with high blood sugar have less ability in their white blood cells to fight pathogens compared to normal people. It means that the higher concentration of glucose in the bloodstream, the lesser ability white blood cells have to fight off pathogens. In prediabetic and diabetic patients with a blood glucose level of 117-137 mg/dL, approximately in the first half hour of sugar intake, their white blood cells' ability to fight off germs and foreign substances is reduced by 12%.[17] And those with a blood glucose level greater than 137 mg/dL, their white blood cells' ability will be reduced by 20%. This means that sugar makes white blood cells less able to fight infections. All of this is consistent with the fact that infection in people with diabetes is more common and severe than in normal people.

Sugar is a calcium killer

Sugar can lead to a decrease in calcium levels in the body. Typically, a person excretes 2-23 mg/L or 20 to 300 mg of calcium per day through urine. However, when sugar is consumed, more calcium is excreted in the urine.[18] The consumption of soft drinks and coffee is similar, as they both can increase the amount of calcium excreted in the urine. This amount can be around 25-80 mg for a single serving of soft drinks and 2-3 cups of coffee. After five hours of consuming soft drinks or coffee, the average amount of calcium excreted in urine is doubled or even tripled with high levels of additional carbohydrate intake.[19,20]

Consuming fructose is also linked to lower levels of calcium and vitamin D in the body, leading to a deficiency in calcium and vitamin D.[21] Moreover, frequent consumption of foods containing white, refined flour and sugar can lead to a bone loss rate of up to 1% per year. In addition to soft drinks and coffee, a high salt intake can also increase the amount of calcium excreted in the urine. Studies have shown that a high salt intake can cause a daily increase in urinary calcium of about 40-60 mg per day. If you don't replace lost calcium, sugar and salt can cause calcium loss in bones, leading to thinner bones and osteoporosis, also known as porous bone.

Sugar consumption is the path to atherosclerosis and high blood pressure

There are scientific evidence linking sugar to the development of atherosclerosis—hardening of the arteries. For example, a scientific study, published in respected medical journal, found that sugar thickens the walls of blood vessels, which is a common symptom of atherosclerosis. Mice fed glucose had thicker blood vessel walls than mice fed water.[22] This suggests that mice fed sugar are more likely to develop arterial plaque and fatty deposits than mice fed water. Because feeding mice glucose repeatedly mimics a person's sugary drink behavior, providing insight into the role of sugar in atherosclerosis development. If applied to humans, glucose intake could accelerate the formation of plaque, causing the blood vessel walls to thicken and leading to atherosclerosis.

Why does sugar cause high blood pressure? Experts in this field have long known that people with diabetes often have high blood pressure. This is exemplified by data from 5 million Thai people with diabetes, of whom one third have high blood pressure.[23] The reason these two diseases occur together is that when the blood glucose level rises beyond the control, it causes inflammation and damage to vital organs like the walls of blood vessels and kidneys, which are the most important organs for maintaining normal blood pressure. When both organs are damaged, their function is impaired simultaneously. This makes people with diabetes or kidney disease prone to high blood pressure.[24]

Sugar is fat

Sugar can make you gain weight and lead to health problems. Table sugar contains both glucose and fructose, which are found in many foods with added sugars. I will give examples of how sugar, especially fructose, can cause weight gain in both mice and humans.

When mice were fed a diet containing fructose, they developed fatty deposits in their liver and became obese.[25] In humans, overweight people who consume 150 g of glucose or fructose a day for 10 weeks can gain weight and increase their visceral fat.[26] Visceral fat wraps around vital organs and can be dangerous if it accumulates around the heart. In healthy men, eating 250 g of fructose or glucose a day for a week can increase liver fat.[27] Drinking a 12-oz can of soft drink every day for a year can also lead to a weight gain of 6 kg due to the high sugar content.[28,29] Some scientists even call fructose an "obesogen."

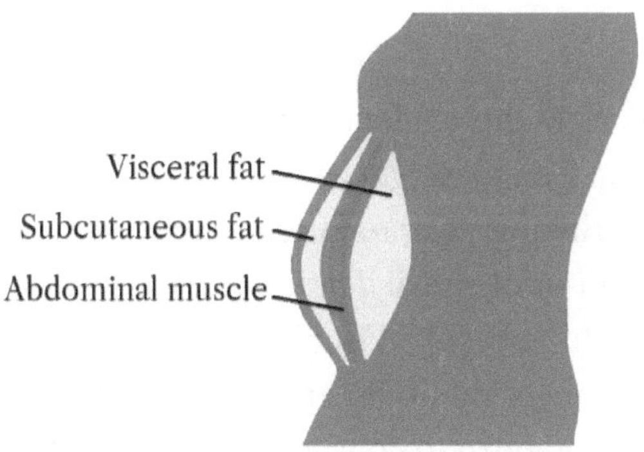

Visceral fat is the fat that wraps around the internal organs located inside the abdomen. This type of fat is harder than the fat that accumulates under the skin, or subcutaneous fat. A large amount of visceral fat can lead to a hard, big belly.

Not many people know that excess sugar in the body can cause the liver to produce more LDL cholesterol and triglycerides, which are stored in fat tissues and can lead to weight gain. Contrary to popular belief, cholesterol and triglycerides in your bloodstream don't come from eating excess fat but from consuming sugars such as glucose and fructose. If the sugar you eat is fructose, it can only be broken down by liver cells and is directly used to replenish liver glycogen and fuel the production of triglycerides. Triglycerides can build up in liver cells, causing a fatty liver, or be released into the bloodstream and cause plaque to build up in arteries. In short, fat comes from sugar, and it's important to be aware of this fact.

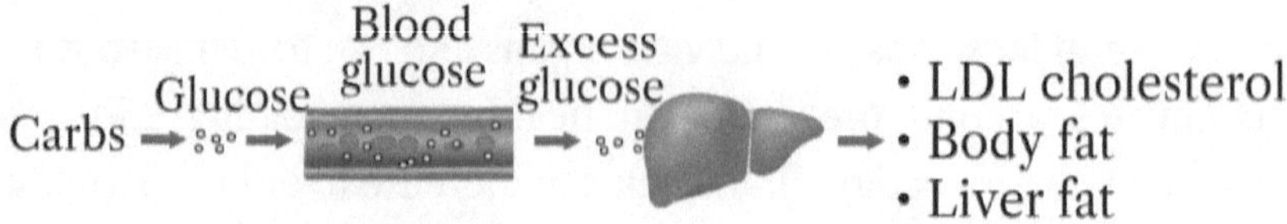

Excess sugar becomes body fat and can contribute to the formation of LDL cholesterol.

Indeed, all of this evidence points to the fact that excess sugar consumption can lead to weight gain and obesity. These days, people are eating and drinking sugar to fatten themselves up. Obesity is one of the leading causes of global death, at least 4 million people died in 2017 as a result of obesity. Visceral fat is a major contributor of obesity. If you can get rid of visceral fat, you will gain a healthy life. Actually, there is no need to consume more sugar. If you were aware of the sufficient carbohydrate intake obtained from bread, pasta and rice, deaths related to obesity could have been prevented.

Should we place the blame on the decades-long popularity of a type of sugar, fructose, as an obesogen? Fructose can be derived from corn, as corn is a common source of high-fructose corn syrup. Fructose is inexpensive and six times sweeter than sugar, making it a popular ingredient in syrups used in the food and beverage industries. Did you know that countries that sale fructose-rich sweeteners also have a higher incidence of diabetes.[30] Fructose is utterly deadly that should be avoided. The number of deaths caused by diabetes is significantly higher than those caused by crime. Today, we live in an environment where unhealthy food is disguised as regular food that appear to be healthy but actually contain ingredients that can lead to diabetes, resulting in approximately 1.6 million deaths each year.

The sugar traps

Since 2014, WHO recommended that adults and children consume no more than 5% of total energy from sugar, or no more than

25 g of sugar per day, which is equivalent to 6 teaspoons of sugar (1 teaspoon sugar weighs about 4 g).[31] The shocking fact is that 6 teaspoons of sugar can lead to 0.5 kg of weight gain per year.[32] If 6 teaspoons of sugar become excessive to your body, first the kidneys have to excrete the extra sugar through the urine, and then the leftover sugar is stored as glycogen and fat.

Certain foods, such as fruit and flavored yogurt, may contain up to 12 g of sugar.[33] Sugar in yogurt can be disguised under unfamiliar names such as corn syrup. Young children who have a tub of yogurt may already be getting half of the recommended daily sugar intake. Parents should be cautious about consuming certain food products. It's important to read the label before buying. If not, some healthy foods can become sugar traps, and yogurt may become "yo hurt."

Tooth decay and dental caries can serve as warning signs of excessive sugar consumption, as they are directly linked to high sugar intake. In fact, if you have dental caries, it's likely that you are consuming more than 25 g of sugar per day.[34] Mexico, which has one of the highest rates of obesity in the world, also has a prevalence of dental caries, with more than 90% of Mexican children between the ages of 6-12 affected.[35] This highlights the strong association between sugar intake and both dental caries and obesity.

Consuming excessive amounts of sugar has been associated with various health concerns in addition to dental caries and obesity. Studies show that individuals who consume high amounts of sugars are 20% more likely to have high triglycerides, which can be detrimental to heart health. Women who consume excessive amounts of sugars also have higher levels of LDL, the bad cholesterol. In a similar way, a diet that is high in sugar can cause chronic inflammation throughout the body and make cells less sensitive to insulin, increasing the risk of type 2 diabetes and heart disease. It's also important to note that sugar is not only hidden in yogurt but also in other foods such as salad dressings, energy bars, and snack bars.

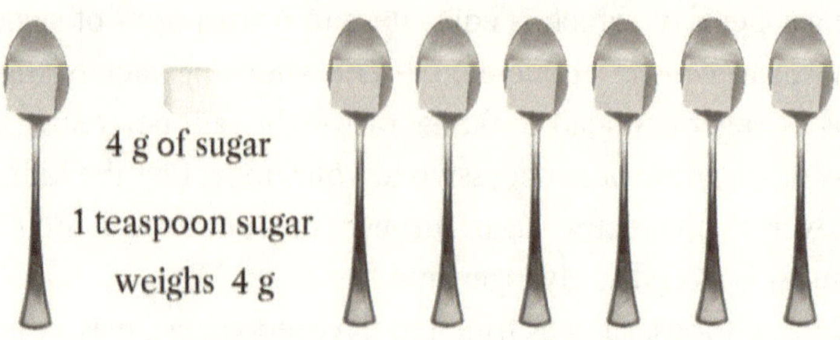

(the recommeded daily sugar in take by WHO)

25 g of sugar

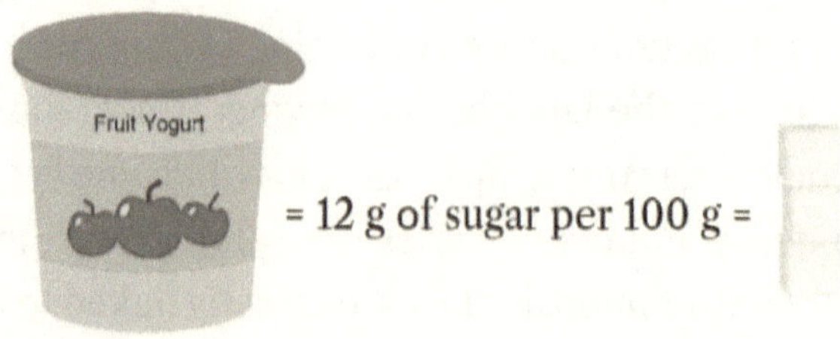

WHO guideline recommends adults and children reduce their daily intake of sugar to roughly 25 g (6 teaspoons) per day. But many fruit and flavored yogurt brands contain around 12 g of sugar, half of the sugar recommendation.

***

Foods with a bitter taste that can lower blood sugar levels

AGEs (advanced glycation end products) are compounds that form when excess sugar combines with proteins or lipids in the bloodstream. AGEs can also be found in foods such as bread and meat that were cooked at high temperatures. The browning or charring of these foods during cooking can lead to the formation of AGEs. When AGEs are formed in our body due to sugar consumption, they bind to different parts of the body, causing the body to deteriorate over time. For example, if AGEs bind to the collagen in the skin, that part of the skin will start to degrade, develop into wrinkles, and even cause the body to age faster. Apart from skin aging, abnormally large amounts of AGEs in the body can also lead to health conditions in vital organs such as the blood vessels, liver, kidneys, bones, nervous system, and heart.

However, nature has been a source of resources to us. There are natural foods that can be used to combat sugars and AGEs. The natural foods that can manage your blood sugar and AGEs are often bitter. One such natural food is bitter melon (*Momordica charantia*), which is loved by the people of Okinawa in Japan. Some Okinawans are among the oldest old people on the planet. Bitter melon is believed to have several health benefits, including blood sugar regulation, which may contribute to the longevity of the Okinawan population. Moreover, it seems that Okinawans have long known that blood sugar and AGEs can be control by intake of bitter melons.

According to a study, participants who received 6 g of dried bitter melon daily (equivalent to 70-80 g of fresh bitter melon) for 4 months saw a reduction in their AGEs.[36] What's more, recent clinical study, patients with type 2 diabetes who took 2 g of bitter melon a day, their blood sugar could be reduced slightly. However, this amount is equivalent to taking 1,000 mg of metformin, an oral anti-diabetic drug.[37] Two grams of bitter melon is as potent and effective as 1,000 mg of metformin, and wouldn't lead to unwanted results. It's worth considering this result seriously.

However, if you've never eaten bitter melon before, start by eating half of a fresh bitter melon. Eating too much of it can lower your blood sugar and make you feel tired and hungry. Alternatively, you can prevent sugar absorption into the bloodstream with natural foods like Thai gurmar (*Gymnema inodorum*), which inhibits the intestinal absorption of glucose.[38] Thai gurmar leaves are edible either raw or cooked as a vegetable, and is not bitter. Gurmar is Hindi for "sugar destroyer." Experiments in guinea pigs and rats showed that Thai gurmar reduced the rate of oxygen consumption in the intestinal muscles and inhibited bowel movement and glucose absorption from the intestine.

There is also an Indian species of gurmar (*Gymnema*

sylvestre) used to treat type 2 diabetes in Indian Ayurvedic medicine for over 2,000 years. But, this kind of gurmar is bitter. In diabetic mice, Indian gurmar can restore the pancreas function by improving the pancreatic function of sugar control and lower blood sugar. The diabetic patients who received a daily dose of 1,000 mg of dried Indian gurmar (this amount is about a few fresh stem tips or leaves of gurmar) for 30 days reduced blood sugar levels by 37%. A gram of dried Indian gurmar also reduced LDL, cholesterol and triglycerides in the bloodstream by 19%, 13% and 5%, respectively.[39] However, for people with type 2 diabetes or underlying medical conditions, eating gurmar should under the general supervision of a physician because too much gurmar can cause your blood sugar levels to fall very low.

Scientists now know that the main active ingredient in gurmar that stimulates the production of beta cells and insulin is gymnemic acid.[40,41] Gymnemic acid can stimulate beta cells in the pancreas to multiply. Thus, it has a high potential for the treatment of diabetes. The gymnemic acid contents in stem tips and leaves of gurmar were found to be 54 and 27 mg/g of dry weight respectively.[42] Likewise, as fresh weights, 1 g of stem tips or leaves of Indian gurmar may contain up to 2 mg of gymnemic acid. In a mouse, gymnemic acid dose of 13.4 mg/kg decreased blood glucose levels by 60% within 6 hours of administration.[43] Humans need a larger quantity of gymnemic acid. The 13.4 mg/kg of mouse dose is equivalent to about 1 mg/kg of human dose. A few fresh stem tips or leaves of gurmar may contain up to 70 mg of gymnemic acid.

Aside from its potential to lower blood sugar levels, gurmar has also been studied for its possible effects on weight loss. A study conducted on rats showed that gurmar extract reduced food intake and body weight gain. It was also found to have an effect on the levels of certain hormones involved in appetite regulation.

Garlic can lower your blood sugar
If you look through data, you will find that about 1.5 g of garlic supplement, which is equivalent to about 2 fresh cloves of garlic a

day, can lower blood glucose levels within 2 weeks.[44] And it can even lower blood glucose levels further, if a person take garlic for 12-24 weeks. Next time you cook, consider adding two smashed garlic cloves to your dishes to help lower blood glucose levels.

Garlic is not only a food staple, as garlic is a popular ingredient used in many cuisines around the world, but also has been utilized for its medicinal properties for centuries. Some countries that are recognized for their high consumption of garlic are Italy, Korea, and China, which are also known for having a large number of centenarians. Garlic can also be taken in supplement form, which is a convenient way to get the benefits without the taste. However, it's important to speak with a healthcare provider before starting any new supplement regimen. Garlic is a flavorful addition to any diet, and can be a natural way to support overall health and well-being.

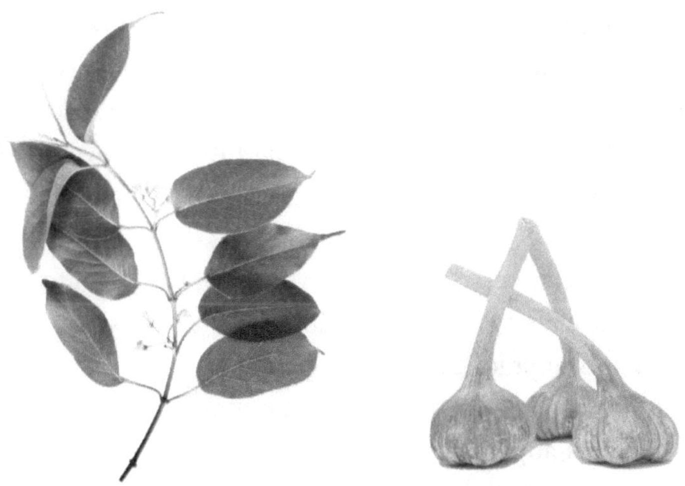

Thai gurmar has the ability to inhibit intestinal glucose uptake with just a single shot tip or leaf. Indian gurmar can also significantly lower blood sugar levels by up to 37%, while consuming 2 cloves of garlic can have a similar effect.

Taking curcumin can prevent the onset of type 2 diabetes

What if you could avoid the onset of type 2 diabetes, would

you do it? Well, there might be a method. A randomized, double-blinded, placebo-controlled study found that when 119 prediabetic participants took 750 mg of curcumin twice daily for nine months, they successfully staved off type 2 diabetes.[45] Meanwhile, 19 out of 116 participants not taking curcumin developed the condition. None of those in the curcumin-treated group were diagnosed with type 2 diabetes after the nine-month period.

Here is where it gets interesting. Curcumin from turmeric extract not only prevented type 2 diabetes in prediabetic participants, but it also boosted their pancreatic beta-cell function. After another year of monitoring, none of the 119 prediabetic participants who took curcumin developed type 2 diabetes. Importantly, there wasn't any report of serious side effects except for mild stomachaches.

In Asia and India, turmeric root is a culinary spice that is a staple in food dishes such as curries and cooked rice. People in these regions often grind dried turmeric roots into a fine powder and use it to favor their foods. Turmeric that contains the most curcumin is the turmeric found in the southern part of Thailand that is rainy throughout the year. A gram of the Thai turmeric powder from the south contains 90 mg of the active ingredient curcumin. Therefore, if you want to take 750 mg of curcumin twice daily to prevent type 2 diabetes or even reverse it, as in the research, you need to take 8.4 g of turmeric powder twice a day, or about 100 g of fresh turmeric root. This amount is impractical for most people.

Although an effective dose of curcumin for the prevention of type 2 diabetes appears to be about 500 mg per day, some clinical studies even report success with a mere 250-300 mg per day, helping to lower blood glucose levels and boost pancreatic function.[46,47,48] That is like taking 2.8-3.3 g of Thai turmeric powder or roughly 30 g of fresh turmeric root. Again, for some people, it's still too much.

Now let's talk about strategies that you can use to increase the bioavailability of curcumin, so that you don't have to consume too much turmeric. One way to increase the bioavailability of curcumin is to consume 150 g of avocado or a table spoon of extra virgin olive oil with curcumin, which can increase its bioavailability up to 7-8 times. For an even more impressive effect, add 20 mg of piperine (roughly 5-7 black peppercorns) to increase curcumin's bioavailability by 2,000%. But be cautious not to exceed 20 mg of piperine, as it might hinder curcumin's activity.[49]

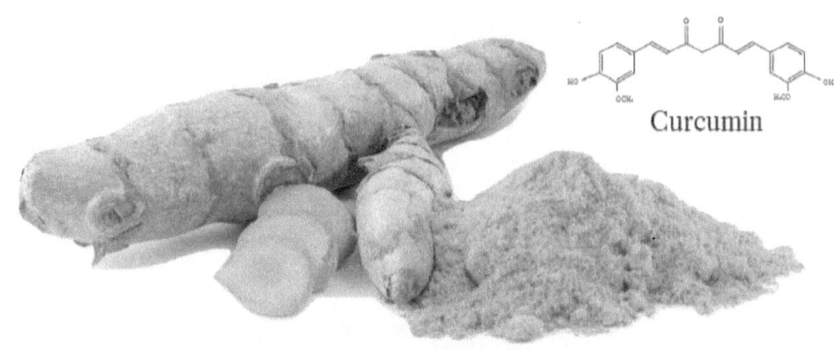

Turmeric, which is a root from the plant *Curcuma longa*, is a popular spice in traditional cuisine in India and Asian countries. Curcumin, a compound found in turmeric, can help to prevent people with prediabetes from developing type 2 diabetes.

It's worth noting that when participants who took 2 g of curcumin, an average concentration of curcumin in their blood was only 0.006 mcg/ml. However, participants who took 2 g of curcumin in combination with 20 mg of piperine, the concentration of curcumin in participant's bloodstream was increased to almost 0.2 mcg/ml. This means more than 20 mg of curcumin is absorbed into the bloodstream. And, for the first hour, a person taking curcumin has the highest level of curcumin in the bloodstream, and after 3 hours curcumin will be eliminated completely.[50] I believe that consuming a combination of curcumin, black pepper, and a source of healthy fat can further improve the bioavailability of curcumin. This means you can slash the amount of curcumin or turmeric required in half.

It's important to note, however, that while increasing the bioavailability of curcumin can be helpful in reaping its benefits, it's also essential to not overdo it with supplements or high doses of turmeric. Too much curcumin or turmeric can cause gastrointestinal distress and interact with certain medications.

For me, diabetes runs in my family. I believe that eating turmeric root will bring me close to being diabetes-free. So, on a regular basis, I consume a 125-mg dose of curcumin, or about 15 g of fresh turmeric root in the form of food. Here is my favorite 15 g of fresh turmeric root in food—boiled chicken with turmeric:

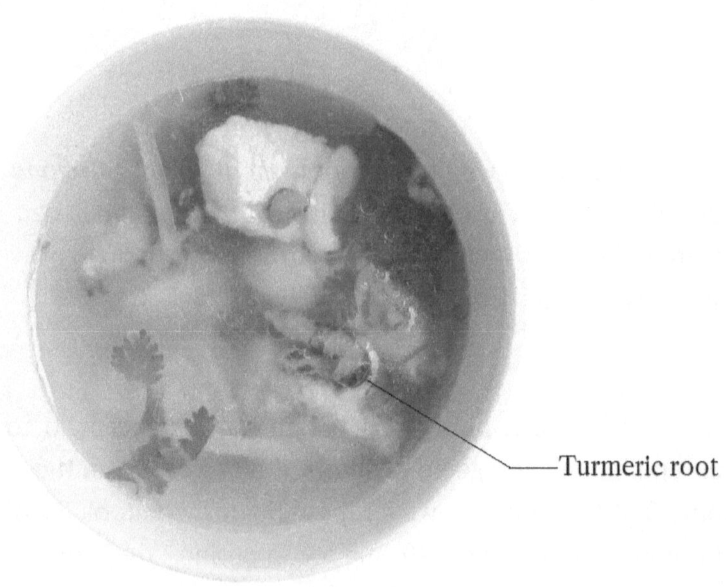

If you have a family history of type 2 diabetes, it's important to be mindful of your diet and sugar intake. For people who want to reduce excess sugar in their bodies, try to cut back on added sugar. Too much sugar can ruin your health. Alternatively, you could eliminate added sugars from your diet, even if it means giving up some of your favorite foods.

Stabilize blood sugar, live longer

Sugary drinks, candies, and processed foods high in refined carbohydrates can cause rapid spikes in blood sugar. High blood sugar levels can be harmful to your health. Sugar can cause issues like inflammation and damage to your tissues, nerves and organs, which can lead to serious health problems. High blood sugar can also lead to insulin resistance and type 2 diabetes, making it harder to live a long, healthy life. When you get close to your late 40s, it's crucial to watch out for type 2 diabetes. This is because research shows that this condition often affects Americans after they turn 45. In fact, a shocking 50% of Americans over 45 have prediabetes or type 2 diabetes.

Some other things that can cause high blood sugar levels, like having too much body weight, which can make your body resistant to insulin and raise your blood sugar levels. Constant stress can be harmful too, as it can negatively impact your blood sugar levels. Additionally, not getting enough sleep can mess up how your body controls blood sugar.

But if you manage your blood sugar levels well, you can slow down the aging process and possibly avoid or delay age-related diseases. Keeping your blood sugar in check is one of the most important things you can do for your longevity.

Two simple ways to keep your blood sugar levels stable are eating healthy foods and exercising regularly. These habits also help your body use insulin effectively, and maintain insulin sensitivity. You can also use a gadget to monitor your blood sugar after eating, so you can make changes if needed. Our bodies' genes work best when our blood sugar stays stable. By doing these things, you're on the right path to maintaining balanced gene activity, leading to a longer and healthier life. Otherwise, imbalanced gene activities can cause aging.

I also believe that lifestyle and dietary habits play important roles in your overall health. If you lead an unhealthy lifestyle and have a poor diet, maintaining your blood sugar levels and consuming curcumin may not be as effective as the damage may have already been done. It's also important to remember that lifestyle changes take time, and it may require patience and persistence to see the full benefits. At the end, the positive impact on your health and quality of life can be well worth the effort.

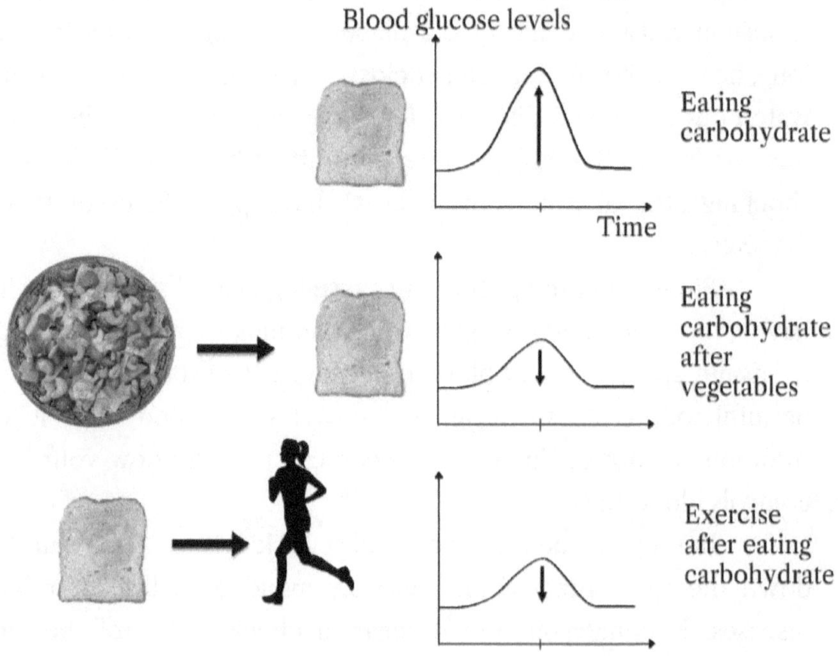

Blood sugar levels typically reach their highest point about 90 minutes after eating. However, when protein and vegetables are consumed before carbs, studies show a roughly 30% decrease in these levels.[51] Also, a brief 3-minute walk half an hour post meal can stabilize blood sugar. Exercise is beneficial as it enables muscles to take in glucose without needing insulin, which in turn lessens insulin production.

Ultimately, when you incorporate foods like gurmar and bitter melon into your diet, which are known to lower blood sugar levels and impede glucose absorption, your body may experience some adjustments. This reaction can be likened to the effects of quitting sugar. These symptoms may last for several days or weeks as your body tries to get accustomed to the healthier alternatives. However, once this adjustment period is over, you may experience positive changes such as more radiant skin, a brighter complexion, healthier hair (less prone to falling out), improved sleep, a stronger immune system, and overall better health. Reaching this point will be a source of great joy and satisfaction. If not, you may end up having to get up at night, wetting yourself before you can make it to the bathroom, and in the end, becoming another person with diabetes.

CHAPTER 5

Karma of eating

The food we eat has a powerful impact on our health and well-being. It's no secret that "you are what you eat", and in today's globalized world, certain foods can be just as harmful as smoking or excessive drinking. The choices we make today will shape the life we live later on, and it's up to us to decide whether we want to nourish our bodies or harm them.

Let me share a story with you. Once, I attended a seminar in a remote province of Thailand. After a long day, it was time for the much-awaited get-together dinner. As I looked around the table, I noticed that many of my fellow attendees were piling their plates high with roast beef, fried chicken, fried vegetables, and sushi, along with tempting desserts and ice cream. But I made a conscious choice to load up half my plate with veggies, and the other half with a mix of rice and meats. And since I tend to eat less, I finished my plate well before anyone else.

As I looked around the table, I noticed one particular attendee whose plate was piled high with fatty foods like roast beef, fried chicken, and squid sushi, yet it lacked any veggies. He turned to me and asked, "How come you eat so healthy?" I just smiled and didn't give an answer.

Years later, I heard from a friend that the same attendee had become overweight and developed high cholesterol. Our choices truly matter—the food we enjoy today can influence our health for years ahead. Also, the type and amount of food we eat can have an effect on many bodily functions, including metabolism, heart health, and immune system. So, choose wisely and prioritize your health!

How bacon, ham, and sausages negatively affect your health

In the production process of bacon, ham, and sausages, curing agents like nitrates and nitrites are added in the form of potassium nitrate, potassium nitrite, sodium nitrate, or sodium nitrite. These preservatives are added to prevent meat spoilage and the growth of bacteria that spoil the products. Nitrates and nitrites also provide the meat with a beautiful reddish-pink color, which remains even after being exposed to high temperatures.

Nonetheless, the World Health Organization (WHO) has cautioned us for years about the health hazards linked to regular consumption of bacon, ham, and sausages, especially concerning colorectal cancer. That is because a carcinogenic compound, nitrosamine, in these products, forms when added nitrites interact with the amine group in meat protein. Despite these warnings, many people continue to disregard the risks.

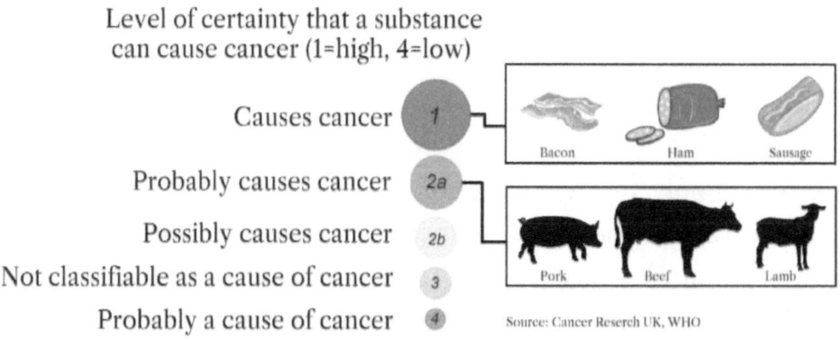

Foods including bacon, ham, and sausages are cancer-causing substances.[1,2]

Health red flag for red meat

Are your favorite meals worth sacrificing your health for? It's time to reconsider your love for red meat like pork, beef, and lamb.

Did you know that consuming too much red meat can increase your risk of getting cancer? Not just any cancer, but esophagus, stomach, and colorectal cancer, the most common ones in red meat eaters. Have you ever wondered why meat is red? The answer lies in the heme iron-containing protein. Red meat contains high levels of heme iron, with a concentration 5 times higher than in white meat like chicken and turkey. Regrettably, heme iron can contribute to carcinogenesis, elevating your cancer risk with each mouthful.[4]

But the risk doesn't stop there. Consistently eating red meat may cause inflammation in the colon's epithelial tissues. Picture this: enjoying your beloved steak or roast beef sandwich could cause a long-lasting inflamed colon, similar to when pathogens attack your body. This ongoing inflammation might even worsen and progress to colorectal cancer.[5,6]

And if that's not enough to scare you, here's another fact: regularly eating red or processed meat can increase your risk of dying from heart disease by 7%.[7] It's time to take a closer look at what you are putting on your plate and consider healthier alternatives.

A little bit of knowledge

Did you know that intestinal epithelial cells have a short lifespan of only 3-4 days and are renewed at a rate of 1 in 10 cells each day? Normally, these cells experience cycles of destruction and regeneration. Yet, in mice, researchers discovered that the cells on the intestinal wall are highly prone to mutations. As the mouse ages, the number of mutations increases, making it more susceptible to cancer.

TMAO—the compound in red meat that can harm your health

Let's explore the world of TMAO (trimethylamine N-oxide), a substance created when red meat is digested. Eating red meat often for just a month can cause TMAO levels in your body to rise more than tenfold. Scientists have found that TMAO plays a role in the development of atherosclerosis that is the hardening of the arteries.

TMAO is usually found in ocean fish like cod, ray, tuna, and mackerel, with levels ranging from 20 to 1,500 mg per 100 g. Interestingly, a fish's tail muscle has more TMAO than its head. In saltwater fish, TMAO plays a crucial role in maintaining balance for urea, salinity, pressure, and temperature.

When you eat red meat, eggs, ocean fish, or foods rich in choline, lecithin, and carnitine, gut bacteria transform these compounds into TMA (trimethylamine), a substance that smells like spoiled fish. TMA is absorbed into your bloodstream and changed into TMAO in your liver by the FMO enzyme. Having too much TMA in your body can cause nausea and dizziness.

Interestingly, gut bacteria composition also significantly impacts TMAO production in people who eat meat. A 2017 study by Cornell University revealed that people with higher TMAO levels after consuming eggs and beef have a greater number of "Firmicutes" bacteria, which are considered harmful gut bacteria and can contribute to obesity. In contrast, those with lower TMAO levels have more "Bacteroidetes," known as beneficial gut bacteria, which can aid in weight loss. People with obesity often have more Firmicutes and fewer Bacteroidetes bacteria in their gut. Interestingly, centenarians who live a very long time—to 100 or more —usually have more Bacteroidetes. Experts believe that having more of these bacteria could be a reason these people live longer.

TMAO promotes atherosclerosis

Let's get back to TMAO. As mentioned before, TMAO is found in the bloodstream after eating foods containing choline, lecithin or carnitine. These substances found not only in red meat, but also in energy drinks and dietary supplements. The bad bacteria in the intestine convert choline, lecithin and carnitine to TMA, which is absorbed into the bloodstream, and into the liver. In this organ, TMA is converted to TMAO. TMAO then enters into the blood vessels. However, as for TMAO in some foods like fish, if we eat fish, about 50% of the ingested TMAO is excreted in urine. Another 50% of TMAO can be depleted by some gut bacteria.

The big problem is that TMAO encourages the buildup of fat deposits and plaque within the walls of blood vessels, causing the arteries to become harder and thicker. As time goes on, the atherosclerosis on arteries can lead to them becoming narrower, more restricted, and possibly even blocked, which can result in heart disease, stroke, or even death.[8,9] In 2016, researchers at the Cleveland Clinic discovered that TMAO can also interact with platelets, which are small blood cells in charge of clotting blood and fixing wounds. However, in this strange situation, TMAO makes platelets extra sensitive to stimuli. This ends up raising the chances of blood clots, heart attacks, and strokes even more.

What's more, TMAO's negative effects go beyond heart disease and stroke, as studies have connected high levels of TMAO with other health issues like kidney disease, liver disease, and even some cancers. TMAO might cause inflammation and oxidative stress in the kidneys, leading to kidney problems and fibrosis. It can also contribute to fat buildup in the liver, causing inflammation and liver damage. TMAO has been linked to DNA damage, which can result in the formation of cancerous cells. TMAO can also cause your blood vessels to age more rapidly. Therefore, it's evident that you should reduce your intake of foods rich in choline, lecithin, and carnitine, especially red meat, to lower your TMAO levels and decrease the risk of these serious health problems.

Moreover, as we age, the number of harmful gut bacteria tends to increase, leading to higher TMAO levels in our bloodstream. Consequently, the older you become, the higher your TMAO levels will be. With increased TMAO levels in your blood, there is a greater likelihood of damage to your arteries, potentially exacerbating health issues related to cardiovascular health.

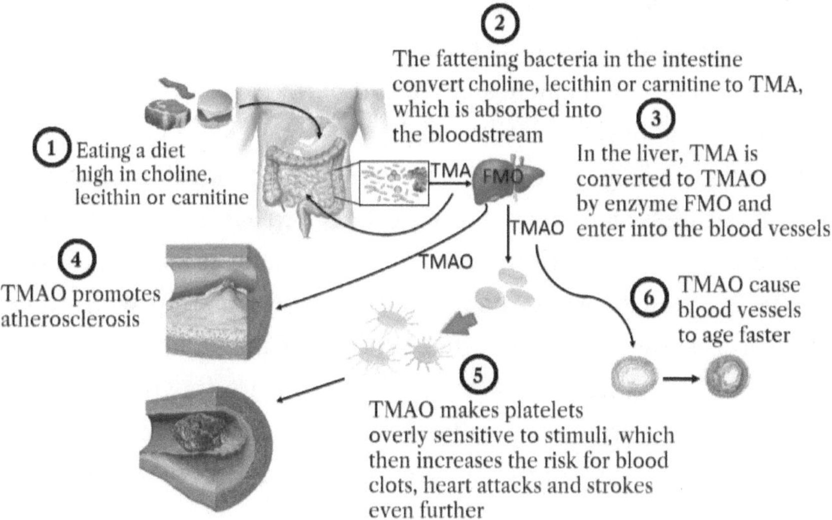

TMAO can cause atherosclerosis and deteriorated blood vessels. It also makes the small platelets overly sensitive to stimuli, raising the risk of blood clots, heart attacks, and strokes, as well as accelerating the aging of blood vessels.[10,11]

Watch out for acrylamide in your food!

Acrylamide is a chemical commonly found in roasted, baked, and deep-fried foods, such as French fries, potato chips, and over-toasted bread and baked goods. The darker the color of these over-toasted products, the more acrylamide they contain. For instance, 100 g of regular toasted bread has 7 mcg of acrylamide, while burnt toast has over 10 mcg. The International Agency for Research on Cancer has classified acrylamide as a "probable human carcinogen."

Once in the body, acrylamide is converted to a compound called glycidamide, which causes mutations and DNA damages. Although the neurotoxic effect of acrylamide intake is 500 times higher than the average acrylamide intake or 75 mcg per day,[12] the WHO has recommended that a liter of drinking water should contain no more than 0.1 mcg of acrylamide. This is a reason to be cautious with acrylamide in our diets. Without even realizing it, you might be consuming foods high in acrylamide, such as French fries, potato chips, toasted bread, baked snacks, and burnt foods. Regularly eating certain types of foods with high acrylamide levels, sometimes exceeding 75 mcg, can increase your risk of developing cancer. Multiple studies have suggested a link between acrylamide intake and an increased risk of various types of cancer, such as kidney, ovarian, and womb cancer. About half of the people diagnosed with cancer often don't show symptoms until it's too late. Cancer develops slowly, like a perfect storm, until it suddenly appears in your life. The following chart provides a rough idea of the amount of acrylamide present in various foods, so you can be more aware of your consumption.

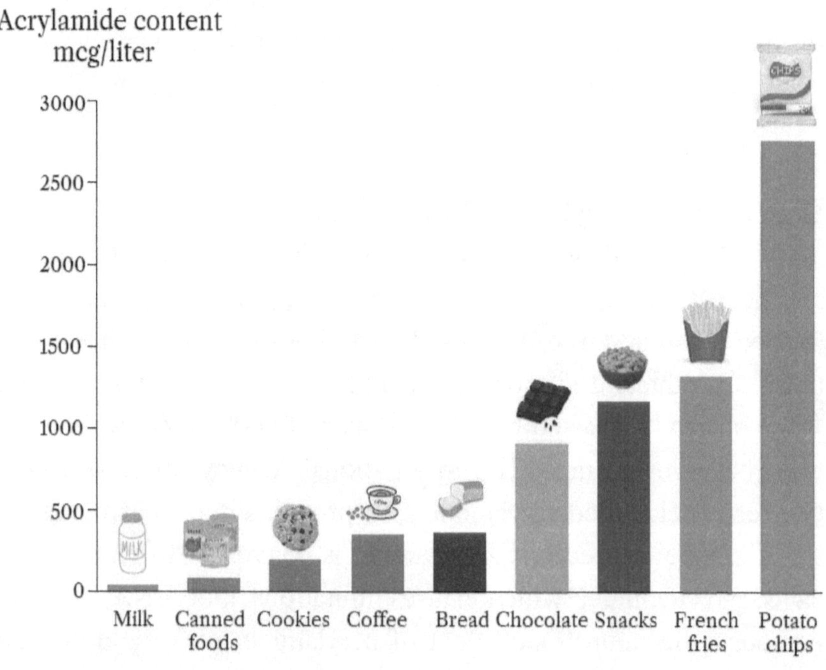

The high levels of acrylamide content found in various foods.[13,14]

Without phosphate, colas will turn black

Foods high in protein and calcium such as milk, tofu, eggs and beans are usually high in phosphorus. In these foods, most of the phosphorus is bound to calcium, and the leftover phosphorus is in the form of phosphate. Therefore, natural foods rarely contain phosphate.

In contrast, processed foods contain much higher phosphorus from phosphate additives. In the European Union, phosphate additives like sodium phosphate (E339), potassium phosphate (E340), calcium phosphate (E341), diphosphates (E450), triphosphate (E451) and polyphosphate (E452) can be used legally as a preservative, acid regulator, buffer or emulsifier. Phosphate salts are also used in many foods to preserve color or enhance flavor, and extend self-life. An example of a well-known phosphate-containing beverage is a cola. Cola is brownish because of inorganic phosphate, without added phosphate, colas will turn black.[15]

Regarding the socio-economic status, processed foods laden with phosphate-containing food additives are popular among people belonging to the middle and lower classes. These foods tend to take over their kitchens. Many lower-class citizens especially often find it difficult to manage time because their work lives are hectic. Therefore, for them, cooking seems like too much trouble. Buying processed and ready-to-eat foods is easier and faster. But, "comfort can be addictive." The most important driver to consume ready-to-eat foods is convenience.[16] And those who buy ready-to-eat foods just can't see the health impacts these junk foods will bring.

Food items with significantly greater phosphorus content that people in the middle and lower classes buy includes frozen foods, dry food mixed, packaged meat, bread and baked goods, soup and yogurt, which contain an average of 67 mg of phosphorus per 100 g.[17] This amount of inorganic phosphorus is similar to that of a 12-oz can of Pepsi.

Although Pepsi actually says that "phosphorus levels in all their beverages are well within the reference daily intake amounts set by the U.S. Food & Drug Administration (FDA) and are safe for consumption by people of all ages." Here the image displayed on the website provides a visual representation of this concept.[18]

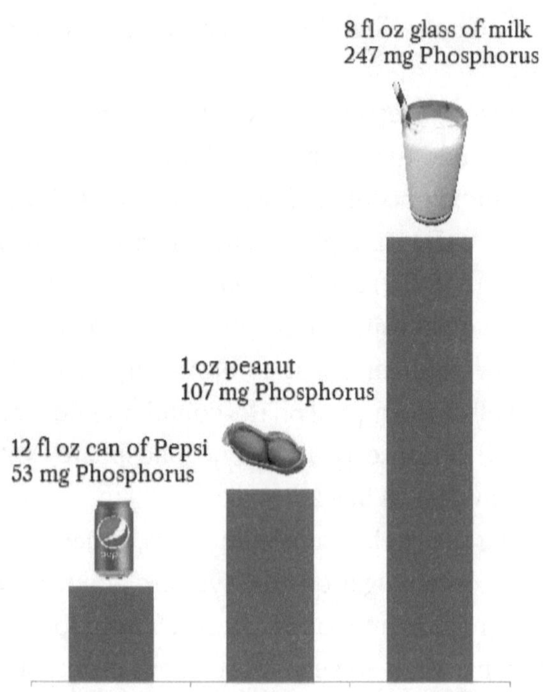

Although our bodies absorb only about 50% of the phosphorus from natural foods, phosphorus added as an additive to processed foods is absorbed more easily, up to 100%. This is a concern, as normal blood phosphorus levels range from 2.5 to 4.5 mg/dL, but can vary slightly from 1.6 to 6.2 mg/dL in healthy people with normal kidney function.[19] The reason for this variation is unclear, but it may be due to differences in kidney function. It's important to note that high blood phosphorus levels have been linked to an increased risk of heart disease, cardiovascular disease, and death, so doctors recommend that levels should not exceed 4 mg/dL.[20,21,22]

These days, there is a battle between healthy and unhealthy foods. Eating natural foods is associated with better health outcomes. In contrast, consuming unhealthy foods such as bacon, ham, sausages, red meat, soft drinks, energy drinks, French fries, snacks, and processed foods with added phosphorus can lead to an early death.

It's observed that people with lower socio-economic status tend to consume more of these unhealthy foods. On the other hand, those who opt for a healthier diet may have a longer life expectancy. It's true that research has shown that the wealthiest 1% of Americans live up to 14 years longer than the poorest 1%.[23] This life expectancy gap is due to variations in health habits. Therefore, if you choose to eat healthy, you can expect to live up to 10 years longer.

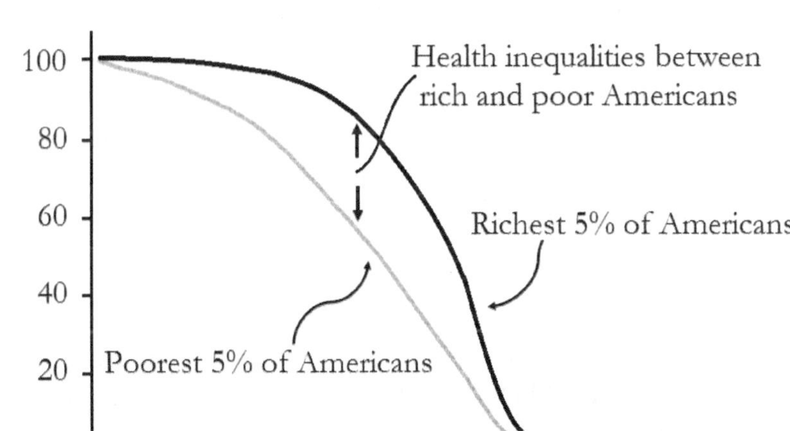

The diagram shows health inequality among the richest and poorest 5% of Americans. Being wealthy adds more years to life while extreme poverty has the opposite effect. Inadequate preventive care and nutrition knowledge may cause the poorest 1% of Americans to have a 14-year shorter life expectancy than the richest 1%.[23]

The 14-year health inequality between the richest and poorest Americans may be due to the lack of preventive care and nutrition knowledge among the poor. To reduce health inequalities, eating more natural foods can make a big difference in overall health and quality of life. For middle and lower classes, prevention and education play vital roles in reducing these health disparities. Initiatives like community gardens, farmers markets, and nutrition education programs can help improve access to healthy food options. By working together, we can create a healthier and more equitable society for everyone.

***

Getting enough fiber each day keeps bad karma of eating away

Developed countries are currently taking steps to address the issue of unhealthy eating habits, particularly the lack of dietary fiber in people's diets. In the European Union, for example, the advised fiber intake for its people is at least 30g a day.[24] Nevertheless, most people fall short of their recommended fiber intake. Some people in Europe are able to eat only 3-4 g of fiber a day, which is far from the recommended amount.

Some scientists suggested that we should eat at least 25 g of dietary fiber a day. People who consume more fiber had significantly lower body weight, blood pressure, and cholesterol compared to those who ate less fiber. But, if you can eat 25-29 g of fiber a day, it will give you even better results. Higher levels of fiber lower the risk of developing serious illnesses such as cardiovascular disease, type 2 diabetes, colon cancer and breast cancer.[25]

But in Japan, the recommended fiber intake is 20 g a day .[26] Why the daily fiber intake of Japanese is set at about 20 g? This magic number is based on studies of the daily dietary fiber intake of Japanese people with colon polyp, colon diverticulosis and colorectal cancer. Interestingly, in a particular region of Japan, Aomori, where the prevalence of colon diverticulosis—a condition where pouches protrude through the colon—was at its lowest, people consumed more than 20g of dietary fiber.[27]

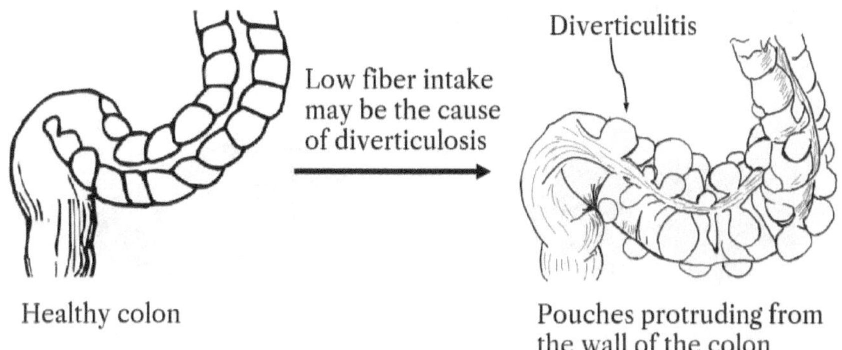

By the age of 60, about 50% of people in Western countries develop diverticulosis. However, a daily fiber intake of more than 20 g reduces your risk of developing diverticulosis.[28,29]

Eating lots of dietary fiber can do wonders for your health because it helps fight off chronic diseases. In one study, they found that having a fiber-rich diet can actually lower your chances of getting serious diseases such as type 2 diabetes, stroke incidence, heart disease and cancer, and boost your survival rate by 15% to 30%.[30]

Why is important to downsizing the risk of death and chronic diseases? Let me explain it. Consider the United States, where 15 young Americans are diagnosed with type 2 diabetes and almost 1,800 Americans die from heart disease every day. By improving their chances of survival from 50% to 60%, one person can be saved from type 2 diabetes, and 180 Americans can avoid death from heart disease daily. Similarly, if you can find a slight improvement in the treatment of a disease, you can raise your chance of survival by 10% or even more.

Natural foods that are high in fiber content include red or black beans, Japanese purple sweet potatoes, apples, carrots, cabbage, and broccoli. These foods contain between 20-30 g of fiber per specific amounts, making them excellent choices for boosting your fiber intake. However, it's important to consume a variety of high-fiber foods to maximize the benefits.

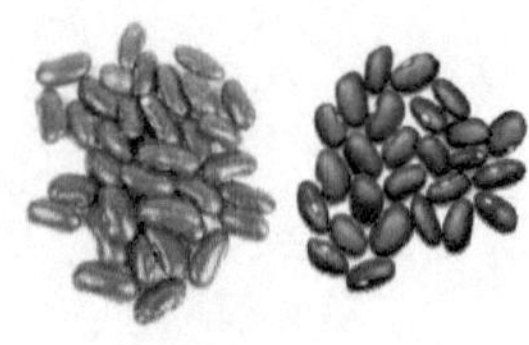

500 g of red or black beans contain 20 g of fiber

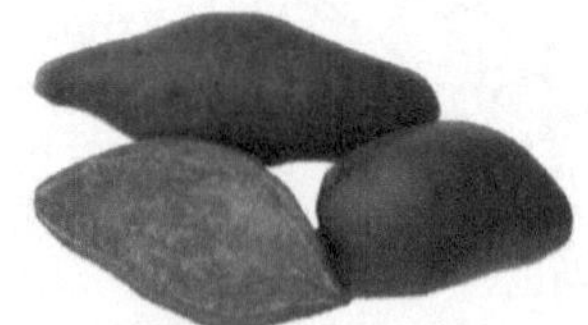

1,000 g of Japanese purple sweet potatoes contain 30 g of fiber

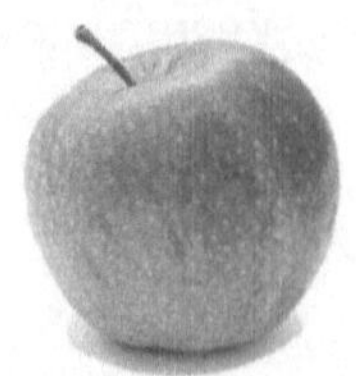

1,000 g of apples contain 30 g of fiber

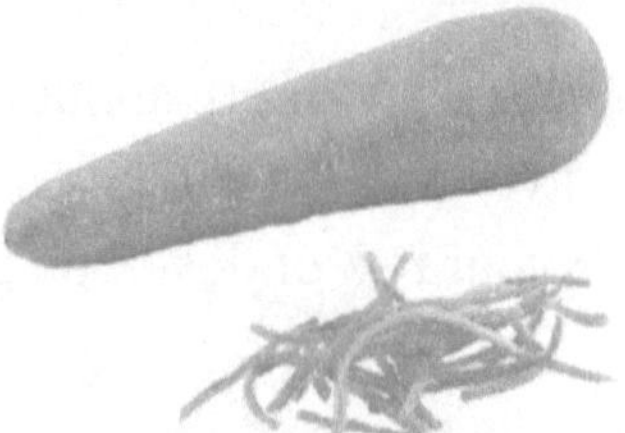

1,000 g of carrots contain 28 g of fiber

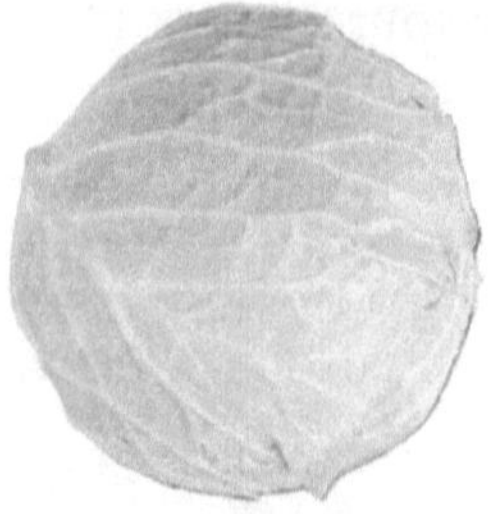

1,000 g of cabbage contain 25 g of fiber

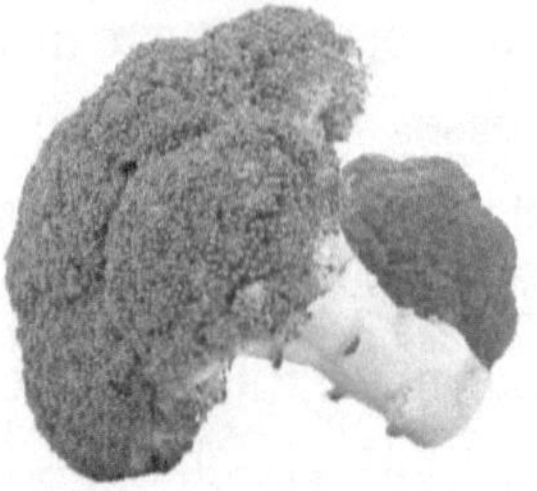

1,000 g of broccoli contain 20 g of fiber

Alternatives to junkie foods, these are high-fiber foods that you can eat each day for health benefits and to prevent chronic diseases like heart disease, stroke incidence, type 2 diabetes and cancer.[32]

It's time to nix the bad food habit and focus on eating healthier. If you want to know how much fiber in your diet is. You can find it on the FoodData Central website at https://fdc.nal.usda.gov. Eating more fiber is a way to prevent chronic diseases and increase the chance of survival. In the context of public health, even small percentage increases can have a massive impact on large populations, ultimately saving countless lives and reducing the burden on healthcare systems.

Foods that may help reduce the negative effects of red meat

If you still crave the taste of luxury red meat, adding orange peel, oolong tea, extra-virgin olive oil, and garlic to your diet may help inhibit TMA production in your gut. Studies conducted on mice showed that eating orange peel or oolong tea extract significantly reduced blood levels of TMAO in mice fed carnitine.[33] Additionally, extra-virgin olive oil, which is a main component of the Mediterranean diet, contains DMB (3,3-dimethylbutan-1-ol), an active ingredient that has a chemical structure similar to choline commonly found in Western diets. DMB can inhibit TMA production in the gut.[34] In mice fed choline or carnitine diet in the presence of 0.18 mcg of DMB every day for 14 days, the reduction of TMA production was 50% compared to mice fed choline or carnitine diet alone. Some brands of extra-virgin olive oil may contain up to 250 mg of DMB per 100 ml. It's possible that consuming red meat with extra-virgin olive oil can reduce TMA production and blood levels of TMAO in humans.

In addition to extra-virgin olive oil, consuming a high-fiber diet may also help inhibit TMA production in the gut. Fiber-rich foods, such as fruits, vegetables, and whole grains, can promote the growth of beneficial gut bacteria that produce less TMA. When the good bacteria in your gut are thriving, the bad bacteria won't be able to take over. A high fiber diet can aid in weight management too. High fiber foods are more filling and take longer to digest, which can help prevent overeating and reduce the risk of obesity. Overall, incorporating these foods and ingredients into your diet can potentially reduce the negative effects of red meat consumption, lower obesity risks, and improve overall health.

What's more, garlic contains one of the major active components, allicin, which also inhibit gut microbial TMA production.[35,36] Allicin is most commonly found in the soft-necked garlic (*Allium sativum* var. Sativum), which its neck is generally soft and has more cloves per bulb. One hundred grams of soft-necked garlic contains 1,465 mg of allicin.[37]

Also, regular intake of garlic is linked to a lower death from any cause .[38] If you eat garlic 5 times a week, it could add a year to your life. In addition, about 1.5 g of garlic supplement or about 2 cloves of garlic a day can also lower blood glucose levels within 2 weeks and improve blood lipid levels by 12 weeks.[39]

As science advances, we could, in the future, see the use of garlic, oolong tea and extra virgin olive oil as better drugs than synthetic drugs to inhibit the production of TMA and TMAO for the prevention of atherosclerosis and cardiovascular disease.

Some cuisines already use vegetables, fruits, extra virgin olive oil, and garlic as staples. Our ancestors may have known that these foods can mitigate the harmful effects of red meat. However, in some cultures, meat-based foods such as bacon, ham, and sausages are not paired with natural foods like vegetables, fruits, extra virgin olive oil, and garlic.

Cooking meals at home is a great way to add vegetables, fruits, extra virgin olive oil, and garlic to your diet. However, it can be challenging to access healthy foods because of complex systems that have been created to prevent it. Additionally, people often opt for convenient foods over natural foods due to busy schedules. Ready-to-eat foods that are widely available can also be an obstacle to healthy eating. As a matter of fact, convenience foods aren't the healthiest, but makers excel at providing them. You should resist the urge for easy options and choose healthier alternatives.

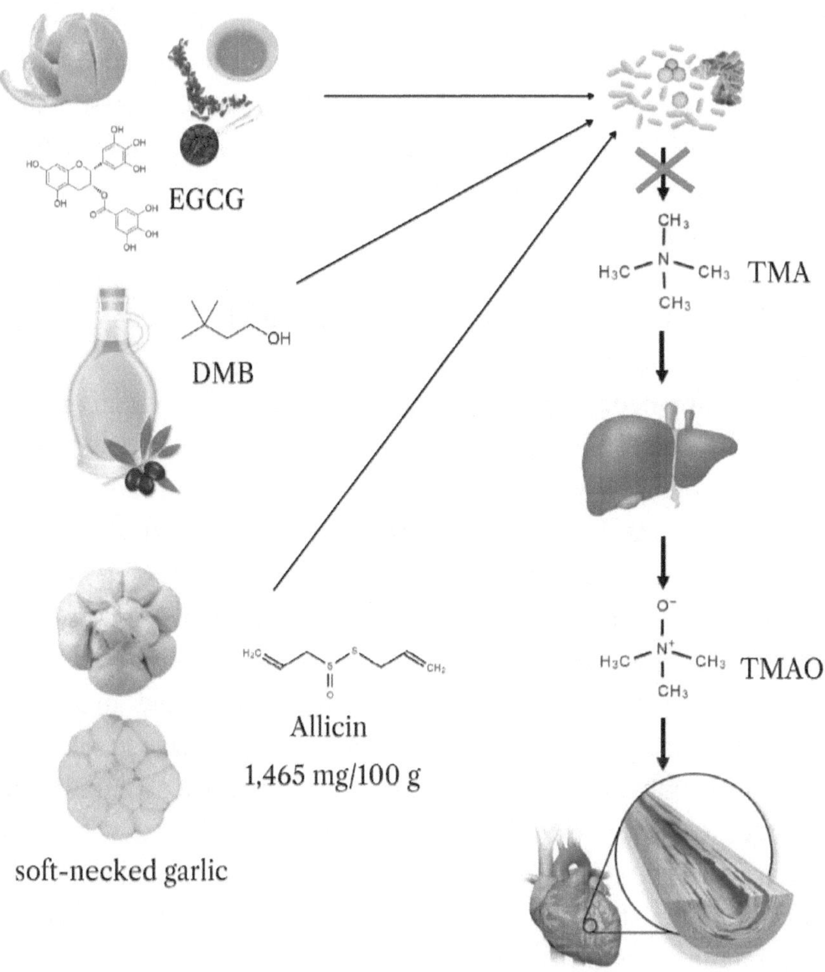

Oolong tea, extra virgin olive oil, garlic and orange peel extract inhibits bacterial TMA production in the gut and reduces TMAO levels in the bloodstream that causes atherosclerosis and cardiovascular disease.[33,36,40]

One way to overcome the obstacle of ready-to-eat foods is by keeping natural foods like fruits, vegetables, nuts, sweet potatoes, extra virgin olive oil, onions, and garlic in your kitchen and fridge. Encouraging your family, especially children, to eat these foods instead of processed foods and drink water instead of soft drinks is crucial. Processed foods are major causative factors of maladies like obesity, type 2 diabetes, heart disease, and cancer, so it's essential to avoid them. Our ancestors ate a diet that was predominantly fruits and vegetables, with very little fat and no dairy. Turning away from your traditional diet can negatively impact your health. Our modern diet is making us sick and filling society with diseased people. Prioritizing the consumption of fruits and vegetables can help you avoid falling ill.

Many people are eating unhealthy because, when it comes to choosing foods, their decision is clouded. Especially when your stomach is empty, you tend to choose high energy foods that are cheap and foods that require no preparation—even though they are less healthy. In modern days, it seems that our bodies urge us toward consumption whatever food that is the highest satiety value and available during that time. However, these types of foods can alter your gene expression, cause you to age faster, and make you susceptible to serious diseases earlier in life. As you have learned, the foods you choose can have a significant impact on your future health. As you get older, your body's ability to fix and deal with aging decreases. The aging process can even speed up if you eat unhealthy foods. The time to act is now. The health you'll enjoy in the future is built on the choices you make today, not when you retire.

In a nutshell, the way we eat can either help or harm us. When you eat things like bacon, ham, sausages, and other red meats, foods high in a substance called acrylamide, or processed foods packed with phosphate, you're doing more harm than good. On the flip side, you can boost your health by eating lots of fruits, veggies, nuts, and legumes, making sure you get more than 20 g of dietary fiber each day, adding garlic to your meals, and enjoying oolong tea and meals cooked with extra-virgin olive oil. So, make the choice today, swap out the bad for the good, and let the healthy eating habits steer you towards a vibrant and long-lasting life.

Part 3

Fight Chronic Diseases with Natural, Anti-aging Foods

CHAPTER 6

Reversible type 2 diabetes

My grandfather died from type 2 diabetes when he was 75 years old. From my experience, I can tell you that type 2 diabetes is a horrible disease that you don't want to have. Though I don't have diabetes yet, I know how much fear a person feels about diabetes and its consequences. When you have diabetes, your life seems to come to an end. Every day you have to worry about what you can and can't eat. You have to be careful not to consume too much sugary and starchy food. Many times, you have to wake up in the middle of the night to go to the bathroom; otherwise, you have to wear adult diapers. Even a small cut or an insect bite is a major concern for people with diabetes, as it can turn into something much worse and lead to the loss of an arm or leg. Nobody would want to live like my grandfather did. It's hard to live in a broken body. Yet, that is the life of a diabetic.

Diabetes is a chronic disease, meaning a condition in which the symptoms of the disease last for a year or more, or persist throughout a person's life, depending on the condition of the disease. A chronic disease is not passed from person to person. Generally, chronic diseases like asthma, arthritis, heart attack, stroke, cancer, and diabetes can't be cured. Although chronic diseases do not fix themselves, they can be controlled or even reversed.

Thailand is my country. Although it's not among the top 5 countries for people with diabetes, as mentioned before, Thai people eat rice as their staple food and have a sweet tooth. These eating habits are similar to those of Indians. The vast majority of Indians, 70-80%, eat carbohydrate foods such as rice, wheat, millet, beans, and corn.[1] What's more, Indians enjoy eating sugar, nectar, bread, crisps, and crunchy snacks more than necessary. It has been reported that Indians consume almost 18 kg of sugar/person/year,[2] making India the world's second-largest consumer of sugar,[3] but less than Thai's intake of sugar, which is 29 kg/person/year on average.[4] As the second-most populous country in the world, India has the second-largest population of diabetics globally—second only to China. In fact, 1 in 6 people with diabetes worldwide is from India.

The prevalence of people with diabetes

When counting the number of people with diabetes between the ages of 20 and 79, the top three countries with the highest diabetes populations in the world are China 116 million, India 77 million and the United States 31 million respectively.[5] To investigate the cause of diabetes in this modern era, one could examine a country that has abruptly changed its people's eating habits and has the highest prevalence of diabetic patients in the world. For instance, that is the Republic of the Marshall Islands.

As of 2018, despite having a population of just 58,413, the Marshall Islands has been reported to have 30% of its citizens with diabetes.[6] However, back in the 1950s, the people of Marshall Island had to have been happier since the Marshall Islands had only 3 people with diabetes. One of the reasons for the Marshall Islands having the highest prevalence of diabetes in the world is due to the dependence on imported foods such as rice, white flour, and foods high in salt, sugar, and fat. This dependence has been present since the 1990s. Another reason is unhealthy lifestyle choices made by the people of Marshall Islands who are more likely to shop for white rice, refined flour, chicken, ramen, and canned meats for their own satisfaction.[7,8] Imagine adults and kids in Marshall Island having ramen noodles, donuts, or pancakes with a cup of syrup, white rice, and meats. Imagine they are having soft drinks, sweetened beverages, and coffee with creamer and sugar like this almost every day. How could they not develop diabetes?

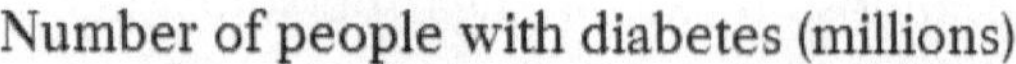

Number of people with diabetes (millions)

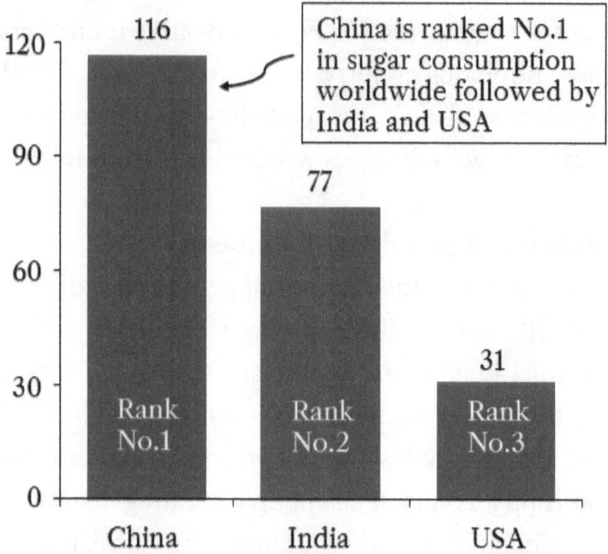

Top 3 countries with highest diabetes population

The top three countries with the highest diabetes populations in the world are China, India, and the United States. It's worth noting that these countries are also among the largest consumers of sugar worldwide.[3,5]

Know your blood sugar numbers

Diabetes is a condition that occurs when blood glucose level stays abnormally high. Generally, a normal blood glucose level before breakfast is 70-100 mg/dL or between 3.9-5.6 mmol/L.[10] Throughout the day, your body must maintain blood glucose level at about 5.5 mmol/L (100 mg/dL) or equivalent to 5 g of sugar in the bloodstream. But if one's blood glucose level before breakfast was 100 to 125 mg/dL or between 5.6 and 6.9 mmol/L, this person can be considered at high risk for developing diabetes. However, the fasting blood sugar level of people with type 2 diabetes is 126 mg/dL (7 mmol/L) or higher.

As for insulin, the normal range of fasting insulin levels is less than 25 mIU/L or 174 pmol/L. Both blood glucose and insulin levels increase after meals and return to normal during periods of fasting, such as during sleep. Carbohydrates are also sugars. The carbohydrates you eat turn into blood glucose. The more carbohydrates you eat, the higher the levels of glucose you will have in your bloodstream. For example, consuming one slice of bread, which is equivalent to 15 g of carbohydrate, can raise your blood glucose level by about 50-60 mg/dL within 15 minutes.

Another way to measure blood sugar levels is through the hemoglobin A1C (HbA1c) test, which measures the percentage of hemoglobin in red blood cells that is bound to sugar. It indicates a person's ability to control blood sugar levels. The higher your blood sugar level, the more HbA1c becomes glycated or sugared. And the higher the HbA1c level you have, the more you lose your ability to control blood sugar and the higher your risk for diabetes. The normal HbA1c level is below 5.7%.

Blood sugar is regulated by the hormone insulin, which is produced by the pancreas. Insulin guides cells to absorb glucose from broken-down carbohydrates, which is used for energy. When there's excess glucose, insulin signals cells to store it as glycogen, with 25% deposited in the liver and 75% in muscles.

Knowing your blood sugar numbers is an essential step in managing diabetes and preventing its complications, especially as we age. As we get older, our bodies can become less efficient at regulating blood sugar levels, making it even more important to monitor them regularly. Everyone's blood sugar levels can fluctuate throughout the day, depending on various factors such as food intake, physical activity, stress, and illness. Maintaining a healthy diet, staying active, and monitoring blood sugar can help older adults reduce diabetes risks. Regular check-ups with a healthcare provider also aid in early detection and prevention of complications.

A picture is worth a thousand words. Let's see what the following diagram says.

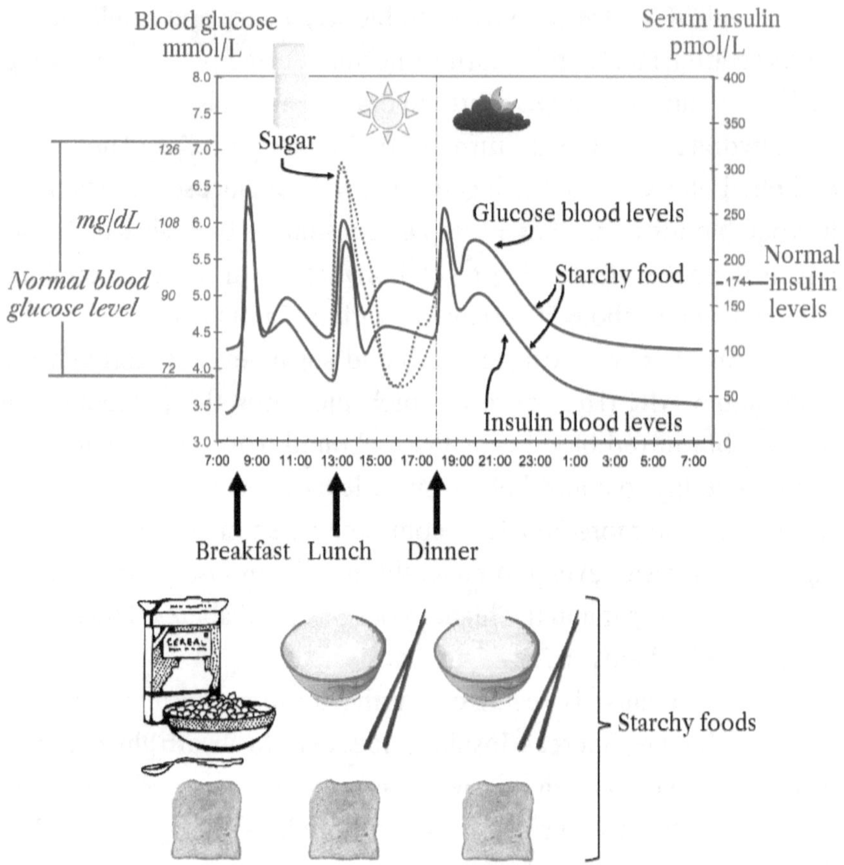

Here, the normal fasting blood glucose levels should be between the ranges of 70-100 mg/dL or between 3.9-5.6 mmol/L. The fasting blood glucose level for people with type 2 diabetes is typically 126 mg/dL (7 mmol/L) or higher. Both blood glucose and insulin levels increase when we eat breakfast, lunch, and dinner, and return to normal when we sleep. The normal fasting insulin level is no more than 25 mlU/L or 174 pmol/L. However, consuming added sugar can cause a slight increase in your blood glucose and insulin levels.[10]

There are two main types of diabetes

Diabetes is of two types: Type 1 and Type 2. Type 1 diabetes is caused when the pancreas is not able to produce insulin due to the immune system attacking and destroying the insulin-producing cells in the pancreas, resulting in a lack of insulin production. On the other hand, Type 2 diabetes is caused when the pancreas doesn't produce enough insulin, or when the body is not able to use insulin properly. Type 2 diabetes is mostly associated with overweight and obesity. When a person is obese, fat accumulates inside liver cells turning them into fatty liver cells, which release fatty acids and signaling molecules that promote inflammation. This inflammation can disrupt insulin's function, making it difficult for insulin to regulate blood glucose levels, leading to type 2 diabetes. This means that the more a person weighs, the less responsive their cells become to insulin, and the more insulin their pancreas has to produce to compensate.

People with prediabetes

Many individuals have blood sugar levels that are higher than normal, but not high enough for a diagnosis of type 2 diabetes. If your fasting blood glucose level is between 100-125 mg/dL or 5.6-6.9 mmol/L, you may have prediabetes. In fact, people with prediabetes can have this level of blood sugar for many years before developing type 2 diabetes, which is likely to happen. Research indicates that within five years, 10-20% of individuals with prediabetes will develop type 2 diabetes, and 70% of those with prediabetes will ultimately have diabetes.[11,12]

Type 2 diabetes is beating us

Type 2 diabetes is a serious health issue that can affect people of all ages, including younger adults. It's hypothesized that excessive sugar intake is a significant factor in the development of this disease. Sugar is thought to be as addictive as cocaine and it can be harmful, causing over 180,000 deaths annually.[13,14] When you eat too much sugar, it gets converted into fat and accumulates in vital organs such as the liver and pancreas. Over time, this may cause a fatty liver that poorly responds to insulin and a fatty pancreas with impaired insulin production, potentially leading to type 2 diabetes.[15,16]

While some researchers argue that high sugar consumption is not the sole cause of type 2 diabetes, being overweight is a recognized risk factor. Other contributing factors, like exposure to specific chemicals or products, might also be involved. For instance, scientists are investigating the potential link between titanium dioxide in the form of micro or nanoparticles and the development of type 2 diabetes. It's been reported that small particles of titanium dioxide are found in the pancreas of some people with type 2 diabetes but not in healthy individuals.[17] These particles can penetrate cells and cause inflammation, which can lead to damage and death of pancreatic cells that produce insulin. However, more research is needed to confirm this theory.

Tissues of the pancreas of type 2 diabetes patients that titanium dioxide particles were detected.[17]

Non-diabetic pancreases (detected titanium dioxide particles per gram)	Diabetic pancreases (detected titanium dioxide particles per gram)
0 of 3 (0)	8 of 8 (200-2,900 million)

Where does the titanium dioxide found in the pancreas of the people with type 2 diabetes come from? Titanium dioxide is a common ingredient in cosmetics, sunscreens, and toothpaste. It's also used as a bleaching agent in the food industry to give certain products a white or opaque color. In the food industry, it's known as E171. Examples of food products that use titanium dioxide as a bleaching agent include candy, chewing gum, and certain beverages. In the pharmaceutical industry, titanium dioxide is used in sunscreens. Additionally, titanium dioxide is a common coloring agent added to pharmaceutical products like gelatin capsules, supplements, and syrups. Currently, it's not known what causes the accumulation of titanium in the pancreas of people with type 2 diabetes.

***

Fasting and exercise are better drugs than metformin

I used to think that modern medicine was the most effective way to prevent and cure illnesses, but my opinion has changed now. In some cases, traditional medical therapies may not be effective for certain diseases. These days, many diseases are difficult to treat and impossible to cure. Some diseases like type 2 diabetes, Alzheimer's, arthritis and cancer aren't a single health condition but an array of health conditions, which has multiple contributing factors and can present differently in different individuals. Sometimes diet and exercise can be more effective in treating these diseases than medication.

The George Washington University study in 2002 provides evidence that supports the idea that diet and exercise can be more effective than medication in preventing type 2 diabetes. In this study, researchers recruited 3,234 people with prediabetes who had blood glucose levels about 106 mg/dL and divided them into 3 groups: group 1 (placebo group) made up of 1,082 people was given a placebo; group 2 (metformin group) made up of 1,073 people received a drug metformin to control blood sugar; and group 3 (lifestyle change group) made up of 1,079 people was to make lifestyle changes in order to lose 7% of their body weight and keep that weight loss by eating fewer calories and exercising at least 150 minutes a week. After nearly 3 years, the researchers found that lifestyle changes did a better job in preventing the incidence of type 2 diabetes than using the diabetes drug metformin. That is because only 14% of the participants in the lifestyle change group had diabetes, while the participants in the metformin group had 21% of the participants with diabetes compared to the placebo group that had 28% of the participants with diabetes.[18]

The findings are consistent with the previous Finnish study in 2001[19] that is lifestyle changes can prevent or delay the onset of type 2 diabetes.

Let's have a look at the following diagram.

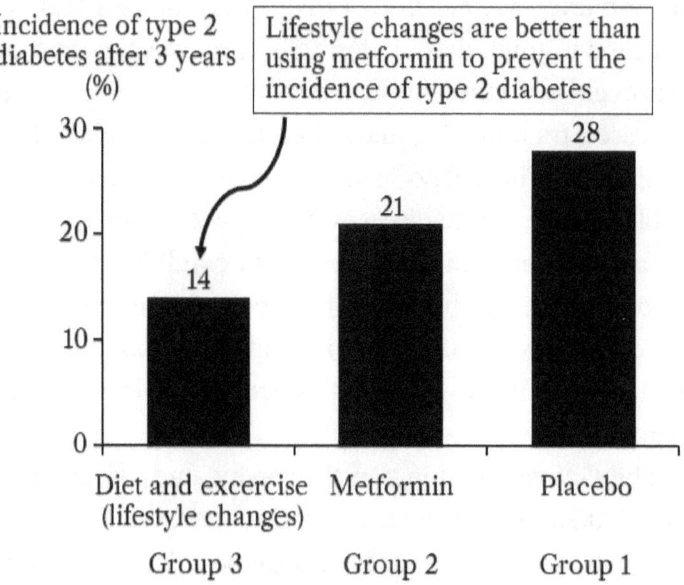

A study was conducted to determine the effectiveness of lifestyle changes and the oral diabetes drug metformin in preventing type 2 diabetes among 3,234 prediabetic volunteers. The participants were divided into three groups: Group 1 received a placebo, Group 2 received metformin to control their blood sugar levels, and Group 3 was instructed to reduce their daily food intake and limit their consumption of high-fat foods in order to lose 5-7% of their body weight. This was combined with regular exercise by brisk walking for 30 minutes a day, 5 days a week. The study found that Group 3 had the lowest incidence of type 2 diabetes compared to the other groups, indicating that lifestyle changes were more effective than metformin in preventing the disease.[18]

Building on the findings of the 2002 George Washington University study and the 2001 Finnish study, it becomes evident that lifestyle modifications play a crucial role in preventing or delaying the onset of type 2 diabetes. These studies highlight the importance of integrating healthy habits into our daily lives to combat this growing health concern.

Weight loss can reverse type 2 diabetes

Despite the belief that type 2 diabetes is a long-term medical condition that can't be cured, calorie restriction can reverse it. If you're familiar with the approach of calorie restriction, you've probably heard of the 800-calorie diet that celebrities and influencers on social media share. This fasting technique reduces food intake to 800 calories a day. The diet is inspired by the Oxford University experiment called DROPLET (Doctor Referral of Overweight People to Low Energy Treatment) and Newcastle University's experiment called DiRECT (the Diabetes Remission Clinical Trial).[20,21] Both experiments were created by medical professionals to fight type 2 diabetes. Unlike a 1944 Minnesota study, they reduced food intake but tried to maintain adequate amounts of essential nutrients to preserve muscle mass during calorie restriction. Both studies show that consuming 800 calories a day is a way to reverse type 2 diabetes. Some study participants can even put their diabetes into remission for years without relying on medication or insulin.

The DiRECT study, in which participants ate 800 calories a day for 5 months, also revealed that the longer the participants maintained their weight loss, the longer they could keep their diabetes in remission. Additionally, two-thirds of the participants who lost more than 10% of their body weight were able to put their diabetes into remission for more than 2 years. The findings highlight the importance of weight management and the potential benefits of maintaining long-term weight loss as a crucial aspect of diabetes management.

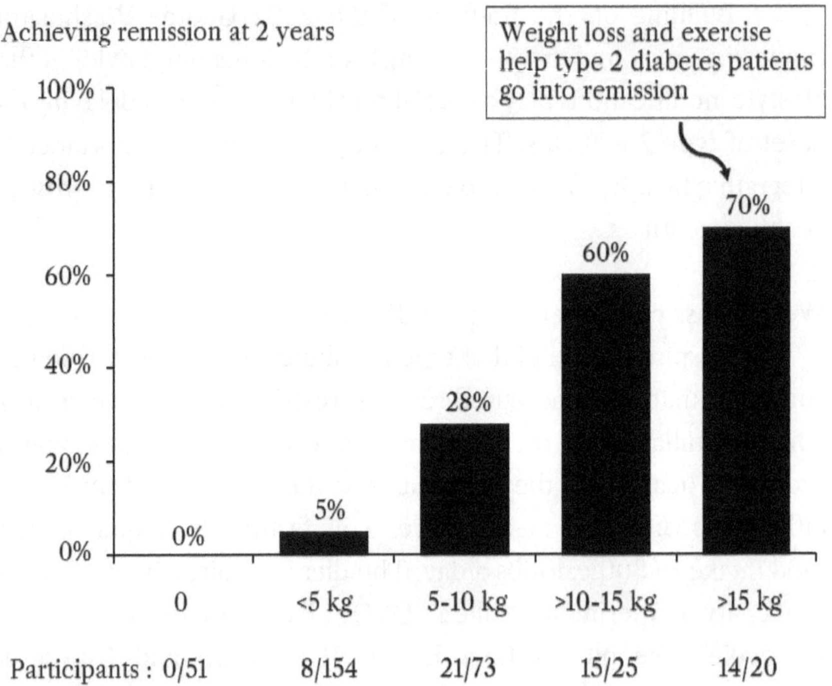

Participants in the DiRECT study lost more than 15 kg in 5 months through calorie restriction and exercise.[21] Over the course of 2 years, 14 out of 20 participants or 70% in this group were able to put their diabetes into remission, which was a higher percentage than the other groups. It's worth stressing that the more weight they lost, the more likely they were to put their diabetes into remission.

It should be noted that eating only 800 calories a day is unsustainable, and most people who attempt it tend to fail. This can be seen in the DiRECT study, where only 16% of the participants lost more than 10 kg of their body weight. Achieving weight loss goals by eating 800 calories a day requires strong determination and commitment. Furthermore, extreme calorie restriction may not be advisable for certain individuals, such as those with specific health conditions or nutritional requirements.

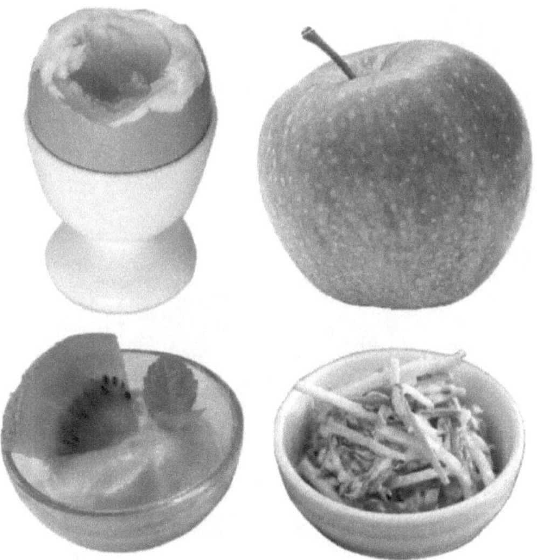

An 800-calorie diet per day typically consists of meals that are less than 300 calories each. For example, a meal could include a large hard-boiled egg (70 calories), plain yogurt with kiwi fruit (150 calories), and a 300 g cabbage and carrot salad (60 calories), or an apple (70 calories). More information on the 800-calorie diet can be found in popular fasting books, such as Dr. Michael Mosley's books. These resources often offer meal options that are more appetizing than the example provided in this photo.

For those who want to lose 10% of their body weight, like in the studies, I would suggest starting by switching to a Mediterranean-style eating plan. This diet is plant-based, with an emphasis on fruits, vegetables, nuts, grains, olive oil, and fish. You can start by incorporating more fruits and vegetables into your diet, and serving salad as a starter or side dish. While most weight loss diets offer only small effects in the short run and literally zero effects in the long run, the Mediterranean-style eating plan is a scientifically-proven way to lose weight successfully and sustainably.[22]

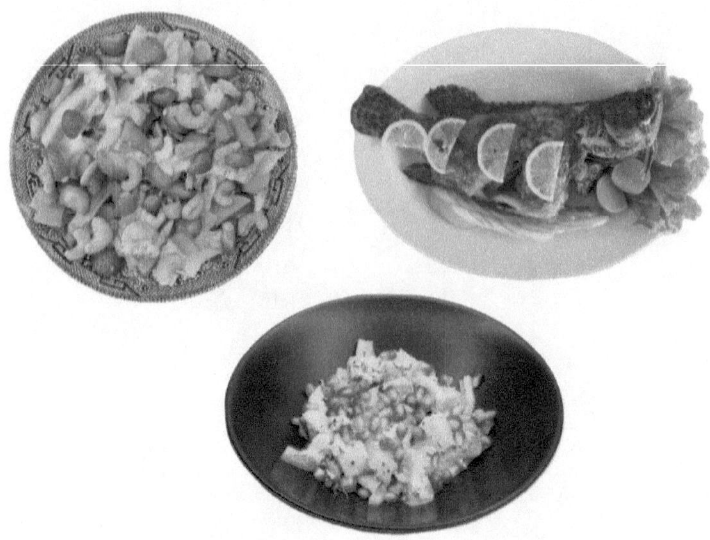

Mediterranean diets emphasized on eating fruits, vegetables, nuts, grains, olive oil and fish are sustainable diets for weight loss in the long run.

Learning to change your eating habits is like riding a bicycle for the first time. Once you've learned it, you'll have it for a lifetime. Developing healthy eating habits is similar to a fisherman getting used to the smell of fish and not being able to sleep in a hotel room filled with the scent of flowers. It takes time and persistence to adjust to a new way of eating. Changing your eating habits requires perseverance, and you must be willing to start over every day until you succeed. You may face challenges, but the key is not to give up. It's important to remember that dietary changes can't be accomplished in a single day. You must strive to consistently make healthy choices until it becomes a habit. Once you have successfully changed your eating habits, it becomes a lifelong habit that you don't have to think about anymore.

Using exercise to lose weight and prevent diabetes
If you have prediabetes, meaning your blood glucose level is

between 95-125 mg/dL, you have less than 10 years to make lifestyle changes before developing type 2 diabetes.[23,24] One of the keys to ending diabetes before it even occurs is to lose weight and to increase daily physical activity. For instance, by losing 7% of your body weight and incorporating 30 minutes of brisk walking into your daily routine, you can cut your risk of developing type 2 diabetes in half within 6 months.[25] Studies from Finland also back up this concept.[19,26] Because shedding pounds is a gradual process, it's crucial to begin applying changes as soon as possible before the 10-year window of opportunity closes.

Also, for individuals with type 2 diabetes and obesity, losing 10-15% of body weight and incorporating 30 minutes of brisk walking daily can aid in managing diabetes. If those with type 2 diabetes can achieve and maintain this healthier weight for two years, there's a 30% chance their diabetes will go into remission. Weight loss helps eliminate excess fat that hinders insulin activity in the liver and pancreas.[27] If lifestyle changes lead to the reversal of type 2 diabetes, medication may no longer be needed. Keep in mind, healthy weight loss involves gradual and consistent lifestyle changes that include exercise.

Additional benefits of exercise for weight loss include. Not only does exercise stimulates the metabolic activity, circulatory system, muscle growth, and hormonal and calcium balance in the body, but it also causes an increase in the production of the hormone fibroblast growth factor 21 (FGF21). FGF21 has an anti-diabetic effect, allowing the body's cells to use blood glucose more effectively. Also, FGF21 is able to stop sugar craving by sending a signal to the brain, which then suppresses your appetite for starchy or sugary foods. In fact, studies show that mice lacking FGF21 become sugar addicts, while boosting FGF21 in obese mice led to a 20% weight reduction in just two weeks.[28,29] Regular exercise is also widely acknowledged as an effective anti-aging strategy across various research fields.

What's more, as a problem, people with type 2 diabetes often experience muscle weakness. However, exercises like brisk walking, jogging, cycling, and swimming can't restore their muscle strength. This is because glucose in their bloodstream interferes the muscle building process.[30] Such exercises can only increase the metabolic rate and burn fat in people with prediabetes or diabetes. To restore their muscle strength and mass, they need to rely on strength training exercises like weight lifting, in addition to taking medication or consuming foods that can reduce blood sugar levels.

Natural foods fight type 2 diabetes

Besides bitter melon and gurmar, which can inhibit glucose uptake, research indicates that for prediabetic individuals, consuming 750 mg of curcumin twice daily for 9 months can help prevent the onset of diabetes.[31] While this research can't be compared with the George Washington University study or the Finland study, it's very likely that turmeric extract can delay the onset of type 2 diabetes as effectively as calorie restriction and exercise. If a person can eat less, exercise more, and take the turmeric extract together, it might even be better in delaying the onset of type 2 diabetes, but no one knows for sure

Curcumin and curcuminoids are related, and both are yellow substances extracted from the root of turmeric. About 3-9% of curcuminoids are found in the rhizome of turmeric, and about 70-80% of curcuminoids are curcumin. Dried turmeric powder containing the most curcuminoids, 90 mg per gram, is Thai turmeric, which is native to southern Thailand.[32] Twenty milligrams of piperine in combination with turmeric powder will increase the bioavailability of curcuminoids by 2,000%. Therefore, taking 2 g of turmeric powder with 20 mg of piperine may provide enough curcuminoids to reach blood levels sufficient to exert its activities.[33] Clinical trials in humans have shown that curcuminoids are safe even at doses of 10-12 g a day. However, taking more than 20 mg of piperine is not recommended, as it may interfere with the biological activities of curcuminoids. Another way to boost your absorption of curcuminoids is to eat fresh turmeric roots or powder with 150 g of good fats like avocado or a tablespoon of extra virgin olive oil, which can increase the bioavailability of curcuminoids by 7-8 times.

Some studies also suggest that regular consumption of small amounts of turmeric may also aid in preventing type 2 diabetes. Additionally, it's equally vital to reduce intake of starchy and sugary foods. Consuming turmeric daily without reducing intake of these foods would render the efforts futile. Starches and sugars can lead to the accumulation of fat and AGEs in blood, bones, muscles, and other vital organs, accelerating the aging process in the body. Moreover, sugars and carbohydrates can interact with curcuminoids, nullifying their anti-diabetic effects. This is the reason behind the increasing incidence of type 2 diabetes among Indians. The harm caused by excessive consumption of sugary and starchy foods is challenging to reverse. Turmeric is a popular cooking ingredient in India, but the country has become home to 77 million diabetics due to its citizens' second-highest sweet tooth in the world, despite its usage of turmeric. That is unfortunate.

Eat to repair the pancreas

This is a key point. Before you begin to repair the pancreas, excess fat must be removed from the liver and pancreas. This step is taken to maximize your body's repair. Fat that covers the liver and pancreas is the cause of inflammation of the liver and pancreas. That, in turn, interferes with the regeneration of pancreatic cells. It's like repairing a road. If the road is not closed, but allowing the cars to run around in chaos, the bumpy road will never be completely repaired. This is the initial step in activating the body's maintenance and repair mechanisms for other vital organs too. To achieve this, it's suggested to lose 7-10% of body weight through either fasting or a duo of fasting and exercise. Human studies have shown that fasting or fasting combined with exercise, such as 30 minutes of brisk walking 5 days a week, can also stimulate the regeneration of beta cells that produce insulin in the pancreas.[34,35] At this stage, fasting and exercise may help repair the pancreas to some extent.

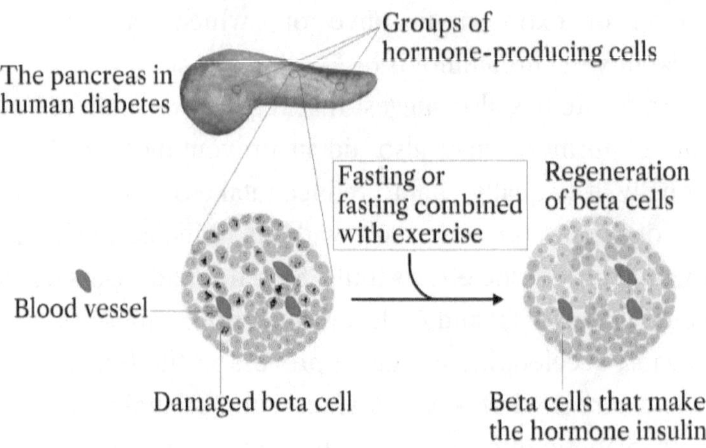

Fasting and fasting combined with exercise such as brisk walking can stimulate the regeneration of beta cells in the pancreas.[34,35,36]

Prolonged high blood sugar levels can also damage and impair the function of beta cells, eventually leading to a decrease in their number. At the beginning of diabetes, if the number of beta cells in the pancreas decreases, the amount of insulin produced and secreted also decreases. This can exacerbate type 2 diabetes and lead to additional health issues, creating a vicious cycle. Common diabetes symptoms, such as tiredness, increased thirst, hunger, and frequent urination, often occur due to elevated blood glucose levels.

Great news! It's possible to boost the number of insulin-producing cells in the pancreas using natural compounds found in certain foods. A promising study published in Nature Medicine by diabetes researchers demonstrated that substances like harmine can regenerate beta cells in mice, which serve as proxies for humans. The researchers discovered that harmine stimulated a daily increase in beta cell mass and numbers of approximately 1-1.5%. Remarkably, this rate of beta cell growth and regeneration caused by harmine is comparable to that of a newborn baby's.[37] However, it hasn't been proven that harmine can have the same effect in humans. The optimal concentration of harmine is also found to be no more than 10 micromolar (at the part-per-billion level), and higher amounts may have an opposite effect, decreasing beta cell regeneration.

However, to successfully regenerate new beta cells, it's crucial to keep your blood sugar levels in check and maintain a healthy immune system. This is because newly grown beta cells may also be destroyed by high blood sugar levels and the body's immune response. As discussed in Chapter 4, there are natural ways that can help maintain stable blood sugar levels, ensuring that your body functions optimally.

If you're looking to enhance the health of your beta cells, natural substances such as harmine may be helpful. Peppermint (*Melissa officinalis*) is a natural source of harmine, with approximately 0.1 mg found in 100 g of peppermint leaves and stem tips.[38]

Studies also show that consuming peppermint is beneficial for reducing visceral fat in overweight individuals.[39,40,41] Additionally, a recent randomized, double-blind, placebo-controlled clinical trial of 35 cardiovascular patients revealed that those who consumed 3 g of peppermint leaves a day for 8 weeks experienced a 12-16% decrease in triglycerides, total cholesterol, and LDL-cholesterol levels, as well as a 20% increase in HDL-cholesterol, compared to those who did not consume peppermint.[43] With this knowledge, you may use peppermint leaves to reduce excess inflammation-causing fat in your body and help regenerate beta cells at a rate comparable to a newborn baby's beta cell growth.

While peppermint leaves can offer some health benefits, it's important to remember that they may not be as effective on their own in reducing excess fat and inflammation, and stimulating the regeneration of beta cells in the pancreas. Combining a healthy diet, including peppermint, with fasting and regular exercise may be a more comprehensive approach to achieve better results in doing these.

A daily intake of 3 g of peppermint leaves, which is about one stem tip, has been shown to be safe in a human trial, indicating that it's an optimal and secure amount for consumption.

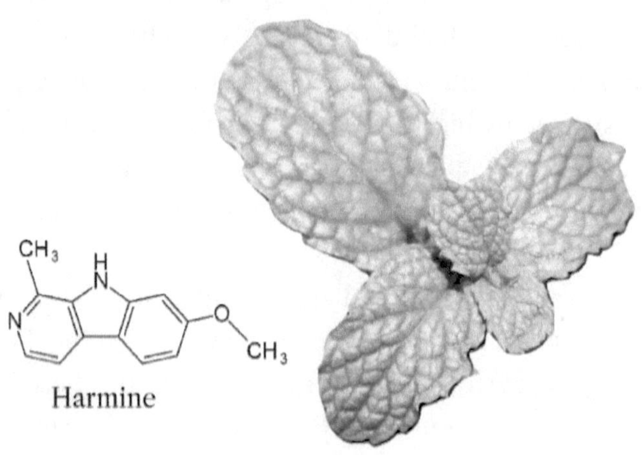

Harmine

Harmine, a compound present in peppermint leaves and stems, has the potential to encourage the regeneration of human beta cells at a rate similar to that of a newborn baby's.[37]

Pomegranate for liver repair

As we age, vital organs such as the liver and kidneys tend to shrink. In particular, the liver can shrink by 20-40% of its normal size, which highly correlates with liver inflammation. Moreover, as we get older, the liver becomes increasingly inflamed and damaged. When inflammation occurs in the liver, white blood cells are sent into it by the body's immune system. If the inflammation becomes chronic, and the number of incoming white blood cells is too high, these cells can accumulate and block the liver. This can lead to inadequate blood flow into the liver and reduce the amount of liver blood flow by up to 35%. In addition, both aging and inflammation can slow the process of liver repair and regeneration.[43,44] Therefore, relying solely on the damaged liver to repair itself can be too slow.

Studies have shown that a unique substance called "ursolic acid" can help damaged liver cells repair and restore themselves faster. Ursolic acid can stimulate faster DNA synthesis in the liver, accelerating damage repair and liver regeneration. This knowledge was obtained from experiments in mice that had their liver partially removed.[45] Ursolic acid may also aid in the release of molecules by gut bacteria to stimulate liver repair. In one study, it was found that when gut bacteria were eliminated, the liver was unable to regenerate.

To repair the liver, it's crucial to first address liver inflammation, as it hinders proper liver function and worsens the condition. Adopting a healthy diet, exercising regularly, and avoiding harmful substances like alcohol and drugs can help reduce liver inflammation and promote healing.

There is currently no clinical trial in humans confirming that ursolic acid can repair liver damage. Therefore, incorporating superfoods like pomegranate into the diet may be helpful in the meantime. Pomegranates contain up to 450 mg of ursolic acid per 100 g and may help damaged liver cells heal themselves faster.

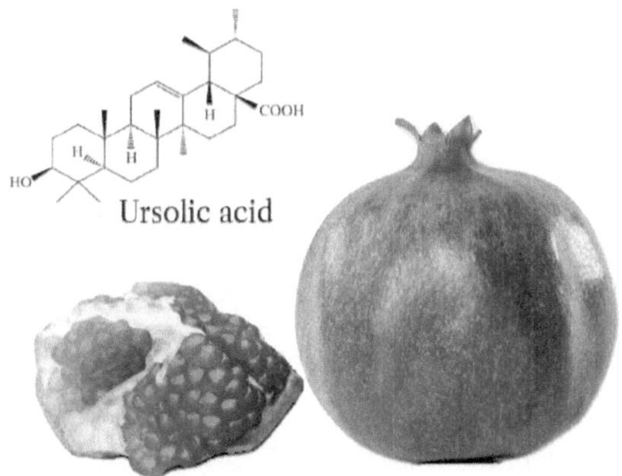

Ursolic acid present in pomegranate, which has a content of up to 450 mg per 100 g. According to animal studies, it may promote the regeneration of liver cells and aid in repairing liver damage.

In conclusion, the power of nutrition goes beyond mere sustenance. Choosing a healthy diet can't only maintain a balanced weight, but also promote cell regeneration and unlock new capabilities for the body. This is particularly important in the fight against aging, as our bodies naturally decline with time. You can halt or even reverse the decline in your health, and change what seemed like your inevitable destiny. By adopting a healthy lifestyle and detecting type 2 diabetes early, reversal is achievable. As more people successfully achieve diabetes remission through natural means, they become role models and inspire others to follow in their footsteps. With more people following this path by adopting healthier lifestyles, such as consuming natural foods and engaging in regular exercise, the prevalence of type 2 diabetes can be reduced over time, leading to improved overall health globally.

CHAPTER 7

Cut out the junk food and maintain healthy weight

You've probably heard it all before: junk food is bad for you, soft drinks are a no-no, and fast food is basically a heart attack on a plate. But even with all this knowledge, why is it so hard to resist those greasy burgers and sugary treats? Let's face it, avoiding unhealthy foods comes down to one thing: self-control.

From soft drinks to potato chips, candy to cookies, fast food to crunchy snacks, unhealthy foods are everywhere. They're ready-to-eat, ready-to-heat, and meant to be served right away. But while they may be convenient, they're also loaded with fat, sugar, and salt, and have little nutritional value. This is especially true for Western-styled fast food. So why are we so drawn to these foods? Well, one reason is that they're energy-dense and can't be found in nature, making our brains crave them even more.

But it's not just that. Fast food is carefully crafted in test kitchens to be incredibly palatable and addictive. And let's not forget that these foods are designed to sell and make profits for the manufacturers, not to promote consumer health. It's a harsh reality, but few companies are truly interested in our well-being when it comes to fast food.

So, the next time you're tempted by that burger or bag of chips, remember that it's ultimately up to you to resist. But also keep in mind that the food industry is not always on your side when it comes to promoting health. It's time for us all to take responsibility for our food choices and prioritize our health over convenience.

Unhealthy diets not only threaten our current well-being, but they can also speed up the aging process. A diet rich in sugar and processed foods can cause an imbalance in gene activities, as well as DNA damage, inflammation, and oxidative stress in the body, which result in causing us age faster. Moreover, an unhealthy diet can result in weight gain, which is a significant risk factor for various age-related diseases.

Ultra-processed foods and drawbacks

The presence or absence of food is essential to people's livelihoods. People can die from hunger. In the old days, if we couldn't eat all of our food at once, we could preserve food for off-season feasts. Again, by using tools and technology, we are able to improve processes used to prevent food from spoiling. These processes are highly efficient, require fewer workers, yet increase productivity and shelf life. Nowadays, humans revolutionized food industry completely, allowing processed food to be stored for longer periods of time without spoiling.

Natural foods can be altered by processes such as removal of seeds, washing, husking, gutting, trimming, shredding and chopping to get rid of germs and to make them convenient for consumption. Foods that have undergone these processes are deemed minimally-processed. The minimally-processed food is then packaged and stored at low temperature, otherwise, spoilage may occur.

However, if you want your food to be kept longer, it has to be processed through a moderate processing by soaking, boiling, steaming, fermenting or getting irradiated. Foods that went through these processes are deemed moderately-processed food.

In addition, there are ultra-processed foods, which are items with added chemical ingredients. Ingredients used to manufacture ultra-processed foods include emulsifiers, preservatives, pH modifiers, flavoring agents, glucose, fructose, MSG, and other substances that you may not be familiar with, but have long and difficult names to pronounce, many of which are completely unrelated to the main ingredient of the food at all. Here are examples of ultra-processed foods sold in grocery stores: processed meats, ready-to-heat meals, canned food, instant noodles, sausages, cereals, soft drinks, crisps, candies and cookies. These ultra-processed foods were heated to very high temperatures during manufacturing and packaged in tight packaging for longer shelf life. They are super easy to find and buy in grocery stores. Manufacturers know that lazy people like us will buy their processed foods because it's convenient. While processed foods are convenient and taste delicious, however, processed foods come with drawbacks.

In fact, you may not know that people who consume ultra-processed foods 3 times a day have 82% shorter telomeres than people who eat real vegetables, fruits and nuts. This means that people who eat a diet high in ultra-processed foods may age faster and be at a higher risk of developing age-related diseases such as cancer and heart disease.

Furthermore, consuming ultra-processed foods accelerates the aging of your cells, largely attributed to their high content of hydrogenated oils containing trans fats that promote chronic inflammation, leading to the breakdown or aging of your cells. People who consume a diet rich in ultra-processed foods also have a higher risk of developing depression, dementia, and other chronic diseases.[3] That is why ultra-processed foods can force you to be hospitalized too early.

Eating ultra-processed foods for 14 days can lead to 1 kg of weight gain

Ultra-processed foods often link to obesity. Why? Because they are typically high in calories, unhealthy fats, sugars, and additives. These foods can negatively affect our metabolism, leading to weight gain, as they are easily absorbed and stored as fat, while also causing hormonal imbalances and inflammation.

The findings, published in Cell Metabolism, from experts at the National Institutes of Health (NIH), indicated that consuming an extra 508 calories of ultra-processed food a day for 14 days leads to 1 kg of weight gain.[4] These findings suggest that ultra-processed foods may be a major contributor to obesity on a global scale. Studies in Italy, UK, Netherlands, Germany and Denmark also showed that consumption of white bread, processed meats, margarine and soft drinks promotes belly fat accumulation.[5] These foods pack a punch to our belly, leaving us with a bulging waistline.

In the study, ultra-processed foods consumed included items like steak, sausages, bacon, turkey meatballs, hot dogs, nuggets, muffins, white bread, sandwiches, biscuits, bagels, French fries, baked potatoes, croissants, cheese, margarine, and bottled orange or lemon juice. On the other hand, unprocessed foods participants ate were baked cod, shrimp spaghetti, oatmeal, salads (lettuce, tomato, cucumber, and carrot), steamed broccoli with olive oil and garlic, spinach, onions, apples, oranges, blueberries, almonds, walnuts, and freshly squeezed lemon juice.[4]

Here you can view the diagram for more information.

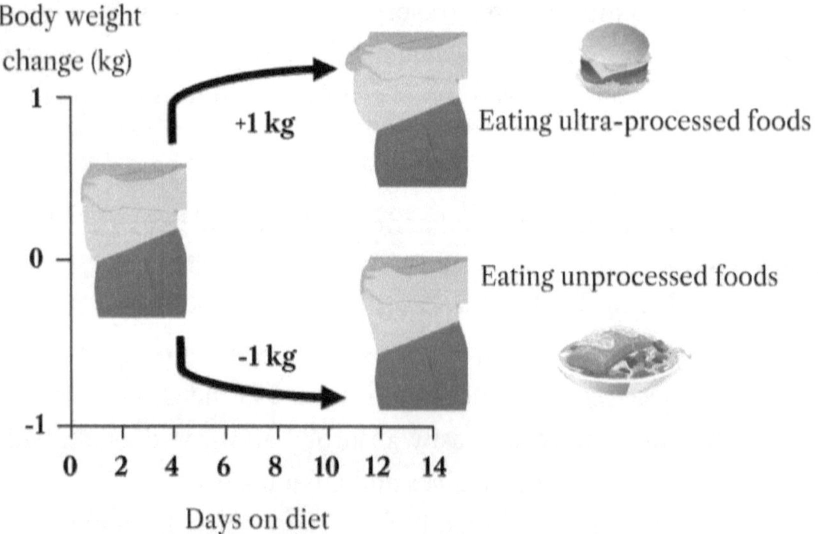

Interestingly, among the European nations the prevalence of obesity is lower in Italy. Speaking of which, research has shown that pasta consumption is related to lower obesity prevalence in Italy.[6] The reason for this may be because Italian people who eat pasta also eat a Mediterranean diet that contains spices like garlic, onion and olive oil. Take a look at the following picture. You might understand why. But you need to be cautious that this research was funded by the food industry. The results may favor the sponsor's interest.

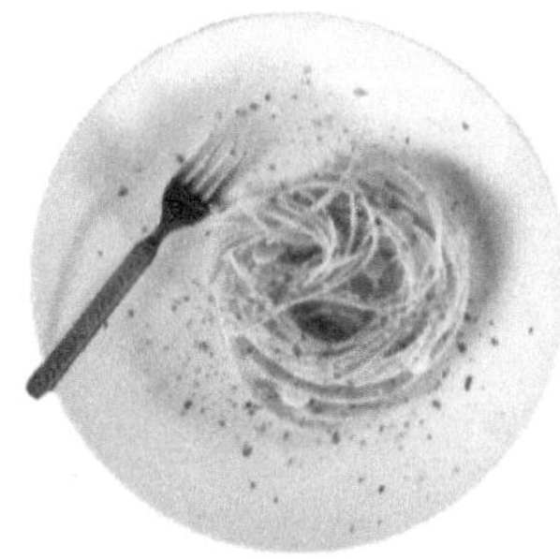

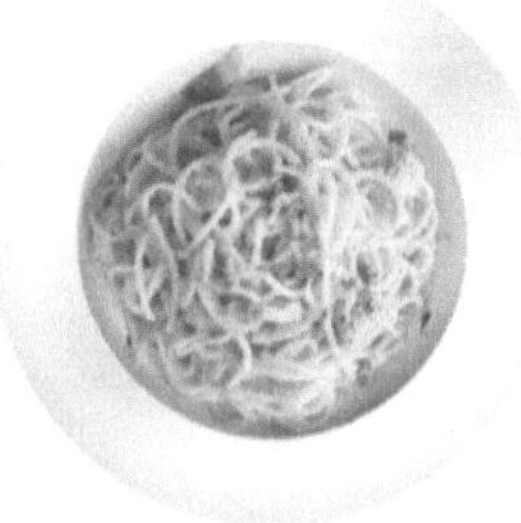

Pasta in Italy   Pasta in other places

In Italy, pasta is usually consumed in moderate portion sizes and is combined with a variety of nutrient-dense and fiber-rich ingredients such as vegetables, legumes, and lean meats, which can lower blood sugar.

The original corn flakes recipe has no sugar

Kellogg's corn flakes, as you may or may not know, were originally invented as a ready-to-eat anti-masturbation meal. But, these days, corn flakes made from toasted flakes of corn is a convenient breakfast cereal. Nearly all corn flake brands have added sugar in the amount that varies from 1% to 40%. When selecting a breakfast cereal, be cautious of the sugar content. Some cereals may contain high levels of added sugar, exceeding 40 g/100 g.

If you eat foods that contain too much sugar, your body will receive more calories than you need. When you eat these foods, they turn into glucose in your body. Any extra glucose your cells don't use gets stored as glycogen in your muscles and liver, and as body fat. Excess glucose can also become triglycerides. Surprisingly, your body can store up to 100 g of extra fat each year in a tissue called adipose tissue. This is why consuming a lot of sugar is linked to weight gain.

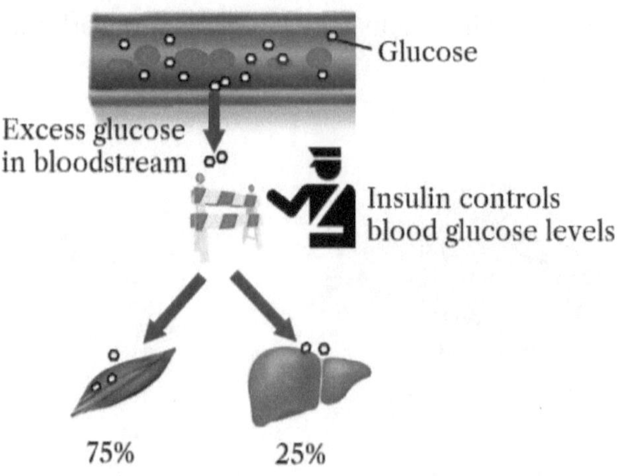

If there is an excess amount of glucose in the bloodstream, three quarters of the body's glycogen formed from glucose is stored in the muscles, while the remaining quarter is stored in the liver.[7]

Secondhand sugar

Keep in mind that carbohydrates and sugars can influence the activation and deactivation of human genes. Nutrients like sugar and ultra-processed foods can easily alter gene expression, leading to imbalanced gene activities that result in accelerated aging. These effects can impact human growth, development, overall health, and may even be passed on to future generations. For example, a pregnant mother who consumes high amounts of carbohydrates and sugars may unintentionally affect her baby's birth weight and height, with these imbalances becoming more apparent when the child is 2-

4 years old. The indirect consumption of sugar by individuals who eat or drink high-sugar foods or beverages is called secondhand sugar. In the case of an unborn baby, this puts them at a higher risk of becoming overweight later in life due to genetic reprogramming associated with obesity resulting from the mother-to-be's diet. Furthermore, the consequences of secondhand sugar and genetic reprogramming due to the mother-to-be's diet can extend beyond childhood obesity. Children exposed to high levels of sugar in the womb may be more prone to developing type 2 diabetes, heart disease, and other metabolic disorders later in life.

Ready-to-eat meals can lead to overeating

While populations in the southern region of the Sahara Desert grapple with food scarcity, Western countries are experiencing an overabundance of food. Food processing industries in these countries enable the rapid preparation of meals. Refined flour and sugar are inexpensive and easily accessible, while ready-to-eat and ready-to-heat meals are both widely available and relatively affordable. However, these factors can lead to overeating.

In Western nations like France, Germany, Italy, the US, and the UK, it's estimated that people consume over 3,500 calories per day on average, nearly double the caloric intake of people in developing countries, such as those in the southern region of the Sahara Desert.[9,10] Consuming excess calories can lead to weight gain and obesity. In fact, an additional 1,000 calories per day can result in a weight gain of 4-13 kg over 100 days.[11]

The food processing industries have significantly altered the global landscape, promoting overeating, sedentary lifestyles, and obesity for millions of people. Although processed foods and ready-made meals offer convenience, it's crucial not to compromise one's health for the sake of expediency.

What is obesity?

When you turn 40, you'll know that it's easier to gain weight.

Weight gain is a common cause of overweight and obesity in people over 40. Obesity is defined as having a body mass index (BMI) of 30 or higher. It's a major global health problem. People with overweight or obesity increase the risk of developing chronic diseases such as high cholesterol, high blood pressure, heart disease, type 2 diabetes, cancer and more. BMI is the ratio of weight to height. A person who is overweight, or BMI of 25 to <30, has too much body weight for his height. The following BMI chart, made by NHS UK, can help you quickly determine your BMI.

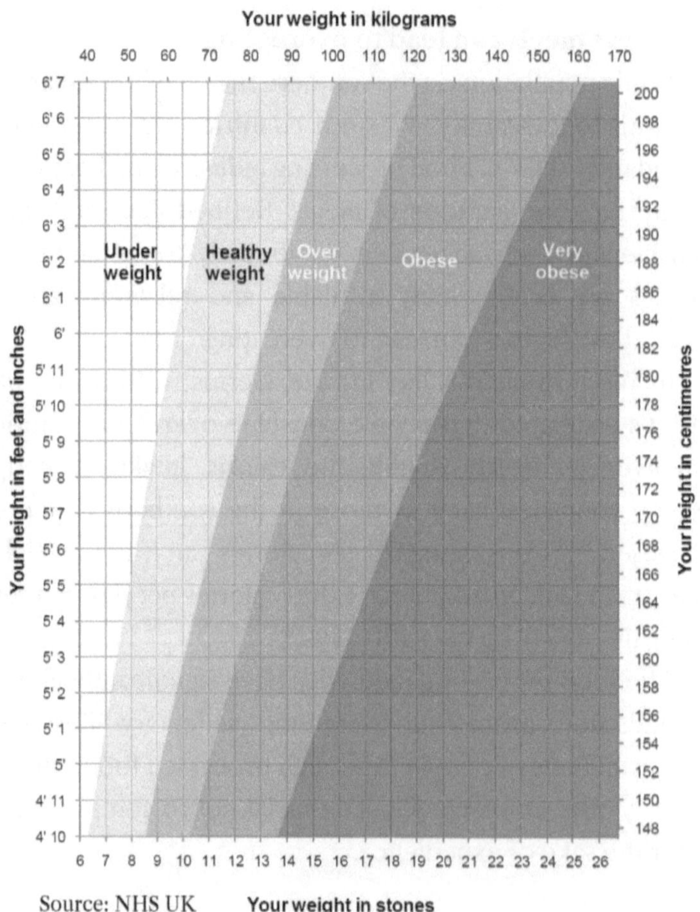

Today's humans resemble androids

There are 3 different types of fat cells in your body: brown, white and beige. Mitochondria-packed brown-fat cells help you burn more energy to maintain body temperature when you get cold. Brown fat cells are located in the sides of the neck, the collarbone area, surrounding the kidneys and along the spinal cord. While white fat stores calories and are found in different parts of the body, beige fat is in between white and brown fat cells. Beige fat cells develop within white fat tissue in response to cold exposure and other stimuli. If beige fat cells are activated, they can become brown fat cells and metabolize lipids to generate heat. In adults, beige fat cells are beneath the skin near the collarbone area and along the spinal cord.

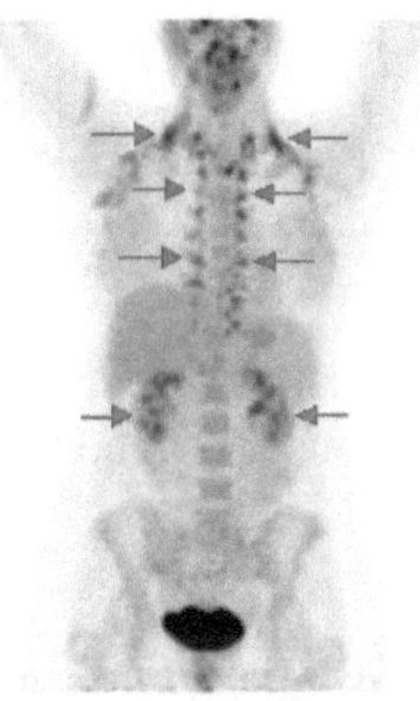

Brown fat is displayed (arrows) as the volunteer was cold during an imaging test.[12]

Body fat is composed of fat cells. Fat is distributed unevenly in different parts of your body depending on your genes, age, sex and hormones. In 1956, Marseille University's John Vague, published his observation about his patient bodies.[13,14] Vague noticed that men have a lot of upper body fat, while women have a lot of lower body fat. He coined the terms "android" to describe those with excess upper body fat and "gynoid" to describe those with excess lower body fat. A person who was very overweight was more android than a person with a healthy weight. And older people are more android than younger ones. Today, Vague's research on fat distribution is considered an important predictor of the health risks associated with obesity, as well as other diseases like diabetes and cardiovascular disease. In contrast to the past beliefs, corpulence is no longer seen as superior to thinness, and is now considered a sign of illness.

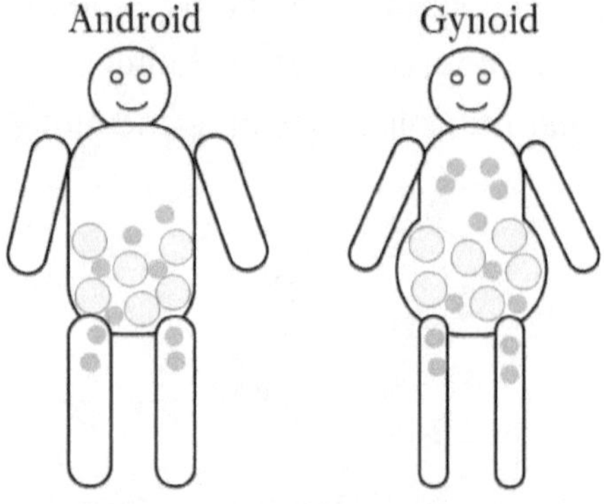

○ Visceral fat surrounds abdominal organs
● Subcutaneous fat found under the skin

Men with obesity often have an android body shape, while women with obesity tend to have a gynoid body shape. Visceral or abdominal fat, which accumulates around internal organs, is responsible for the appearance of a big belly. On the other hand, subcutaneous fat can be found in various parts of the body, including the hips, waist, chest, and neck.

The growing prevalence of android and gynoid body types is worrisome. As Our World in Data reveals, nearly a third of the global population is affected by obesity and being overweight. Developing countries are especially at risk due to the rise of inexpensive processed foods and sedentary lifestyles. Thailand exemplifies this trend, with 1 in 4 people being overweight or obese. The escalating obesity crisis, which plays a major role in chronic diseases like diabetes, heart disease, and some cancers, is a pressing health issue.

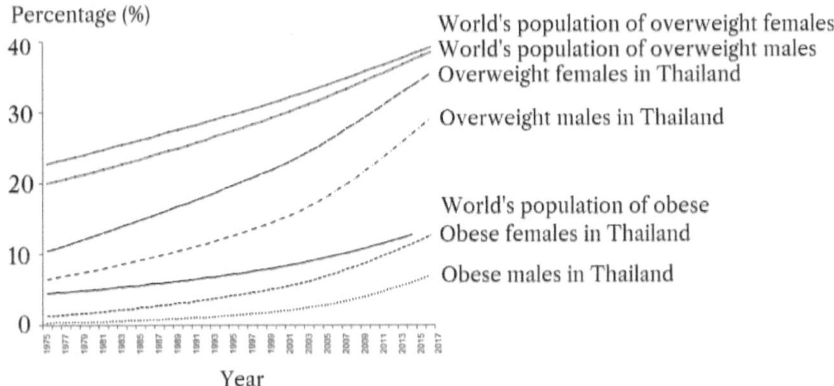

An increasing number of people are now classified as overweight or obese compared to the past. Currently, over 60% of men and women fall under the category of overweight or obese.

Economic growth contributes to obesity

It's unreasonable for developed countries to equate economic growth with an increase in obesity. Why do prosperous nations experience high rates of obesity? How does wealth contribute to poor health? It appears that in affluent societies, an abundance of unhealthy foods and economic growth together drive obesity.

Economic growth refers to the increase in the production of goods and services within an economy. Governments aspire to achieve continuous economic growth, which requires encouraging citizens to create and consume more goods and services. Consumerism fuels the economy, and the faster it grows, the more goods are sold, including processed foods that are cheaper and easier to produce in large quantities. These foods have longer shelf lives, making them ideal for mass distribution and sale.

What's more. The restaurant industry's growth has long been considered a crucial economic indicator. The more restaurants sell, the faster the economy grows. Plus, the widespread availability of restaurants can also contribute to overweight and obesity.[15] In the United States, economic growth has been a driving force behind the rise in obesity since the early 1980s.[16] The expansion of superstores, retail stores, and restaurants has led to a 23% increase in obesity.[17] Inexpensive foods from these establishments, often cheaper than fruits and vegetables, are likely to be responsible for the surge in obesity. However, other factors, such as lifestyle and culture, also play a role in obesity and should not be overlooked.

Interestingly, the benefits of economic growth are not only reaped by many individuals but are also spent on obesity. In 2005, the United States spent an estimated $190 billion on treating obesity and obesity-related conditions, equivalent to Thailand's gross domestic product for the same year. A country's wealth doesn't always translate into the improved health of its citizens. Obesity has a substantial economic impact on the United States and other developed countries. Thus, nations should not solely focus on economic development but also address the obesity issue, recognizing it as an economic concern as well.

Chemicals in plastic can make you fat

Besides eating too much and not moving enough, there is a link between gut bacteria and obesity. People who are overweight often have lots of bad bacteria in their gut. If you don't want to gain weight, you need to eat more high-fiber foods, fruits, and veggies to help good bacteria grow in your gut.

Chemicals and tiny plastics can also make you gain weight. Many food and drink containers have something like bisphenol A and phthalates that can move from the container into the food or drink.[18] Eating processed food from plastic containers might lead us to take in more chemicals found in plastic. In studies with mice and humans, these chemicals have been tied to obesity. In fact, a 2017 study in the

Lancet Planetary Health showed that bisphenol A exposure was linked to obesity in the American population.[19] This chemical can act like hormones and mess with the body's metabolism, leading to obesity. It's also believed that Americans who drink water from plastic bottles swallow about 70,000 tiny plastic pieces each year. To cut down on exposure to these chemicals, try to eat fewer processed foods and drinks stored in plastic containers.

Obesity can cause fatty buildup in the respiratory tract

Recent research indicates that overweight and obese individuals tend to accumulate more fat in their airways compared to those with a healthy weight. This fat can adhere to the respiratory tracts and cause inflammation, similar to a response to a pathogen attack, resulting in respiratory problems.[20] In addition to breathing difficulties, individuals with respiratory problems may experience fatigue. Given these factors, it's understandable why those with obesity may appear more tired.

Furthermore, the accumulation of fat in the respiratory tract can also lead to sleep apnea, a sleep disorder characterized by interruptions in breathing during sleep. Sleep apnea can cause snoring, daytime sleepiness, and difficulty concentrating, all of which contribute to the feeling of tiredness in obese individuals.

***

What should we do next?

Scientists have just proposed perhaps a way to solve the obesity problem and develop a sustainable economy concurrently. The proposed solution is to encourage more people to work in the agricultural sector. Based on 40 years of data from 147 countries around the world, a country's agricultural production was inversely related to the prevalence of obesity.[21,22] In other words, countries with high agricultural productivity tend to have lower rates of obesity. Thus, engaging in agricultural activities may be a lifestyle intervention to prevent and reduce overweight and obesity.

Undoubtedly, fast lifestyle with fast food intake makes us look like androids or gynoids. In the future, if more people switch to a healthier diet, the prevalence of obesity could gradually decrease. If people eat more fruits and vegetables, more people will be needed in agriculture sector. People who switch their occupations to ones in agriculture will also be healthier as they are busy, planting, growing, and harvesting fruits and vegetables to feed those who consume healthy foods. Encouraging individuals to engage in physical activity through agriculture could also have a positive impact on mental health, providing an opportunity to connect with nature and engage in meaningful work.

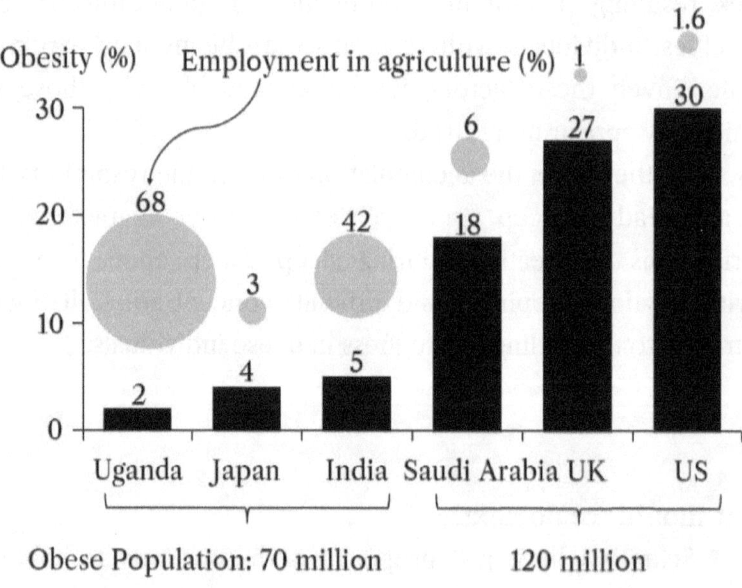

The prevalence of obesity in certain countries is linked to a lower number of people employed in the agricultural sector.[23] Promoting employment in the agricultural sector can be a potential solution for addressing obesity and fostering a sustainable economy.

Revolutionizing the diet: Brazil's stand against processed foods

Brazil may be the only country in the world that its government criticizes the production and deceptive advertising of food companies that have caused significant cultural, environmental, and lifestyle changes. Currently, Brazil has one of the best dietary guidelines in the world. This guideline suggests that industrially processed foods such as snacks, soft drinks, sausages, cakes, instant noodles, ready-to-heat meals and high-sugar breakfast cereals are unhealthy. It recommends that the people of Brazil consume natural or minimally processed foods. Additionally, the Brazilian government recommends cooking meals from scratch, which involves using basic ingredients such as brown rice, nuts, steamed vegetables, soups, and curries, as well as fresh fruits like tomatoes, bananas, and oranges, to feed hungry family members. The guideline also advised Brazilians to beware of false advertising from food manufacturers.[24] False advertisements contain hidden messages that promote products, which should be carefully scrutinized by consumers.

Hopefully, in the future, we will see that Brazilians can stop bad habits from taking hold in them. Brazil's fight against processed foods can serve as a model for other nations. You too can start cooking from scratch at home and eat real foods. View your cooking as a good therapy; and eating healthy as a good investment. Investing in your health is one of the best returns on investments that even Wall Street investments can't match.

Eat your way to a healthy weight

When you grow older, you may witness your loved ones or friends suffering physically and mentally from age-related ailments that can't be cured. Eating junk food is like feeding a disease. Unhealthy diets can only worsen a person's health condition. Obesity is prevalent in all population groups, regardless of age, gender, and economic status. Building a good relationship with natural foods is crucial to sustain your body's well-being. The human body deserves foods that are better than pizza, soft drinks, and chips.

Here are some keys to achieving and maintaining a healthy weight:

Consuming fruits and grains regularly can help prevent the accumulation of belly fat and reduce waist size, aiding in maintaining a healthy weight.[25]

Drastic weight loss methods may seem quick and effective, but studies show that around two-thirds of people who try to fast and accelerate weight loss within 3-5 days experience yo-yo weight cycling and a negative impact on their heart. Therefore, this is not a sustainable way to maintain a healthy weight.

The reason why cutting calories while providing adequate intakes of essential nutrients is more favorable is that it can increase sirtuin enzymes. Sirtuins play an essential role in aging, repair, rejuvenation, and extending lifespan.[26] Sirtuin enzymes can also lower blood sugar. Scientists have long known that calorie restriction stimulates the production of sirtuins and increases lifespan in animal models and humans.

Some people try to reduce their calorie intake by eating less than 1,800 calories a day, a few times per week or month. However, I personally believe that the key to maintaining a healthy weight is to eat within 10-hour window. For instance, I start eating breakfast at 07.00, lunch at 12.00 and dinner at 17.00. There must be no food before 07.00 and after 17.00. And I don't snack or eat outside of the meal times. More importantly, if you have diabetes, high blood pressure or obesity, limiting eating to a 10-hour window can reduce your weight, belly fat, blood pressure and cholesterol.[27] Indeed, eating food for a limited time is beneficial for the body's metabolism and the repair process. Eating at the wrong time can disrupt biological rhythms, such as altering the biological clock of the liver. As a result, the nutrients eaten can't merge with the protein or enzyme that required them, causing the liver to send those nutrients on to other parts of the body.[28]

In addition, as you are on a diet, you should lose no more than 2 kg of your weight a month. Since our bodies need time to adjust to newly acquired body weight, composition, and metabolism. In other words, losing a kilogram of weight a month requires another month for the body to adjust, which is believed to be a truly sustainable approach.

Importantly, combining calorie restriction with exercise is a most effective strategy for losing weight. What's more, to burn more fat in your body, you can exercise before breakfast.[29]

Again, I would like to remind you that if there is too much glucose in your blood, you can't get your body to burn stored fat. Actually, to use fat for energy, your body first needs to deplete glucose in your bloodstream, and then burn glycogen stored in your liver and muscle. After the blood glucose depleted, about 80 g of glycogen stored as liver glycogen will be used to replenish the 5 g of glucose circulating in the blood quickly to ensure that your heart and brain has adequate energy stores.[30] After glycogen was used up, your body will turn to burn your fat in your bloodstream and then your body fat.

For instance, during exercise, you can burn about 1 g of glycogen stores per minute by cycling along, 2 g per minute by riding harder and 3 g per minute by cycling at higher intensities. These glycogen stores are used to keep your muscles fueled. What it means is that you can deplete glycogen stores after 1.5 hour of riding a bike. After that it's a bonus—you can then burn fat.

Another way to deplete glycogen stored in the liver before burning fat is to lower your carbohydrate intake. Interestingly, low-carbohydrate diets even lead to significantly greater weight loss than low-fat diets.[31] This means you have to take in fewer calories than you burn to lose fat. Remember that you can burn fat but only after glycogen stores are used up.

Getting enough sleep also can help you reduce body fat. When you sleep, your body's energy needs are lower, which causes it to burn a higher percentage of fat for energy. As a rough estimate, a person weighing 70 kg may burn around 4 to 7 g of fat during a sleep cycle. Consider this information and apply it to your routine.

Two cups of yogurt daily can aid in fat loss

Reducing body fat can be achieved not only by combining calorie reduction and exercise but also by increasing calcium intake, which can be an additional way to improve fat loss. Research has shown that people on a calorie-restricted diet who consume calcium supplements or foods that are high in calcium, such as 2 cups of yogurt, for 6 to 12 months can experience greater weight and fat loss.[32,33,34] In a study, men who consumed 2 cups of yogurt daily for 12 months lost approximately 5 kg of body fat, while others did not. Another study revealed that calcium intake accelerated weight and fat loss during calorie restriction in adults with obesity. In summary, increasing daily calcium intake from 400 mg to 1000 mg can help lose more body fat than diet alone. Therefore, those on a weight loss diet should consume 2 cups of yogurt a day as each cup contains about 450 mg of calcium.

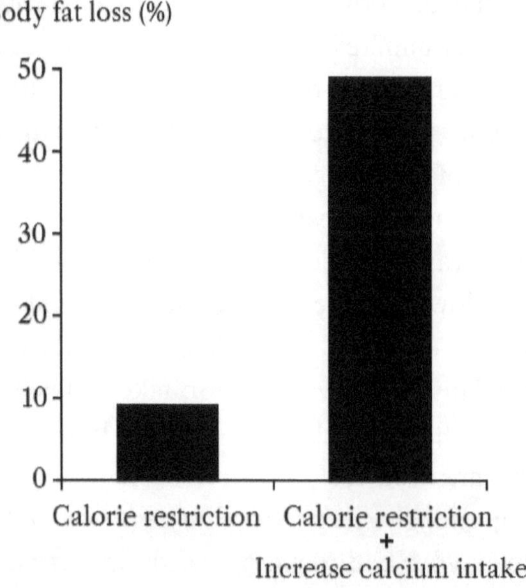

Higher calcium intake aids weight and fat loss in overweight and obese people on calorie-restricted diet.[32,33,34]

Noted that while increasing calcium intake may aid in fat loss, it should not be relied upon as the sole method for weight loss. A balanced diet and regular exercise are still essential for overall health and weight management. Additionally, it's important to choose yogurts that are low in added sugars and fats, as these can negate the potential benefits of increased calcium intake. Adding yogurt to a well-rounded, healthy diet and exercise routine may be a helpful tool in achieving and maintaining a healthy weight.

Eat the Mediterranean diet to beat obesity

The Mediterranean diet is a healthier and more sustainable option compared to other diets.[35] By eating fruits, vegetables, nuts, cereals, extra virgin olive oil, and fish like in Mediterranean countries, such as Italy, Greece, and Turkey, you can lose weight, lower LDL cholesterol, and reduce the risk of chronic diseases. Following short-term diets, such as Atkins, low fat, or Paleolithic diets, only provide temporary weight loss. To maintain a healthy weight, a lifelong pursuit of a healthy lifestyle is necessary. But, if you don't like fish, you can opt for a vegetarian diet that emphasizes fruits, vegetables, nuts, grains, green tea, and walnuts. This diet can help you lose 5-8 kg of weight over six months and maintain it.[36,37] Additionally, if you're looking for tips on curbing food cravings and forming new habits, check out "The Power of Habit" by Charles Duhigg, a self-help book with valuable insights. Lastly, remember, the weight you lose is not as important as the process of losing weight itself.

Resveratrol helps clear off fat in your body

As mentioned earlier, brown fat cells or brown fat is good fat cells. Calorie restriction, exercise, and exposure to cold temperatures can increase the activity of brown fat cells in the body. That, in turn, helps to increase calories burning and speed up weight loss. White fat is bad fat located on our waist, hips and thighs, and it stores excess energy in fat droplets. The accumulation of white fat cells is behind how you gain weight.

Phytonutrients like resveratrol can turn white fat cells into brown fat ones.[38] Resveratrol not only reduces the accumulation of fat but also helps to remove fat from the body.[39,40,41] What resveratrol can do is much like cutting calories through diet and burning calories through exercise. A suitable resveratrol dosage is 1.25 mg per serving, which is equivalent to consuming 1,000 g of red Merlot grapes from Japan or mulberry. Taking resveratrol with breakfast or lunch can help dilute the effects of stomach acid. However, grapes contain high levels of sugar, making them unsuitable for some individuals with certain health conditions. Thus, you can take 125 mg of resveratrol that comes in the form of supplements, which is probably the effective dose for humans.

Give up sugar and refined flour for a healthier life

Overeating contributes to the leading causes of death in the United States, affecting more than 100 million people.[42] If you're overeating, you're malnourished and harming your health. Unhealthy diets can also exacerbate existing health conditions. Unfortunately, the US has the highest rate of diabetes and obesity in the world.[43] Is it time for Americans to cut out bad carbohydrates like sugar and refined flour from their diets?

In 2013, a research team from Australia conducted a study on lab mice and found that the life expectancy of mice fed a low glycemic index (GI) diet increased by an additional 18% compared to mice fed a normal diet.[44] Mice fed a low GI diet also had significantly longer telomeres than mice fed a normal diet. However, data shows that people who cut out bad carbohydrates and opted for low GI foods only slightly lowered their risk of developing cardiovascular disease, diabetes, and colorectal and breast cancer.[45] This could be because other factors are involved and responsible for these illnesses. Nonetheless, people with low blood sugar levels tend to have longer and healthier lifespans.[46] Therefore, I believe that the best way to achieve a healthier and longer life is to say goodbye to all foods that contain added sugar.

After eating carbs in the form of starches, your blood sugar will rise a little. The more carbs you consume, the higher your sugar levels will be. It's important to eat just enough carbs, about 350 g per day, and pay attention to your body's needs to eat only what's necessary. Processed foods are often high in starch, especially refined ones that don't occur naturally, so it's best to avoid them. If you are overweight, have high blood pressure, or diabetes, eating processed foods rich in carbs can increase your risk of heart disease.[47] People can survive and even live longer without added sugar. Naturally sweet fruits with a low GI, like apples, bananas, kiwi, prunes, cherries, grapes, and strawberries, raise blood glucose levels much less than foods with added sugars. Glucose and white bread are reference foods with the highest GI of 100. To check the GI of your diet, visit the international GI database at www.glycemicindex.com.

Examples of foods with varying glycemic index, comparing them to blood glucose levels when consuming sugar.[48]

Food	Glycemic index	Serving size (g)	How it raises blood glcose levels compared to 4 g of table sugar?
Rice, boiled	69	150	10.1
Potato, baked	86	150	8.2
French fries, baked	64	150	7.5
Spaghetti, boiled	39	180	6.6
Whole meal bread ×2 slides	74	60	6.0
Banana	62	120	5.7
Apple	39	120	2.3
Pea, boiled	51	80	1.3
Broccoli, boiled	54	80	0.2
Chicken, egg, fish, mushrooms, almonds	0	60	0

= equivalent to scooping 4-g teaspoon of table sugar into your mouth

Previously, experts recommended choosing wholemeal bread instead of white bread because this can have a slightly better effect on blood glucose levels. However, new research led by specialists at Weizmann Institute of Science in Israel found no significant differences in blood sugar levels after eating wholemeal bread or white bread.[49]

For countries in Asia, in which rice is the staple food, cooked white rice 150 g is equivalent to 10 teaspoons of table sugar. If white rice is your staple food, switching from white rice to brown rice or Riceberry rice can help lower blood sugar levels.[50] And people who eat less white rice have a lower risk for type 2 diabetes. If you feel unfamiliar with brown or Riceberry rice, you can start by consuming 50-70% white rice mixed with 50-30% brown rice or Riceberry rice.

As mentioned before, one way to kill sugar in the body is to eat bitter foods like bitter melon or gurmar. A 2012 study also shows that eating 4.8 g of bitter melon extract, equivalent to 90 g of fresh bitter melon, a day for a month can actually reduce a person's waistline up to an inch.[51]

In addition, we should avoid eating junk food, processed food and sugary food altogether. If our ancestors can survive without eating these types of food, so can you. A life without junk food, processed food and foods with added sugar is possible. Today, the world's biggest problem is not a food shortage, but how not to die from eating certain foods. Obesity has already been a bigger global problem than infectious disease. It's a noticeable trend in developed and developing countries. Countries with higher obesity rates spend hundreds of billions annually to tackle obesity. This is a development trap. Eating junk food is a form of malnutrition that we shouldn't allow our children, grandchildren and our future generations to continue to get a share. Humans should provide their loved ones with the best possible nutrition. Like introducing a solid food to a baby for the first time, now it's time for you to explore new and healthy foods for your kids and yourself. You can take gradual steps towards this. Even small adjustments in your eating habits can lead to significant improvements in the long run.

In conclusion, shedding pounds might take more time than anticipated, so staying patient and persistent is crucial. If you tend to overeat, reduce your food intake. Avoid snacking or eating outside of regular meal times and limit eating to daylight hours. Crucially, cut back on the foods you love most and exercise consistently. Ultra-processed foods can change your gene actions in harmful ways, making you age faster, while natural foods keep your gene actions balanced, keeping you healthy. Centenarians who live to be 100 years or older, typically maintain healthier lifestyles, which includes maintaining a healthy weight and consuming healthy diets consisting of whole, natural foods, rich in fruits, vegetables, whole grains, and lean proteins. This eating habits, along with regular physical activity and other healthy lifestyles, keep their gene expression in balance. It's time to embrace natural foods, for nourishing your body with essential nutrients. These nutrients found in natural foods play a big role in stem cell proliferation, DNA repair, and inflammation reduction, helping you fight aging. By fueling your body with the right nutrients, you can promote regeneration, unlock anti-aging abilities, and ward off age-related diseases—especially when you choose fresh, unprocessed, and real foods.

CHAPTER 8
Real atherosclerosis begins in childhood

Taking care of your health is really important. One way to do it is by paying attention to what your body says. Your body can give you clues about how you're doing. Sometimes, your body might drop hints about any hidden health problems. If you spot these hints and take action, you can stay healthier and avoid big health problems later on. Let's explore some of these signs your body can give you.

Corneal arcus: white cholesterol deposits around the cornea, which is a dome-shaped tissue covering the front of your eye, may be a sign of high blood cholesterol levels. It can be found in 60% of people aged 50-60 years and over. In people aged over 80 years, this cholesterol built up in the cornea is usually associated with high blood cholesterol levels.[1] However, a white ring around the cornea is not necessarily an indication of high blood cholesterol. But, if this abnormal sign appears in someone younger than 50, it's likely associated with high blood cholesterol in the body with increased risks for cardiovascular disease and atherosclerosis. That's what you should be concerned.

Ear lobe crease refers to a deep wrinkle or furrow that appears on the earlobe. Some studies have suggested that the presence of this crease may be a predictor of coronary artery disease, a condition in which the arteries that supply blood to the heart become narrow or blocked due to the buildup of plaque.[2] However, having an ear lobe crease doesn't necessarily mean that a person has coronary artery disease, and other risk factors such as high blood pressure, smoking, and high cholesterol levels should also be taken into consideration.

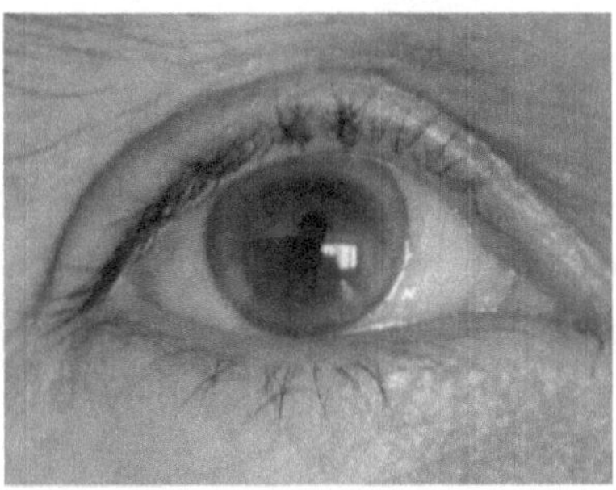

A ring that appears white in color on the front of the eye resulting from the accumulation of cholesterol and other lipids surrounding the cornea is associated with high blood cholesterol. This telltale sign may be an indicator of coronary artery disease or atherosclerosis.[1,3]

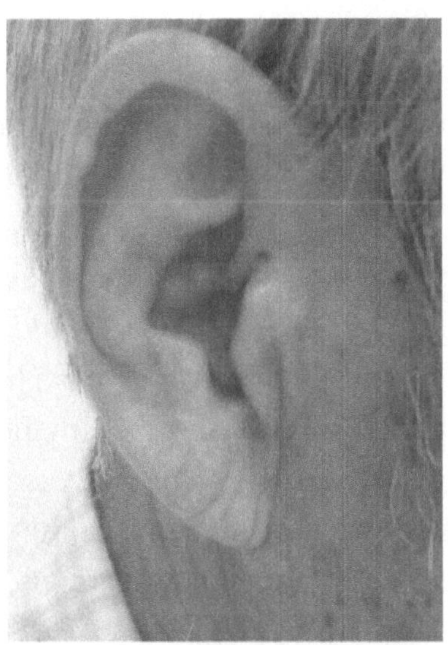

A deep wrinkle on your earlobe may be a predictor of coronary artery disease.[2,4]

Let's talk about the endothelium, the largest organ in our body. This single layer of cells, which lines the walls of blood vessels, is essential for regulating blood flow. It makes substances that can either dilate or constrict the vessels. The endothelium, weighing about 1 kg and equivalent in size to 4 tennis courts, is responsible for maintaining our circulatory system. Surprisingly, around 10 g (0.1%) of the endothelial cells of the endothelium are removed and replaced every day.[5] Importantly, if this single layer of cells inside the artery blood vessels that carry blood away from the heart becomes damaged, it can lead to the development of atherosclerosis and heart problems.

What's destroying your blood vessel walls?

The most important enemy of the blood vessel wall is cigarette smoke. The chemicals in cigarette smoke cause the lining of your blood vessels to become swollen and inflamed. Additionally, smoking or inhaling someone else's smoke causes blood platelets to become sticky and more sensitive to stimuli, which increases your risk of developing a blood clot. Furthermore, the nicotine in cigarette smoke causes high blood pressure and increases heart rate, both of which can affect your heart. If you take a look at the data, you will find that countries with higher rates of heart disease, like Afghanistan and Turkmenistan, are also countries where people smoke the most.[6] However, if you don't smoke, you are as lucky as a person who has a certain type of FOXO3 gene, a human longevity gene that can maintain telomere length and protect you from heart disease.[7,8]

In addition to cigarette smoke, anything that can cause inflammation can also contribute to blood vessel wall damage. This includes high cholesterol levels, diabetes, obesity, sedentary lifestyle and consuming a diet high in processed foods, saturated fats, and sugars. If left unmanaged, this inflammation can lead to the hardening and narrowing of arteries, ultimately causing atherosclerosis. As we age, our risk for atherosclerosis also increases. An easy way to understand this is by comparing the artery on your wrist to that of your grandparent's. You may notice that your grandparents tend to have harder arteries, indicating the development of atherosclerosis over time.

Atherosclerosis

Atherosclerosis is a condition in which the arteries become narrow and hardened due to the accumulation of plaque. People with atherosclerosis tend to have plaque deposits inside the arterial walls of large and medium-sized arteries in the heart, brain, kidney, and legs.

Chronic low-grade inflammation is linked to the development of atherosclerosis. While inflammation typically occurs in response to invading pathogens, chronic low-grade inflammation is actually caused by the slow buildup of fat and calcium in the artery wall. When the body attempts to destroy this fatty deposit by sending white blood cells to clean it up, they can become trapped in the artery wall. As the fat buildup hardens, it forms calcium deposits called "plaques." Plaque is composed of materials such as fats, cholesterol, calcium, white blood cells, cellular debris, and other materials from the bloodstream. Over time, the accumulation of plaque impairs the structure and stretchability of the artery wall.[9]

What's more, if the plaque tears or ruptures, a blood clot may form and block blood flow. If this happens in a major blood vessel, such as the coronary artery, it can lead to a heart attack. Similarly, if a blood clot blocks a blood vessel in the brain, it can cause an ischemic stroke. Conversely, if a blood vessel ruptures in the brain, it can cause bleeding inside the brain, which is known as a hemorrhagic stroke. Atherosclerosis can also be a silent condition and may not show symptoms until a blood clot or a blockage causes a significant reduction in blood flow.

Apart from chronic low-grade inflammation caused by the buildup of fat and calcium, atherosclerosis can also be influenced by other factors, including diabetes, obesity, excessive alcohol consumption, physical inactivity, a sedentary lifestyle, and unhealthy habits. These factors contribute to the risk of developing atherosclerosis.

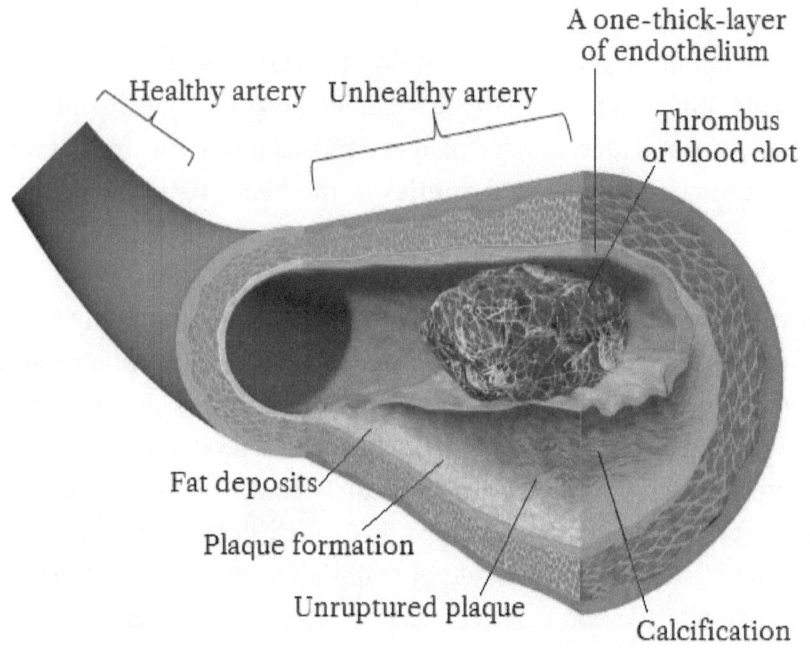

Atherosclerosis is a condition in which plaques, made up of fat (cholesterol), calcium, and cellular debris, build up inside the artery walls.[11] As time goes by, these plaques can narrow or block the arteries, hindering blood flow. If a plaque ruptures, platelets gather at the affected site, forming blood clots. Complete blockage of blood flow due to a large blood clot (or thrombus) can lead to fatal events. In the coronary arteries, it may cause a heart attack, while in the brain, it may result in a stroke.

Plaque buildup inside artery walls is a key feature of atherosclerosis. These deposits can accumulate over time, narrowing the lumen of the artery and blocking the flow of blood to vital organs and tissues.

Atherosclerotic plaques can be categorized into 3 different types according to their composition:[10]

1. Calcified plaques with more calcium
2. Fatty or noncalcified plaques with high fat content
3. Mixed plaques with less than 50% calcium and fat

Different plaque structures can influence the pathogenesis of atherosclerosis. Fatty, or noncalcified, plaque is the most dangerous type of plaque. This soft noncalcified plaques are more likely to rupture than calcified plaques, which are stronger and more stable. Therefore, fatty plaques are likely responsible for most heart attacks and strokes.

As you age, plaque buildup inside the arteries, which are blood vessels that carry blood away from the heart, is common. It's estimated that by the age of 45, about half of people will have fatty deposits in their arteries.

However, the vast majority of women (80%) who have plaques have calcified plaques, which is why women are less prone to atherosclerosis than men. This may be a result of the protective effects of estrogen.[12] Sixty percent of men who have plaque buildup in their arteries are often found to have mixed plaques. Cyclists and marathon runners, on the other hand, usually have calcified plaques in their arteries. Experts are still unsure why these athletes have more calcium deposits than normal people. Potential mechanisms for calcified plaques in athletes include increased blood flow that damages the blood vessel walls, free radicals, or inflammation response to prolonged strenuous exercise that gives rise to calcium deposits. It's also possible that exercise is a panacea that makes athletes immune to atherosclerosis by reducing the buildup of fatty plaque. Of course, people who exercise regularly, like marathon runners, tend to have larger, more flexible, and expandable arteries than those who don't exercise.[13] This helps protect athletes from atherosclerosis and heart problems, and helps them live up to 6 years longer than normal people.[14]

Atherosclerosis starts as early as childhood

As people say a person's early years shape their health decades later, poor diets in childhood can have a significant impact on a child's future health status. It's essential to know that atherosclerosis gradually develops during childhood and progresses over time.

When fat starts to accumulate inside the artery walls, it triggers the release of free radicals into the bloodstream, which results in further plaque buildup. As time passes, these symptoms become more noticeable, including chest or leg pain, numbness in the face, arms or legs, and can be an indication of atherosclerosis. Children who gain weight disproportionally to their height and have a sedentary lifestyle are more susceptible to the accumulation of plaque in the arterial wall.[15,16] In people who spend most of their time sitting or lying down while working, watching TV or using a computer, a lack of physical activity can result in weight gain, elevated blood pressure, and increased cholesterol levels. These factors contribute to a higher risk of plaque buildup. The risk of plaque accumulation and atherosclerosis also increases with age, as blood vessels naturally lose elasticity and become more susceptible to damage over time.

Let's discuss the telltale signs of arteries hardening once more. As we age, plaque builds up inside our blood vessel walls, making them thicker and less flexible. This narrowing and thickening of the capillary walls slow down the delivery of oxygen, nutrients, and other essential substances to our body's cells. Consequently, tissues have difficulty obtaining oxygen and nutrients and eliminating metabolic waste products. Stiffened arteries may result in symptoms such as numbness or tingling in the hands or feet and shortness of breath. These changes put additional strain on our organs, leading to further complications. Therefore, these symptoms should not be ignored, as they are critical indications that our body is attempting to inform us of a severe health issue. However, noted that numbness may also be caused by other factors such as vitamin B12 deficiency and nerve damage from diabetes or injuries.

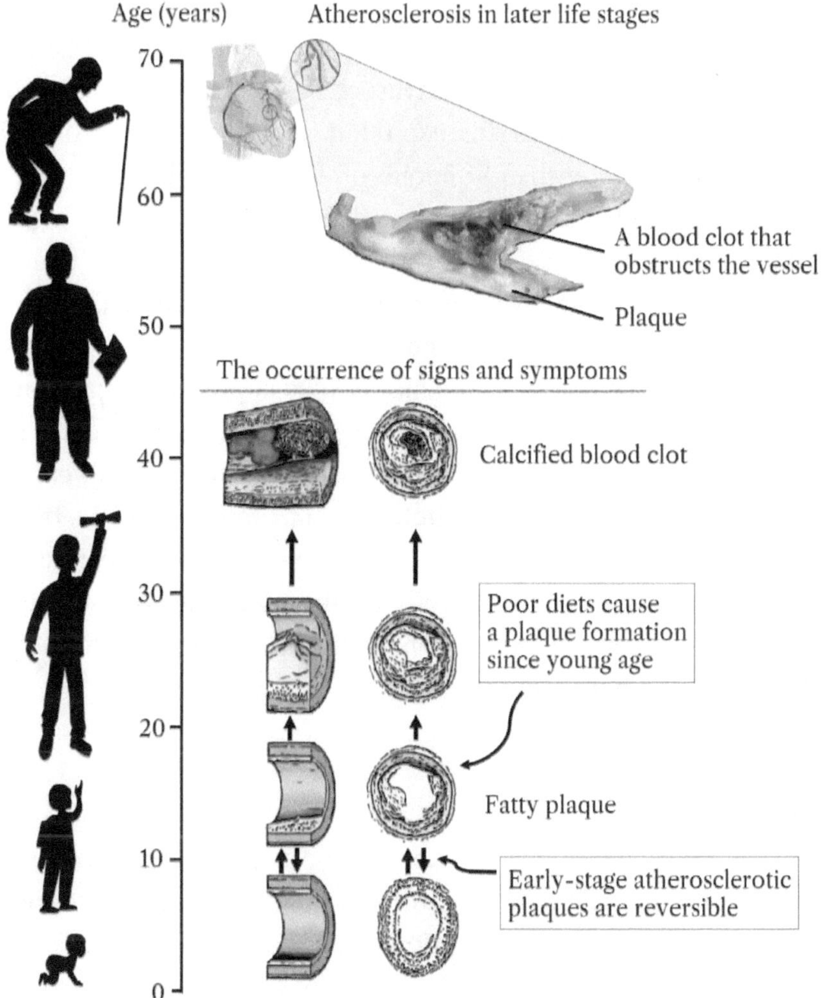

Atherosclerosis is a condition that develops over time as a result of plaque buildup in the blood vessels. This process can begin in childhood and progress throughout a person's life.[11,16,17,18]

A little bit of knowledge: good cholesterol and bad cholesterol

Cholesterol is one of many types of fats in the blood. LDL

cholesterol, also known as "bad cholesterol," and HDL cholesterol, also known as "good cholesterol," are the two main types of cholesterol. LDL cholesterol is water-insoluble and can deposit excess cholesterol in blood vessel walls, causing atherosclerosis. In contrast, HDL cholesterol absorbs cholesterol in the blood and transports it to the liver for excretion. A desirable level of HDL cholesterol is greater than 1 mmol/L or 40 mg/dL, while the level of LDL cholesterol should not exceed 3.4 mmol/L or 130 mg/dL. Additionally, a desirable level of triglycerides is less than 1.7 mmol/L or 150 mg/dL, as high levels of triglycerides can increase the risk of heart disease. While diet and exercise habits can influence cholesterol levels, other factors may also be at play. It's important to know your level of LDL cholesterol to take steps to reduce risk factors before it's too late. For example, if there are four 45-year-old men with high levels of LDL cholesterol (3.7 to 4.8 mmol/L), by the time they turn 75, doctors might only be able to prevent heart failure or stroke in one of them.[19] While atherosclerosis is a common condition that starts to develop in childhood, taking steps to reduce risk factors can help prevent it.

Curved penis

Peyronie's disease is a condition caused by the formation of scar tissue and calcium deposits under the skin of the penis, resulting in a curved penis during erection. Men with a curved penis may experience pain during an erection, which can be uncomfortable during sexual activity. Risk factors such as high blood pressure, high levels of lipids in the blood, diabetes mellitus, and smoking can contribute to plaque formation, which may lead to Peyronie's disease. Experts estimate that more than 1 in 10 men in the United States may have this condition, with prevalence higher in men over 40 and those with diabetes.[20,21,22] However, the exact cause of Peyronie's disease remains unclear. While all men with the condition have a plaque, many may be unaware of it. Atherosclerosis, which is found in up to 30% of individuals with a curved penis, is believed by some experts to be a contributing factor to this disease.

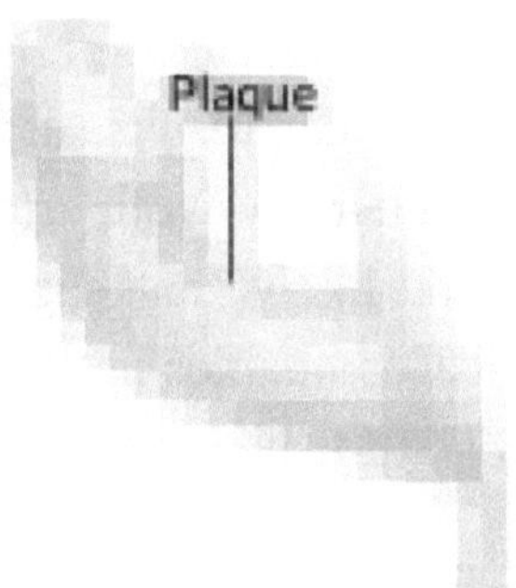

Peyronie's disease

Unveiling the hidden villain behind atherosclerosis

Just as Coca-Cola and other big companies try to shift the blame for type 2 diabetes from sugar to lack of exercise, fat is also claimed to be responsible for atherosclerosis.

What is the actual cause of atherosclerosis? Again, I personally think that it's "sugar." It's because sugar can damage the inner endothelial layer of blood vessels. When a large amount of sugar enters the bloodstream, it causes the artery wall to leak. Glucose at concentrations of 10 mmol/L or more in our blood can allow for the flow of nutrients, water, ions or even white blood cells in and out of, or penetrate, the blood vessels. And this amount of sugar glucose can harden the arteries too.[23,24] In general, this blood glucose level is less common in normal people, but can be found in people with pre-diabetes and diabetes. Actually, blood glucose levels at or above 10 mmol/L can also be found in normal people. That is because our bodies respond differently to starchy and sugary foods. For example, consuming cornflakes, energy bars, or cereal bars containing 20-35 g of sugar can cause some healthy people to experience a 10-12 mmol/L increase in blood glucose levels.[25]

Do you remember that in Chapter 4, glucose accelerates the formation of arterial plaque in lab mice,[26] leading to atherosclerosis? I haven't seen any experiment like this in humans yet, because people would not want to participate in such experiments as test subjects. However, if one were to conduct an experiment on himself, it's likely that he would observe similar results. In fact, the fat and calcium buildup that hardens and narrows your arteries is most likely caused by sugar. Therefore, it's likely that sugar is the actual cause of atherosclerosis, and that companies in the sugar industry have tried to conceal this fact by shifting blame to fat.[27,28]

Phosphates may be a third factor that contributes to atherosclerosis

When it comes to phosphates, I hope you remember the story about phosphates in cola drinks that was mentioned in Chapter 5, Karma of Eating. Normally, phosphate compounds in nature are in the form of organic matters such as energy rich substances and genetic material in living things. But in the food industry, synthetic phosphate compounds like phosphoric acid are used in the production of soft drinks, jams and instant coffee. Tricalcium phosphate, an anti-caking agent, is used to prevent foods such as sugar, milk powder, and cheese slices from clumping or aggregating. Polyphosphate and sodium polyphosphate are widely used in refrigerated and frozen meat and seafood products.

In our body, inorganic phosphates behave completely differently from organic phosphates. Organic phosphates are slowly broken down in the digestive tract and, from the intestine, absorbed only 40-60%. In contrast, inorganic phosphates are absorbed almost 100%.[29] Phosphate blood levels that are too high can also cause calcium plaque buildup that leads to atherosclerosis. If you are a fan of soft drinks or instant coffee, it's not yet known whether consuming these products, which contain both sugar and inorganic phosphates, will double a person's chances of developing atherosclerosis.

You should also be aware that the effects of phosphate

overload are most common in people of low socio-economic status. Among these people, the incidence of kidney conditions and death from heart disease was also associated with an elevated level of phosphate in the blood.[30] A phosphate level in the blood that is more than 4 mg per 100 ml of blood is considered abnormally high. Phosphate blood levels that are too high can cause calcium plaque buildup on the artery wall, which, in turn, causes damage to blood vessels leading to atherosclerosis. According to a study, patients with atherosclerosis had an average blood phosphate level of 4.23 mg/dL, which was significantly higher than the level of 3.68 mg/dL in the control group without atherosclerosis. What's more, higher levels of phosphate in the blood may lead to kidney disease.[31]

You can find the quantity of phosphate or phosphoric acid present in different food items by checking the Open Food Facts website at https://us.openfoodfacts.org.

A little bit of knowledge

Blood pressure is measured using two numbers: the higher (systolic) and lower (diastolic) values. A blood pressure reading below 120/80 mmHg is considered normal. The higher number is the pressure when the heart pumps blood out into the arteries, while the lower number is the pressure that occurs when the heart relaxes and refills with blood. If a person's blood pressure numbers are between 130-139 and 80-89 mmHg, they have prehypertension and are at risk of developing high blood pressure (140/90 or higher) if left uncontrolled. It's important to know your numbers and take steps to manage your blood pressure if necessary.

Gut bacteria keep your arteries young

Let's determine whether you are at risk of atherosclerosis or not, as arterial stiffness can increase the likelihood of developing cardiovascular disease by almost 50%. When comparing the incidence of atherosclerosis between men and women, it was found that men are more likely to have this condition than women. But when women enter the golden age and the magic of estrogen is gone, even hormone replacement therapy won't be able to save postmenopausal women from atherosclerosis.[32] Furthermore, postmenopausal women with atherosclerosis trend to have less gut microbial diversity than women of the same age with healthy arteries.[33,34]

How is reduced gut bacteria richness linked to arterial stiffness? It can be a kind of skepticism, so I would like to share a bit of knowledge. Living inside of the human gut are 300 to 500 different kinds of bacteria. Trillions of them make what's known as gut flora or gut microbiota. The gut microbiota can control whether we become overweight or develop type 2 diabetes. Of course, it can also affect the formation of plaques in arteries.

The gut microbiota produces IPA (indolepropionic acid), which is released in the intestines and then absorbed into the bloodstream at levels that are high enough to be detectable.[35] In the bloodstream of women, IPA can make the arteries more flexible and youthful. There are bacteria in our gut that help create IPA. The only species of bacteria known to synthesize IPA is *Clostridium sporogenes*. Therefore, creating a healthy gut environment is necessary to promote the thriving, division, and multiplication of these good gut bacteria.

But whenever your gut is imbalanced and full of bad bacteria, it will adversely affect your health. There are also bad bacteria in our gut that can use carnitine, choline or lecithin as energy source and excrete TMA as a waste product. The more carnitine, choline or lecithin you eat, the more bad gut bacteria can grow and multiply. As such, they increase TMA and TMAO in the bloodstream and eventually results in hardening of the arteries.[36,37] To avoid this, you can inform your family members and close friends that consuming carnitine, choline, and lecithin-containing foods such as red meat, dietary supplements, and energy drinks may increase their blood levels of TMAO, which is linked to an increased risk of atherosclerosis.

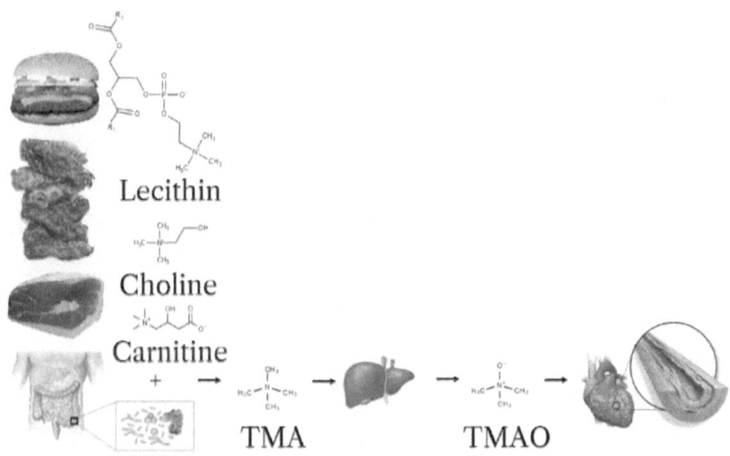

When the gut bacteria digest carnitine, choline, or lecithin in red meat, ham, energy drinks, junk food and dietary supplements, they excrete TMA that is then converted to TMAO via enzyme in the liver. TMAO enters the bloodstream and plays a role in atherosclerosis.[11]

Poor sleep leads to atherosclerosis

Have you ever heard of "food is to hunger as sleep is to weariness?" Sleep is an essential element of human life. Scientists have long known that people who have restless nights increase their risk of cardiovascular disease and atherosclerosis.[38,39]

Moreover, a 2019 study published in Nature revealed that mice experiencing frequent awakenings during sleep developed larger fatty plaques in their arterial walls than the control mice that had a good night's sleep.[40] Because of ethical implications, mice were used as stand-ins for humans. Using mice as a model, scientists were also able to show that when they sleep-deprived mice, orexin—also known as hypocretin, a hormone that regulates sleep and wake cycles—decreased. And somehow, mice that had been sleep-deprived also had higher levels of white blood cells, i.e., macrophages, monocytes, and neutrophils, in their bloodstream. This is because lower levels of orexin in the sleep-interrupted mice resulted in increased production of white blood cells, which normally occurs in response to infection. This led scientists to conclude that orexin loss during interrupted sleep can cause inflammation and thus promote atherosclerotic plaque development. The scientists have also found that, in sleep-interrupted mice, an increase in the hormone orexin can help protect blood vessels from damage. The study suggests that a good night's sleep protects against atherosclerosis, while a bad night's sleep has the opposite effect.

What is true for mice is usually true for humans. People who sleep less than 6 hours or sleep lightly, awakening frequently, are more likely to have a buildup of plaque in their blood vessels.[41] Again, it's true that those who don't get enough sleep have a higher number of neutrophils in their bloodstream. The increased production of neutrophils has also been proven to cause excess inflammation and is linked to the buildup of fatty deposits in our blood vessels.[42] Getting enough sleep is essential for good health, and it turns out that sleep is just as important as a healthy diet. If you are someone who doesn't sleep enough, try to aim for 7-8 hours of sleep per night to reduce the risk of developing atherosclerosis.

***

Nuts, vegetables and fruits can lower your blood cholesterol

When atherosclerosis occurs in the artery that supplies blood to the heart muscle, it's called coronary heart disease. It's a type of thickening or hardening of the artery that you would want to avoid clogging. However, if you develop this condition, it can be reversed by a healthy eating plan that emphasizes fruits, vegetables, whole grains, beans and nuts, as well as avoiding high-cholesterol foods.[43,44] Even if you are taking medication to manage your cholesterol levels, you can still improve your cholesterol levels and reverse coronary heart disease by eating them.

Even though cholesterol is often linked to bad health effects, our bodies actually need cholesterol to create hormones. This complicated connection can be better understood by realizing that our bodies can take in cholesterol through the intestines and into the blood in different ways, depending on our genes. Some people naturally make more cholesterol, while others don't produce much at all.

Actually, about 50% of people in this world have a natural ability to efficiently produce vitamin A from beta carotene, which is found in carrots, sweet potatoes, spinach, and kale, due to their genes. As a result, they can lower blood cholesterol levels, especially LDL cholesterol naturally. Therefore, when beta-carotene is given to individuals with a gene that can efficiently convert it to vitamin A, it may result in reduced development of atherosclerosis lesions or plaques in their arteries and lower levels of cholesterol. On the other hand, the remaining 50% of people don't have this genetic advantage and may have higher levels of LDL cholesterol.

Your body can also make all the cholesterol it requires, but it also absorbs a small proportion compared to the total cholesterol produced by the body. Actually, cholesterol in foods is already absorbed poorly—about 25% of your blood cholesterol comes from what you eat. Some people have gut bacteria like *Lactobacillus* that make cholesterol less absorbed than other people. When these people eat foods high in fat and cholesterol, their blood cholesterol levels won't rise as much as they would for other people, even when consuming high-fat and high-cholesterol foods. But for some people, if they consume foods high in fat and cholesterol, such as prawns, squid, or egg yolk, their blood cholesterol levels rise quickly.

What's more, saturated fat and trans-fat are major contributors to increased blood cholesterol levels for most people. Also, for those who consume alcohol, you should know that the intake of alcohol can lead to an increase in triglycerides and cholesterol in your bloodstream by up to 50%. If you are fond of drinking, it's necessary to be aware of the possible elevation of your blood cholesterol levels.

In fact, a simple trick to lower your cholesterol naturally is to eat 200 g of nuts. One study showed that people who ate almonds, soybeans, oats, fruits, and vegetables for a month could lower their cholesterol by 20%. This is as good as taking a 20-mg dose of a medicine called statin.[46] Doctors usually give statins to patients with heart issues to lower their cholesterol.

Nuts and beans help lower our cholesterol because they have something called phytosterols. These molecules are structurally similar to cholesterol. When we eat nuts and beans, the phytosterols compete with cholesterol for absorption. This means our body takes in less cholesterol. As the cholesterol goes through our small bowel, even less gets absorbed. Finally, our body gets rid of the cholesterol and other waste through feces.

Phytosterol

Cholesterol

Phytosterol is cholesterol analog. In the digestive tract, phytosterol competes with cholesterol for absorption.

For instance, when people ate 450 mg of phytosterols along with food that had 160 mg of cholesterol, like 200 g of pork or chicken, their bodies absorbed 26% less cholesterol. Also, they got rid of 79% more cholesterol in their feces, which was about 1,200 mg a day. Over 1,000 mg of the body's cholesterol was removed daily through their feces. This is a good thing. Eating 450 mg of phytosterols can help our body get rid of 1,000 mg of extra cholesterol every day.

Foods contain the highest amount of phytosterols.[48]

Foods (100 g)	Phytosterols (mg)
Cherimoya	1,770
Pistachio nuts	271
Soybeans	221
Peanuts	206
Almonds	161
Walnuts	143
Brown rice	60-90

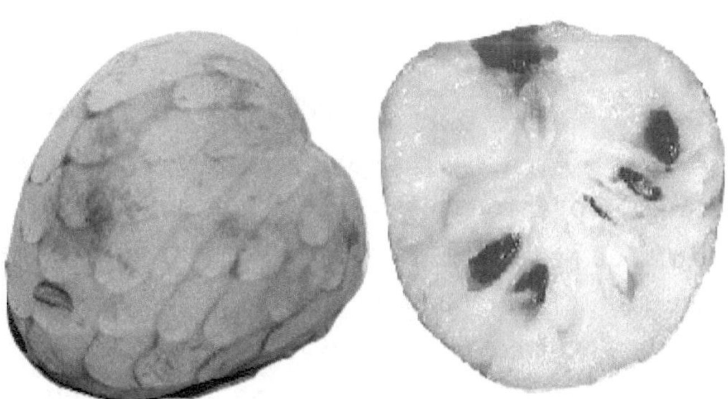

Australian cherimoya or custard apple, *Annona cherimola*, contains up to 1,770 mg of phytosterols per 100 g.

By understanding the benefits of functional food, you can reduce the risk of high blood cholesterol levels by including fruits, vegetables, whole grains, beans, and nuts in your diet as a practical solution.

How a plant-based diet reverses coronary heart disease

I would like to share a story with you about a doctor treating another doctor. In 1996, a 44-year-old male surgeon, who was a patient of Dr. Caldwell Esselstyn, presented as a non-smoker in good physical condition without a history of diabetes. He had no family history of coronary heart disease and, like many Americans, followed a standard American diet. Blood test results indicated normal cholesterol and LDL levels (a total cholesterol of 156 mg/dL and LDL of 97 mg/dL). Despite this, he was diagnosed with coronary heart disease, characterized by a narrowing of the artery supplying blood to his heart muscle. Under Dr. Caldwell's guidance, the patient transitioned to a plant-based diet without cholesterol-lowering medication or fat intake (even avoiding healthy fats) for a duration of 32 months. Subsequently, his cholesterol and LDL levels decreased to 89 and 38 mg/dL, respectively. Remarkably, following an X-ray imaging examination, it was observed that the previously narrowed blood vessel in his heart had been completely reversed.

However, it's important to note that this is just one case study, and more clinical trials are needed to confirm these findings. Interestingly, existing data suggest that a plant-based diet may really protect against both coronary heart disease and other types of heart disease. For example, in Uganda, a country with one of the lowest heart disease rates, the majority of the population consumes a predominantly plant-based diet made up of starchy foods like cassava roots, sweet potatoes, cereals, and bananas. This dietary pattern contributes to Uganda's low death rate from heart-related diseases.

While many people believe that a plant-based diet is challenging to adopt, it could be a worthwhile change, especially if one's life is at stake. For those hesitant to rely on medications, a whole food, plant-based diet offers an alternative solution. The potential of such a diet to dissolve plaque within arterial walls and even reverse coronary heart disease aligns with the views of Dr. Caldwell Esselstyn, a leading supporter of this dietary approach. As he boldly claims in his book, "We can end the heart disease epidemic forever by changing what we eat."

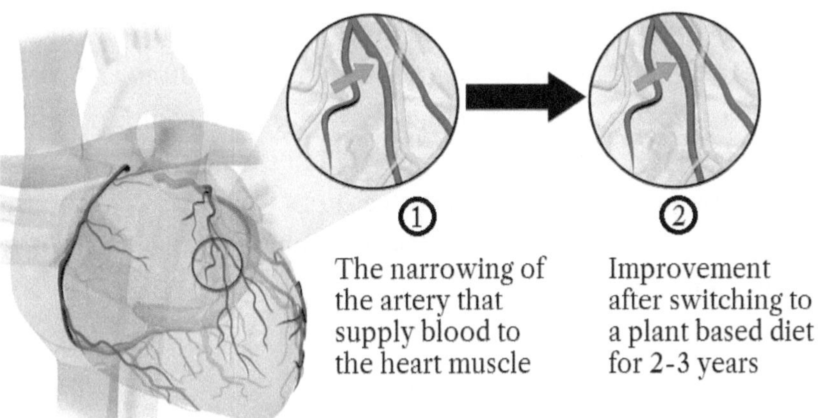

In a study involving six patients with coronary heart disease who were on cholesterol-lowering medications such as cholestyramine or lovastatin, it was found that adopting a plant-based diet effectively arrested and even reversed the progression of the disease. Notably, one patient achieved complete reversal of existing coronary heart disease without the use of cholesterol-lowering drugs.[43,44,49,50]

Vitamin E helps protect against atherosclerosis and curved penis

Along with vitamin A, which can lower cholesterol levels in the bloodstream, vitamin E is effective in preventing the early stages of vascular plaque formation. It does so by stopping white blood cells from adhering to the single-layered endothelium within artery walls.[51] That is why vitamin E may naturally decrease the risk of plaque progression in arteries.

Another one, in humans, vitamin E has been shown to alleviate symptoms of Peyronie's disease, a condition that causes penile curvature. In a study, a daily intake of 600 mg of vitamin E reduced Peyronie's plaque by 50% and diminished penile curvature in almost all participants.[52]

Some natural foods with high vitamin E content include almonds, which contain 25 mg of vitamin E per 100 g, and roselle (*Hibiscus sabdariffa*), which contains 50 mg of vitamin E per 100 g. Whole foods are usually thought to be better than supplements, and natural treatments that don't involve drugs are often the preferred method for improving health. The recommended daily intake for vitamin E is 15 mg.

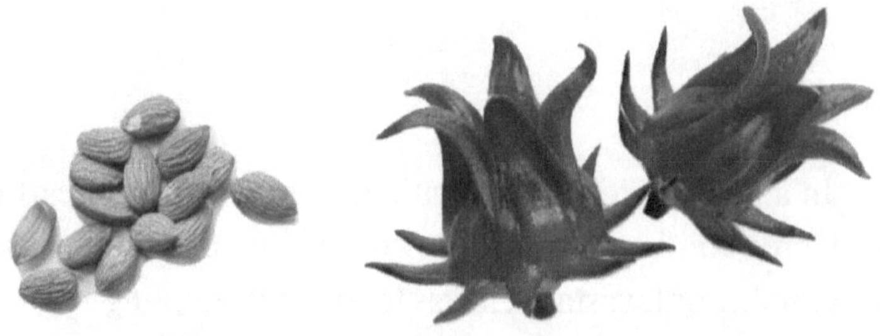

One hundred grams of almonds contain 25 mg of vitamin E, while 100 g of roselle contains 50 mg of vitamin E. The presence of vitamin E in these foods may help protect against atherosclerosis and Peyronie's disease.

Aged garlic extract decreases fat and calcium deposition in arteries by 20%

Both garlic and aged garlic extract can reduce systolic blood pressure by approximately 10 mmHg and lower total cholesterol levels by about 20 mg/dL. A dose of 4 ml of aged garlic extract per day can also reduce arterial calcification and help prevent the progression of atherosclerosis and the development of heart disease by approximately 20%.[53] Aged garlic extract also exhibits antioxidant activity and, importantly, has an anti-AGE activity 1.7 times stronger than fresh garlic.[54,55] It should be noted that these studies were funded by the supplement manufacturer whose product was investigated.

By the way, if you are interested in making your own aged garlic extract, here's how to do it: First, cut and slice the garlic into slivers. Second, macerate the garlic slices in 15-20% aqueous ethanol, which is equivalent to a mixture of half water and half vodka. Finally, seal the container tightly and keep it at room temperature for 18-20 months.[56] The extract can then be concentrated to dryness and stored in a freezer for further use.

Vitamin K inhibits calcium buildup in arteries

Vitamin K, particularly vitamin K2, can inhibit the formation of calcified plaque in artery walls. Vitamin K2, especially in the form of MK-7, stays in the body longer than other forms of vitamin K2, up to two days. In rats, vitamin K2 lowered calcium in arteries by 50%.[57]

In humans, a study found that taking 180 mcg of vitamin K2 a day helped reduce arterial stiffness and increase the elasticity of artery walls in older women who regularly take calcium supplements.[58,59] Research by nutritionists from Erasmus Medical Center Rotterdam, the Netherlands, in 2004, also revealed that people who ate a diet containing just 32 mcg of vitamin K2 could reduce calcium deposits in arteries and risk of death from heart conditions significantly.[60]

Have you ever wondered why your body needs vitamin K2? It's not just a passing thought. Vitamin K2 plays a crucial role in keeping calcium out of the bloodstream and putting it where it belongs—in the bones. This knowledge is nothing short of vital. But here is the catch: when your body lacks vitamin K2, calcium can build up in other tissues, such as your artery walls.[61] That is why vitamin

K2 and calcium work best when they work together. It's a secret worth knowing, one that could ultimately save your life. By incorporating vitamin K2 into your diet, you could halt the progression of atherosclerosis, or even reverse it altogether.

Vitamin K2 is rarely present in junk food. Even in a Western diet full of green leafy vegetables, there is very little vitamin K.[62] However, a traditional Japanese food, one of the most popular breakfast dishes in Japan, called "natto," is rich in vitamin K2. Natto is made from boiled soybeans that have been fermented with *Bacillus subtilis* var. natto. One hundred grams of natto contains 1,034 mcg of vitamin K2, with 930 mcg of vitamin K2 in the form of MK-7. The Okinawans, who regularly eat natto, have a low risk of heart problems, such as heart attacks, and live longer lives. Data also revealed that Japanese people who eat 50 g of natto a day cut their risk of heart attack by 10%.[63]

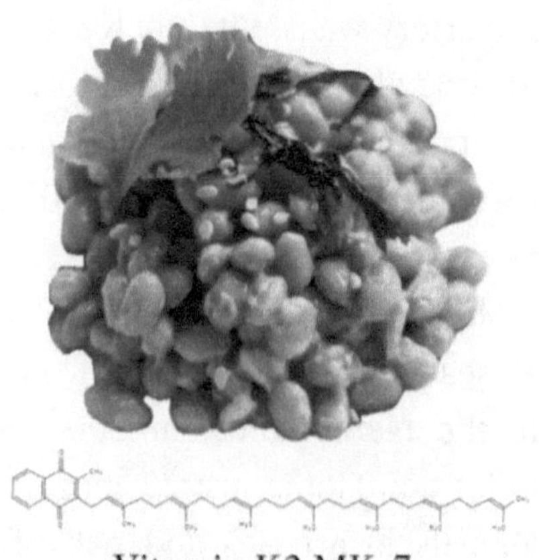

Vitamin K2 MK-7

Eating natto, a traditional Japanese food made from fermented soybeans, is an excellent source of vitamin K2 MK-7, which helps keep calcium out of the bloodstream and inhibits plaque formation in the wall of the arteries. In fact, a hundred grams of natto contains 930 mcg of vitamin K2 MK-7.

Eating a pack of natto a day is likely to keep the artery walls healthy. Natto is rich in vitamin K2 MK-7, which research suggests can enhance the activity of the bone-derived hormone osteocalcin. Osteocalcin is responsible for transferring calcium from the blood to build bone. Therefore, it inhibits the formation of calcified plaque in the arteries and prevents it from getting worse. Natto is rich in vitamin K2 MK-7, which can keep your bones and arterial walls healthy.

Another important point to remember is that natto is made from soybeans. One hundred grams of soybeans contain phytosterols, high amounts of tryptophan, and about 10 g of soluble fiber. Soluble fiber can help trap fat in the intestines and reduce cholesterol absorption, contributing to improved heart health. Eating soybeans, as well as green, red, or black beans, every day for a month can also reduce LDL by 4 mg/dL and increase HDL good cholesterol by 1.4 mg/dL. Adding soybeans to your diet can be beneficial for reducing cholesterol levels and enhancing heart health.[64]

In addition to natto, bitter melon is another popular food among the Okinawan people in Japan. This could be another reason why they have lower rates of heart disease compared to the average Japanese and Americans. Studies have shown that people who consume 9 g of bitter melon per day can reduce LDL, which can cause fat to accumulate in artery walls, by about 5 mg/dL.[65,66]

Gut bacteria that can enhance the flexibility of blood vessels

While unhealthy arteries are stiff, healthy ones are elastic. As previously mentioned, the bacteria in your gut play a role in determining the elasticity of your arteries. Consuming a diet rich in vegetables and nuts promotes the growth and proliferation of gut bacteria called *Clostridium sporogenes*. Studies have shown that women with a significant quantity of *C. sporogenes* in their gut have more flexible arteries.[35] This is because these tiny microbes produce IPA, which enters the bloodstream and circulates throughout the body. The bacterial metabolite IPA is an anti-inflammatory molecule.[67] People with higher levels of IPA in their blood are likely to have improved blood vessel elasticity. What's crucial is that, in our gut, *C. sporogenes* can break down tryptophan and produce IPA.

Tryptophan, which is a precursor to IPA, is found in various foods such as chicken, eggs, soybeans, and Atlantic cod. Other foods with high tryptophan levels include red bell pepper (7,000 mg per 100 g), pistachio nut (142 mg per 100 g), cashew nut (127 mg per 100 g), and almond (106 mg per 100 g). These nuts not only contain tryptophan but also phytosterols that can help lower blood cholesterol levels. Regularly eating these nuts can lead to better artery elasticity and support a heart-healthy lifestyle.

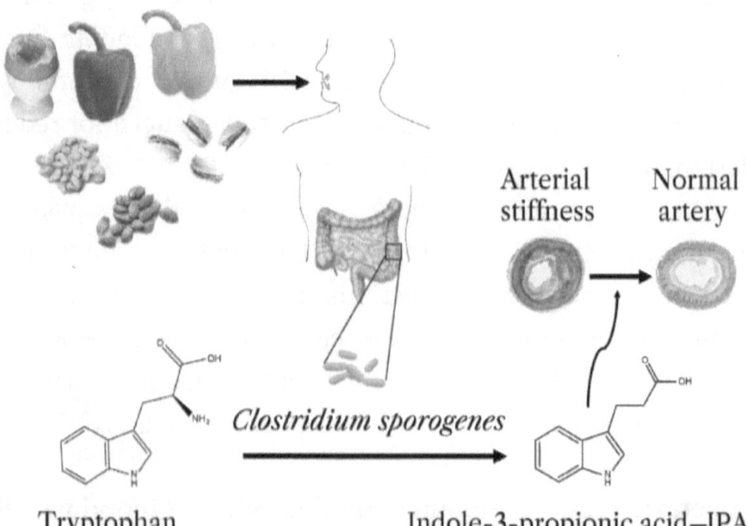

Clostridium sporogenes uses tryptophan to produce IPA, which, then absorbed into the blood, helps to improve and maintain artery flexibility.[11,17,67]

Taking hot baths could help prevent atherosclerosis

For those aged 65 or older, their risk of developing coronary artery disease increases. At this age, even a simple chest pain, caused by restricted blood flow to the heart, could signal a more alarming issue like a heart attack. Although medication and surgery can be used to treat coronary artery disease, lifestyle changes can also be safe and effective. One such change that doesn't require medication is engaging in regular hot water baths.

Frequent sauna or hot baths in 41°C (106°F) water for one hour, four times a week, may protect your heart and lower your risk of cardiovascular disease and heart problems. Current study suggests that the sauna-like heat dilates blood vessels, lowers blood pressure, and boosts circulation, much like the effects of exercise.[68] So, if you want to take care of your heart health, consider soaking in hot water more frequently. Combining hot water baths with additional heart-healthy practices like regular exercise, a well-balanced diet, stress reduction, and quitting smoking—and you can enhance the benefits of these baths. As a result, you can better protect your cardiovascular health, keeping your heart healthier as you clock more years.

Foods with anti-inflammatory properties to combat atherosclerosis

Atherosclerosis often begins in childhood, but its warning signs usually only become evident more than 20 years later. This delayed visibility is why the problem is often discovered too late.

If inflammation primarily contributes to the development of fatty plaques in arteries, finding a way to reduce inflammation is crucial. There are multiple ways to reduce chronic inflammation in the body without medication. Given that inflammation is a natural process, it's only logical that we can counteract it naturally too. This can be achieved through an anti-inflammatory diet or by eliminating inflammatory foods. In this chapter, we'll spotlight these natural inflammation-fighting foods.

Fruits and vegetables are natural anti-inflammatory foods. Some compounds in fruits and vegetables have even demonstrated higher anti-inflammatory activity than other compounds. Natural anti-inflammatory compounds, like lutein and zeaxanthin, appear to be effective in protecting blood vessels from inflammation and damage in patients with coronary artery disease.[69] They can reduce pro-inflammatory cytokines IL-6 and TNF by 20%. IL-6 and TNF are molecules secreted by immune and fat cells and contribute to the dysfunction of the inner lining of blood vessels. Therefore, increasing lutein and zeaxanthin consumption may also benefit patients with coronary artery disease.

Lutein is found in relatively high levels in green leafy vegetables. Foods containing the most lutein per 100 g include tomatoes (31 mg), spinach (12 mg), and egg yolks (520 mg). Other vegetables rich in zeaxanthin are kale (2,000 mg of zeaxanthin per 100 g) and okra (*Abelmoschus esculentus*) (280 mg of zeaxanthin per 100 g). These foods are excellent functional foods that help combat inflammation. In fact, consuming foods high in lutein and zeaxanthin can reduce body-wide inflammation.[70,71] However, those who don't eat enough lutein and zeaxanthin-rich foods may struggle to regulate inflammation in their bodies, potentially leading to chronic inflammation in blood vessel walls, which are comparable to the size of a tennis court. Research shows that people who eat less lutein and zeaxanthin often have higher body weight and fat, leading to inflammation.[72]

To enhance the absorption of lutein and zeaxanthin, research suggests including 3-5 g of healthy fats like extra virgin olive oil or avocado per meal.[73]

There are also other fruits and veggies that help fight inflammation. Things like berries and cherries have anthocyanins, leafy greens are full of flavonoids and carotenoids, cruciferous veggies like broccoli and cabbage have sulforaphane, tomatoes are packed with lycopene, papaya has papain, and beets are rich in betalains. These all have antioxidant and anti-inflammatory powers that help cool down inflammation throughout the body and provide protection against atherosclerosis.

Food high in lutein

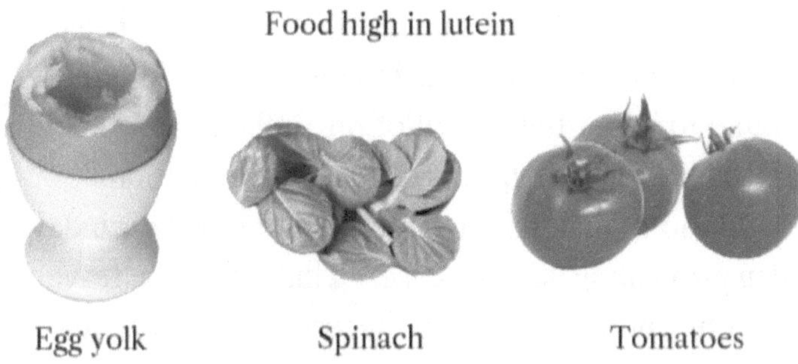

Egg yolk　　　Spinach　　　Tomatoes

Food high in zeaxanthin

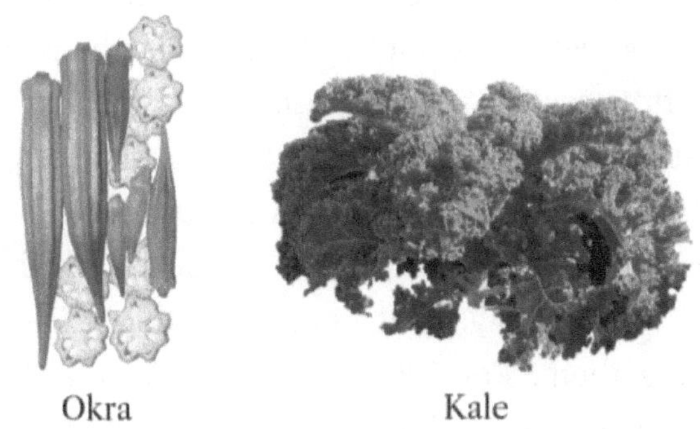

Okra　　　Kale

Foods rich in lutein and zeaxanthin can help reduce widespread inflammation in the body, potentially lowering the risk of coronary artery disease.[70,71]

Resveratrol's role in halting inflammation and atherosclerosis

Another phytonutrient that can help reduce inflammation and slow down atherosclerosis is resveratrol. In fact, it has been known for some time that resveratrol increased oxygen in the bloodstream, making the arterial walls more relaxed and flexible in a mouse model.[74]

In humans, a study at Toho University's Sakura Medical Center, 50 patients were given either 100 mg of resveratrol daily or a placebo for 12 weeks.[75] Those taking resveratrol had less stiff arteries than the placebo group. Resveratrol also acts like an antioxidant, getting rid of harmful free radicals that can harm cells and lead to issues like atherosclerosis and inflammation. Plus, resveratrol has been found to lower the output of pro-inflammatory molecules, like IL-6 and TNF, which helps in reducing inflammation.[76]

On top of that, taking 8 mg of resveratrol each day for a year can aid in preventing heart disease.[77] This is because resveratrol helps produce a hormone called adiponectin from fatty tissue, which acts to protect against hardening of the arteries. Past research has shown that patients with heart disease who took 8 mg of resveratrol daily for a year had a noticeable increase of adiponectin in their blood. Even though this increase was small, it was enough to demonstrate a protective effect against heart disease.

In summary, consuming plant foods rich in phytonutrients that can inhibit the biochemical pathways leading to chronic diseases like atherosclerosis and coronary artery disease is highly beneficial.

Yet, when eating meat, remember that cholesterol content differs among them. Per 100 g, beef, pork, and chicken contain around 60-100 mg of cholesterol, while fish has about 35-65 mg. Make sure to incorporate foods that can lower cholesterol in your diet to maintain healthy blood cholesterol levels.

It's also essential for children to eat foods that combat atherosclerosis and cardiovascular disease for good health. Failing to do so may not reduce their risk of developing these conditions. It's crucial to promote healthy eating habits at an early age to prevent unhealthy patterns from continuing into adulthood. Establishing these habits early on sets the foundation for a healthier life later.

As the saying goes, "children's health is our nation's wealth." Undeniably, we and our children must consume natural foods that reduce widespread inflammation and protect against atherosclerosis, the main factor contributing to cardiovascular diseases. This includes heart attack, heart failure, and stroke. By encouraging a diet full of good nutrients and balance for ourselves and our children, we're investing in long-term health and happiness.

CHAPTER 9

Repairable heart

Currently, we have reached "a turning point in public health," where the leading cause of death worldwide is no longer an infectious disease or road accident but a chronic disease. "The wealth of a nation is changing the way people die all around the world." It may surprise you that developed countries like the United States spend more than $3.3 trillion, accounting for 90% of the country's public health budget, on chronic diseases. Even though Americans spend a lot of money on health, they still often face serious health issues like heart disease, cancer, lung problems, and other diseases related to the heart and blood vessels.

We must ask ourselves, "Is chronic disease the inevitable fate of civilization?" If the future of civilization is not plagued by chronic diseases, why is every country in the world developing into one? As countries around the world develop, they allocate significant resources to combat chronic diseases. This raises the question, "Can our wealth change the course of our health?"

Your body is made up of materials that are constantly broken down and repaired. If you don't provide them with healthy foods and instead consume high-starch, high-sugar, and high-fat diets, you may eventually face a health crisis. Poor food choices in the past can lead to illness in the future, potentially draining your hard-earned savings on medical expenses. From my perspective, our work shouldn't just be a means to pay future medical bills. If you've been saving money for future healthcare costs, it may indicate that you haven't prioritized your body and health. By the time you decide to care for yourself, it might be too late.

These days, health problems such as type 2 diabetes, obesity, high blood pressure, and heart disease are terrifying and dreadful. Every year, millions of people get sick and die from these diseases. And the problem is likely to continue.

Heart and heart diseases

The human heart weighs around 250-350 grams and contains about 3.2 billion heart muscle cells, known as cardiomyocytes.[1] Remarkably, these cells are fully developed just a month after birth and then gradually renew, producing new cells to replace old ones. In the first 20 years of life, heart cell replication occurs at a low rate of 1% per year, which decreases with age. In older adults, renewal drops to 0.5% per year or less. This limited renewal rate cannot repair major damage. As a result, 60% of your heart is formed in the womb, and 40% is newly created. Previously, experts thought that when heart muscle cells die, they aren't replaced. Contrary to earlier beliefs, it's now understood that the human heart can make new heart muscle cells all the time, even in middle or old age. But this cell renewal process is not as effective as it used to be, so it can't completely fix damage caused by a heart attack.

Heart disease includes various conditions affecting the heart function, such as coronary heart disease, myocardial disease, irregular heartbeat, and heart valve disease. But the most common type of heart disease in adults is coronary heart disease. Coronary heart disease involves the narrowing of the arteries that supply blood to the heart muscle. You may know that it's often caused by atherosclerosis. If blood flow to the heart is reduced by such condition, it will cause myocardial ischemia. And if the artery that supplies blood to the heart muscle is completely blocked, it will lead to a heart attack.

Normally, one heart attack can lead to the loss of 1 billion heart muscle cells, accounting for 1 in 10 of heart muscle cells.[2] After heart attack, these 1 billion heart muscle cells are going to just die. The loss of 1 in 10 of heart muscle cells is a very serious problem for the heart. Plus, the replacement of dead heart cells with new ones is not a quick process. Yet for people aged 65 or older, the regeneration of heart muscle cells occurs even less than 0.1% per year. Even worse, after a heart attack, myocardial cells die and a scar permanently takes the place of heart cells in the heart. A person who has recovered from a heart attack, although survived, has lost parts of heart muscle cells. As a result, the person also loses the heart's ability to pump blood and has a higher risk of developing heart failure. Later on, when the heart fails, the heart muscle will lose its function, and finally, unable to pump blood around the body, the person dies.

Besides the narrowing of blood vessels, another risk factor that can lead to heart disease is aging. As we age, there are changes occur in our hearts. For instance, the shape of the heart may change from melon-shaped to ball-shaped. An accumulation of aging cells in the heart is also an inevitable part of growing older. Yet when senescent cells accumulate in the heart, they can cause neighboring cells to become senescent cells as well, leading to the further decline of heart function, which is a contributing factor for heart disease. The longer a person lives, the greater the number of aging cells in their heart. And, in older people, it's extremely difficult to get rid of the old heart cells to slow down the deterioration of the heart.

A sedentary lifestyle turns your heart into a monkey's

Your older body is like an old car; there are lots of problems. As you age, the main engine of your body, the heart, which drives your body, also deteriorates with age.

On the other hand, if you have an old car that has been sitting unused for a long time, its engine will go bad. This is comparable to a normal human heart that is normally elongated, thin-walled, and flexible, having evolved to cope with strenuous and time-consuming activities. However, if you stop using your heart, something will go wrong as well. If you stop doing strenuous activities and opt for a sedentary lifestyle, or sitting in the office like a monkey sitting in a tree all day, your heart will resemble a monkey's heart, which is smaller and thicker-walled.[3] This form and structure of a monkey's heart fit only the daily lifestyle of monkeys.

The reason for this is when you are inactive, your tissues and organs become inactive too. Sedentary lifestyles, such as too much sitting and too little physical activity, reduce blood flow to the heart and allow fatty plaque to build up in the blood vessels. Because there is less blood flow to the heart, the heart works less and becomes smaller than that of people who are more active, such as athletes and a group of amazing people in Mexico and subsistence farmers, the Tarahumara, that can run 200 miles barefoot in 2 days.[3] Not only are the Tarahumara people more active, but they also focus on a diet that mostly consists of plant-based foods like fruits and vegetables. Therefore, it's no surprise that why the Tarahumara runners suffer from zero heart disease.

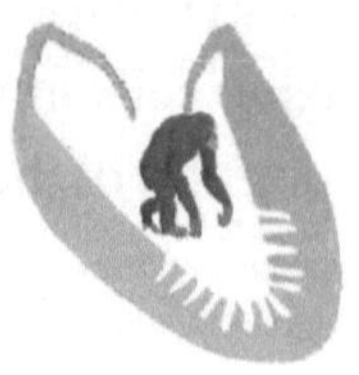

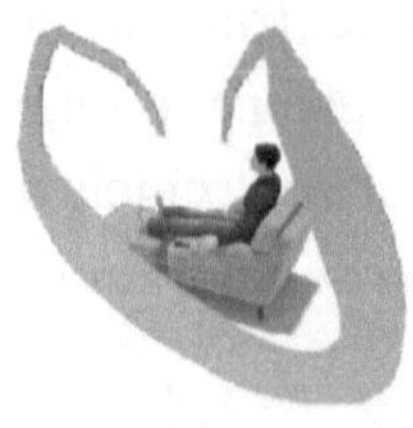

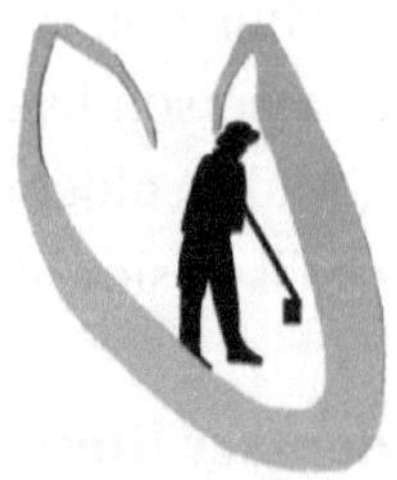

Chimpanzee heart   American lives a   Tarahumara
sedentary lifestyle   farmer and runner

Compare the left ventricular structure of a chimpanzee, an American living a sedentary lifestyle, and a Tarahumara farmer and runner.[3]

A little bit of knowledge

There are around 5 liters of blood in the human body, and an impressive 7 liters of blood flow through our heart each minute. What's more, it's fascinating to consider that during the early stages of human development, heart cells rely on glucose as their primary energy source. However, this changes after a baby is born and begins to consume breast milk, which is rich in fats and provides more energy-giving nutrients than glucose. Once the baby starts consuming breast milk, the heart cells adapt and begin to use fatty acids as their main source of energy. This switch is important because it allows the heart to function more efficiently and meet the increasing energy demands of a growing body. As the baby continues to grow and develop, the heart becomes more adept at using fatty acids for energy, ensuring that it can pump blood effectively throughout the body. This heart's ability to switch from using glucose to fatty acids as its main energy source is a remarkable adaptation that occurs soon after birth.

Alcohol weakens the heart muscle

In addition to being high in calories and potentially causing weight gain, which is a risk factor for health issues, alcoholic beverages can also harm your liver and heart. Continued excessive alcohol consumption can lead to inflammation, damage to liver cells, and cause the liver to develop scar tissue. For the heart, when your blood alcohol level is between 80-250 mg percent (mg/100 ml), it can weaken the heart muscle and reduce the heart's ability to pump blood. Moreover, for older adults, drinking alcohol can be even more harmful, as it can alter the heart's structure and function.[4] Drinking a lot of alcohol can also make your heart beat unevenly, leading to problems like an irregular heartbeat called atrial fibrillation.

Normally, your body can eliminate 10 g of alcohol per hour. However, having 250 mg percent of alcohol in your blood, which is equal to 12.5 g of alcohol, is more than your body can handle in an hour. The longer alcohol stays in your blood, the more likely it's to damage cells in vital organs like the heart, brain, and liver. Too much alcohol can also increase a person's blood pressure. High blood pressure is a major risk factor for heart issues like heart muscle disorders and irregular heart rhythms. As a result, heavy drinking can lead to heart disease and create a vicious cycle.

Moreover, there's a lot to learn from a global perspective. According to information from Our World in Data, a website that offers data about global health, low and moderate drinkers are less likely to develop heart disease compared to heavy drinkers or non-drinkers. However, a study in Japan, published in the journal Cancer from the American Cancer Society, discovered that consuming just one drink a day—equivalent to a 500-ml beer or 60-ml whiskey—is already harmful.[5] Surprisingly, the debate about whether drinking alcohol is healthy or unhealthy is still ongoing today.

Still, how much alcohol people drink can vary from one country to another. This is influenced by different factors like culture, economy, how easy it is to get alcohol, taxes and laws, social norms, weather, and marketing. According to global statistics, the highest levels of alcohol consumption per capita are found in Moldova, Lithuania, and the Czech Republic.

Here are some details on why alcohol consumption is appreciated by people in different countries.

In Germany, the locals are well-known for their love of beer, exemplified by the annual Oktoberfest celebration in Munich. With more than 1,300 breweries, Germany's per capita beer consumption is among the world's highest.

In France, the population is famous for its passion for wine, an integral aspect of their culture and daily life. Wine comprises about 60% of the country's alcohol consumption, making France the 12th heaviest-drinking nation globally.

In the United Kingdom, the pub culture plays a significant role in social life. The UK is also known for its beer, particularly ale, and its gin production. This makes its citizens the 24th heaviest drinkers in the world.

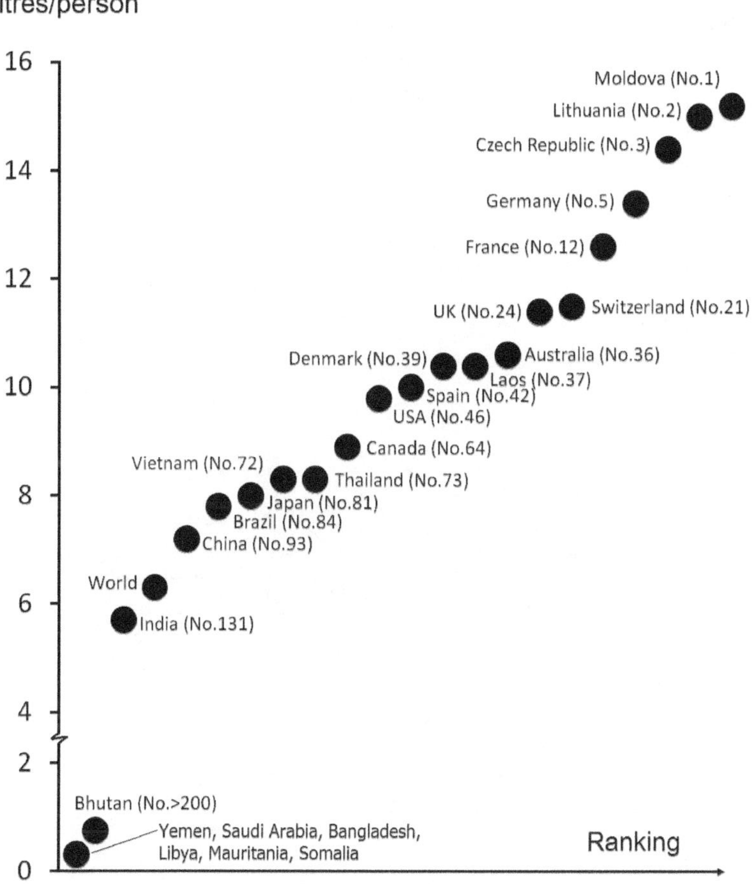

Alcohol consumption per person varies in different countries. It's measured in liters of pure alcohol per person aged 15 or older. In 2016, the Republic of Moldova had the highest average alcohol consumption in the world, with 15.2 liters per person. Meanwhile, the global average alcohol consumption in 2016 was around 6.4 liters per person.[6]

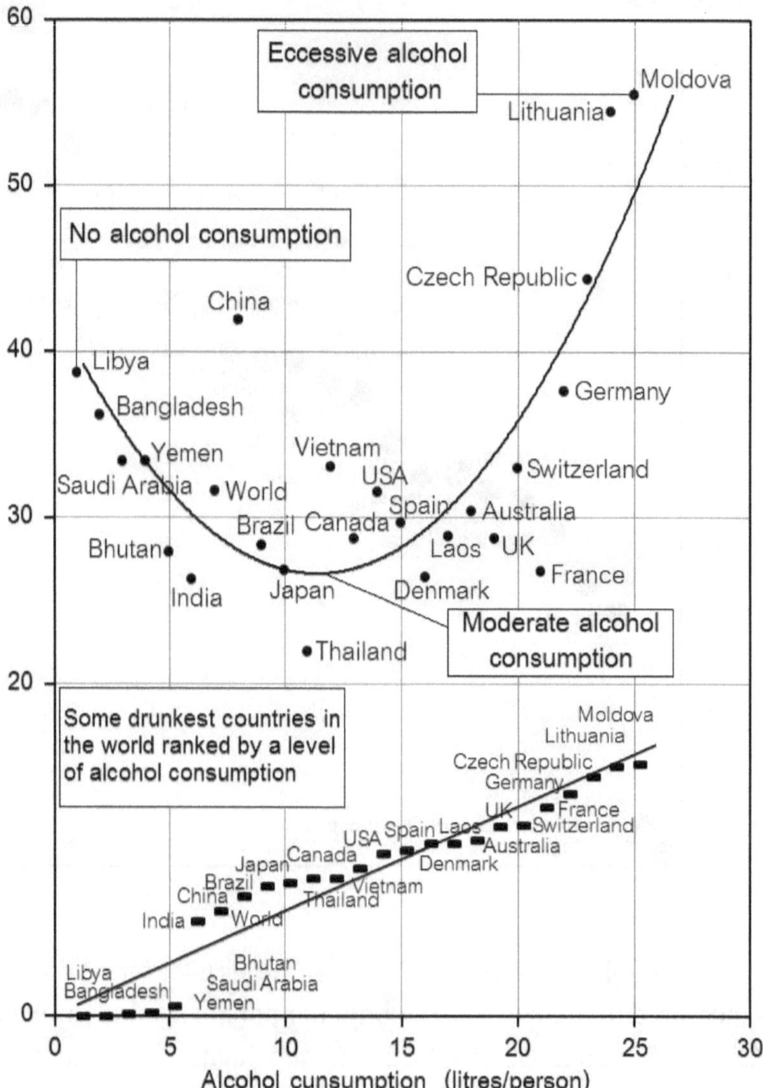

While heavier drinking is associated with a higher risk of heart muscle disorders and heart rhythm irregularities, moderate alcohol consumption is linked to a lower risk of heart diseases. According to the National Institutes of Health (NIH), low to moderate drinking is defined as one drink per day for women and two drinks per day for men.

The self-healing heart of a Mexican fish

When scientists wanted to understand the repair and regenerative mechanisms of the heart, they turned to the blind Mexican tetra cavefish (*Astyanax mexicanus*) and their surface-dwelling relatives. University of Oxford's scientists, led by Professor Mathilda Mommersteeg, discovered that while the blind Mexican cavefish are unable to repair their hearts after injury, their surface-dwelling relatives can regenerate their hearts after damage. The blind Mexican cavefish are comparable to humans in that they lack the ability to regenerate their hearts. By comparing genes from the two types of tetra fish, the researchers discovered two genes—lrrc10, a newly discovered gene, and caveolin—that work to repair the heart.[7]

A caveolin gene encodes caveolin proteins. In the human heart, there are caveolin proteins found in cardiac myocytes (the muscle cells that make up the heart muscle) and cardiac fibroblasts (heart cells that produce connective tissue). However, the content of caveolin proteins in cardiac myocytes and cardiac fibroblasts decreases as we grow older. This depletion of caveolin proteins associated with aging can be a risk factor for heart disease.[8]

In fact, scientists already know that caveolin is an important protein in the heart. If the caveolin protein is deficient in the heart, it could lead to heart conditions like myocardial infarction. In animal models, when the caveolin gene was impaired, the likelihood of mice surviving a myocardial infarction was also reduced.[9] This evidence certainly indicates that the caveolin gene is extremely important for heart repair and regeneration.

Since caveolin is a very important gene, humans have three distinct caveolin genes. The caveolin gene that appears to be the most important for heart function is the "caveolin-1 gene." There is evidence from research on humans at the University of Texas that the activation of the caveolin-1 gene in the human heart leads to heart regeneration. That is when experts studied heart disease patients using a type of artificial heart pump, they found that the device triggered the activation of the caveolin-1 gene, which in turn helped to increase the heart's ability to pump blood.[10] Hence, it's possible that if a person can induce the caveolin-1 gene to work, they might stimulate heart repair and regeneration.

***

Natural nutrients that help repair the heart

You should be providing your health with the best of what nature has to offer. In nature, there is a substance that can raise levels of caveolin-1 gene expression and help repair the heart; that is, chlorogenic acid.[11] In a mouse model, chlorogenic acid increased caveolin-1 gene expression, helping to restore damaged heart and improve the elasticity of the mice's blood vessel walls.[12,13] As these were studies in mice, it's not yet known whether chlorogenic acid has the same regenerative effect in humans.

Chlorogenic acid is found in mulberry, roselle, and in components of the Mediterranean diet such as artichoke (*Cynara cardunculus* var.scolymus), which has been found to contain up to 200 mg of chlorogenic acid per 100 g. A clinical study on human subjects showed that when chlorogenic acid was ingested, only one-third of chlorogenic acid was absorbed in the human small intestine. However, the rest of the chlorogenic acid was transformed into caffeic acid and ferulic acid, which can also improve the elasticity of blood vessels and prevent high blood pressure in human volunteers.[14]

Here is another clue that has been found to suggest that natural nutrients can activate the caveolin-1 gene expression and stimulate heart cell regeneration. Those natural nutrients are bitter melon polysaccharides.[15] A promising study in animal models suggested that a treatment of low concentrations of polysaccharides from a fruit of bitter melon for 25 days was able to repair damaged heart tissue. The dose of bitter melon polysaccharides used in the experiments was equivalent to 1,700 mg for a 70-kg human dose. There is a study suggests that polysaccharides in a fruit of bitter melon are estimated to be about 27-36% of their weight.[16,17] Thus, about 10 g of a fruit of bitter melon contains as much as 1,700-mg bitter melon polysaccharides.

With optimism, chlorogenic acid and bitter melon polysaccharides may trigger the activation of caveolin-1 gene, like an artificial heart pump, to repair damaged heart tissue in humans.

Moreover, to maintain good heart health, it's important to recognize the presence of senescent cells in the heart and blood vessel walls. Senescent cells are damaged cells that can no longer divide, leading to a decline in heart function as we age. Senolytic compounds such as curcumin, luteolin, and quercetin may help remove old cells from the heart and vessel walls. Exercise also appears to play a role in preventing age-related accumulation of senescent cells, in addition to senolytic compounds. Although further research is necessary to understand the mechanisms and potential benefits of these natural compounds, they may offer a safe and effective alternative for treating heart disease.

Green leafy vegetables containing vitamin K1 could prevent heart disease

The left ventricle, which is the heart's main pumping chamber, is the largest and thickest chamber in the heart because it has a vital role in pumping blood to the entire body. If you have hypertension, you may experience thickening of the heart wall, an enlarged heart, or hypertrophy of the heart, which can lead to subsequent heart failure. In addition, insufficient intake of vitamin K can increase the risk of heart enlargement. When the heart becomes unhealthy and enlarged, it makes it difficult for the major heart pumping chamber to fill up with blood and pump out blood. However, a 2017 study shows that taking vitamin K1 can help strengthen the heart muscle and prevent left ventricle enlargement, especially in adolescents.[18] The recommended daily intake of vitamin K1 is 75 mcg.

Green leafy vegetables are found to have the highest content of vitamin K1, with kale containing 531 mcg of vitamin K1 per cup, half a cup of spinach containing 444 mcg of vitamin K1, wild cabbage (*Brassica oleracea*) containing 418 mcg of vitamin K1, half a cup of Swiss chard containing 287 mcg of vitamin K1, and a cup of broccoli containing 220 mcg of vitamin K1.[19] Since vitamin K1 is a fat-soluble compound, consuming these vegetables in a salad with healthy oils such as extra virgin olive oil and avocado can aid in the absorption of it. Additionally, experts agree that the best way to obtain the necessary amount of vitamin K1 is through food.

Resveratrol inhibits the scarring of the heart

The latest clinical research has revealed that taking 10-mg resveratrol a day for 3 months can significantly improve left ventricle function and the heart's ability to contract and pump blood properly in post heart failure patients, in comparison to those who took a placebo. Resveratrol's ability to inhibit scarring of the heart muscle tissue is the reason behind this beneficial effect in post heart failure patients.[20,21]

In fact, resveratrol is believed to prevent heart muscle scarring in several ways. By lowering inflammation, it may stop scar tissue from forming in the heart after injury. Also, resveratrol could safeguard heart tissue by fighting off damage caused by oxidation and by boosting blood flow. Collagen, which is a key part of scar tissue, is kept in check by resveratrol. It also stops the action of fibroblasts, which can limit scar tissue growth within the heart muscle.

In the near future, we may witness an alternative approach to restoring heart function in post heart failure or heart attack patients with the use of resveratrol. In order to maintain a harmonious balance inside your body, it's a good idea to get resveratrol from natural foods. You can get 1.25 mg of resveratrol from 1,000 g of red Merlot grapes from Japan or 1,000 g of mulberries. To ensure the sufficient amount of resveratrol needed for its activity, consume resveratrol with breakfast or lunch. Otherwise, you may take 10 mg of resveratrol in the form of a dietary supplement, as used in the clinical research.

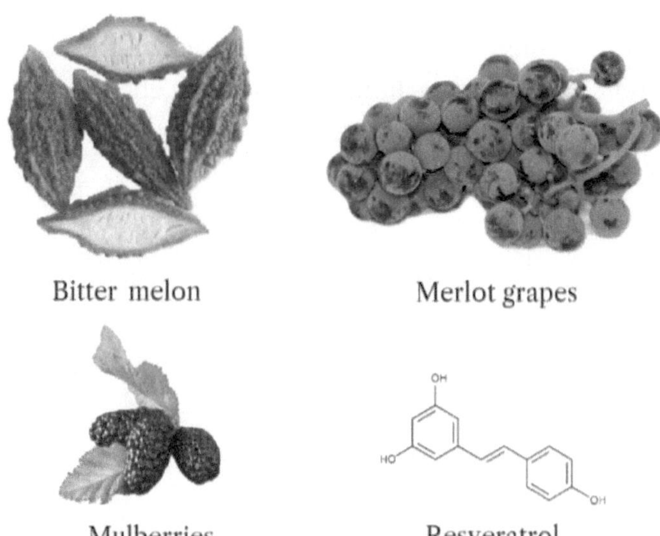

Bitter melon

Merlot grapes

Mulberries

Resveratrol

Bitter melon polysaccharides have the ability to repair damaged heart tissue in animal models, offering a potential therapeutic solution for heart disease. On the other hand, resveratrol, which can be found in red grapes or mulberries, has been found to inhibit scarring of the heart in post heart failure patients, potentially restoring their heart function. It suggests that natural compounds may offer a safe and effective alternative for treating heart diseases.

Eating lots of green veggies and sticking to a heart-healthy diet is crucial, but it's also key to avoid sitting for too long. Even with regular exercise, too much sitting can hurt your heart. To fix this, try to get up and move about every half hour to limit the harm of sitting for long periods. Also, habits like smoking and drinking a lot of alcohol can up your risk of heart disease. If you quit smoking and cut back on alcohol, you can do a lot of good for your heart and lower your risk of heart disease. It's also important to eat less of the foods that cause inflammation, such as processed foods and those high in saturated and trans fats.

Remember, the heart is the main engine that drives the body, and taking care of it's crucial for overall health and well-being. By adopting a heart-healthy lifestyle, you can reduce the risk of heart disease and live a longer, healthier life. So, take charge of your heart health today and make the necessary changes to lead a healthy and happy life.

adopting a heart-healthy lifestyle, you can reduce the risk of heart disease and live a longer, healthier life. So, take charge of your heart health today and make the necessary changes to lead a healthy and happy life.

CHAPTER 10

Pain and inflammation

I had rubella when I was 19. That year was the worst year of my life because after the rubella attack, I developed rheumatoid arthritis. My arthritis symptoms appeared very suddenly; one morning I woke up with intense pain in my knees. They were swollen, red, and difficult to bend. I had to walk with crutches, feeling crippled. After recovering from the illness, I thought my life would return to normal. But something changed forever. I continued to experience arthritis in my knees occasionally. Sometimes it occurred in my right knee; other times, it flared up in my left knee. Until I was 30, I had to deal with flares several times a year.

I once asked one of my doctors, "What caused my arthritis?" He replied, "It's not known exactly what causes arthritis. It may be caused by the body's immune system attacking the joints. Perhaps it has a genetic basis." I thought that I didn't have a family history of rheumatoid arthritis, so the genetic cause seemed unlikely. The most plausible cause was the rubella virus I contracted at the age of 19. The virus probably triggered my body's immune system to attack my knee joints ever since.

Do you know what the worst things about having arthritis are? The answers include painful inflammation in the knee joints and the desire to walk, run, and live like a normal person always on my mind. But those desires weren't possible because my life changed since the rubella virus struck. Plus, living with arthritis since I was 19 hasn't been fun at all.

Over the past 20 years, I've been trying to heal myself and learned that self-preservation is a good thing. Self-preservation allows me to know myself, take care of myself, and recognize the signals my body sends when a part is harmed or damaged. Relying solely on doctors didn't help me learn anything about my archenemy. So, I tried to figure out how to fight this disease that couldn't be cured by any medicine. Eventually, I learned how to manage rheumatoid arthritis without medication. In the end, I took care of myself using nutritional therapy and stopped arthritis flare-ups from time to time. By the way, I'm fortunate that I never took any painkillers that doctors prescribed.

About painkillers

Here's an intriguing piece of information about painkillers. Back in 1886, one of the very first painkillers ever developed was acetanilide. However, a short time later, it was found to have toxic effects on the liver and kidneys of users. Acetanilide was on the market for only a year before it was banned. In 1887, a drug company developed a new painkiller called phenacetin.[1] Interestingly, phenacetin was derived from acetanilide and had a very similar structure, but it was less toxic to the liver and kidneys. It wasn't until 1893 that paracetamol was accidentally discovered in the urine of people who took phenacetin. This led to the realization that, in the body, phenacetin was converted into paracetamol, which then provided pain-relieving properties. This is the history of the paracetamol sold today.

When examining the structures of acetanilide, phenacetin, and paracetamol, it's clear that these three drugs are very similar. Plus, all of them can be toxic to the liver and kidneys, but they have varying degrees of toxicity. With paracetamol, undesirable effects can occur, but they may not always be evident immediately after taking the drug. Instead, liver or kidney damage might only become apparent later. Besides, in older adults, the side effects of paracetamol could be more severe than in others. This is because, as we age, our liver and kidneys shrink, and their functions decline as well.

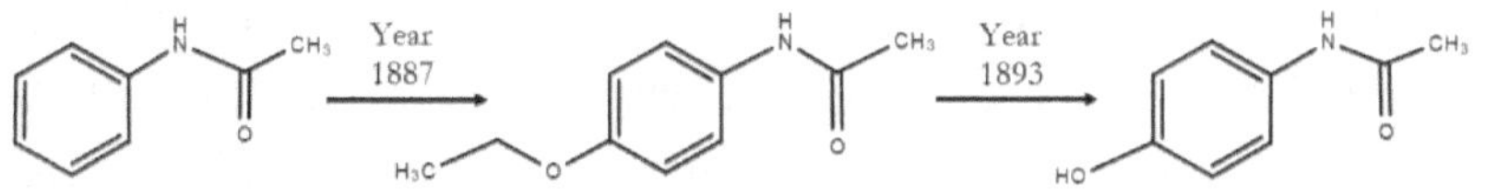

Acetanilide   Phenacetin   Paracetamol

Pharmaceutical companies developed acetanilide, phenacetin, and paracetamol, which all have varying degrees of toxicity to the liver and kidneys. Acetanilide is the most toxic, followed by phenacetin, and then paracetamol. While paracetamol is generally considered safe when used as directed, overuse can lead to liver and kidney toxicity.

People need to know that painkillers like paracetamol can have risks, especially as they age. To avoid harm, it's important to only use these drugs as directed and talk to a doctor if side effects happen or if the pain continues. Remember, your health comes first when managing pain. You might be surprised by the potential side effects of painkillers.

In 2020, following California's listing of glyphosate as a carcinogen in 2017, state regulators attempted to classify paracetamol (known as acetaminophen in the United States) as a carcinogen as well. That year, regulators reviewed paracetamol-related research data published in peer-reviewed academic journals. After examining the data, they concluded that people who take paracetamol might be at risk of developing certain cancers. However, the evidence linking paracetamol to cancer remains weak.[2] Regardless, I believe that even if paracetamol were to be listed as a carcinogen, it would likely follow the same path as alcohol and acrylamide. These substances have been classified as carcinogens for over 30 years, yet many products containing them still don't carry warning labels.

Inflammation affects almost everyone

Generally, inflammation is a process by which the body's immune system responds to irritants, invading pathogens, or foreign elements. For instance, when your skin becomes red, warm, and swells after an injury, or in people with a sore throat. Inflammation often leads to pain, which is one of its main symptoms. We can easily recognize pain because our skin, where pain receptors are abundant, is highly sensitive to the discomfort caused by inflammation.

Sometimes, inflammation occurs because the immune system is overactive and further attacks itself. In the inflamed area, the pH ranges between 4 and 7, which is more acidic than normal compared to the body's pH of 7.4. Inflammation is also more common in older adults than once thought. It's currently estimated that more than 50% of all deaths of people worldwide are due to chronic inflammation diseases.[3] So, it's not surprising that the pharmaceutical industry is so interested in developing anti-inflammatory painkillers.

You also need to know this: inappropriate inflammation in a vital organ is one of the factors that cause the stem cells in that organ to lose their regenerative function, leading to a shorter life expectancy.[4] For example, in the case of patients with osteoarthritis, joint and bone repair is much more difficult in inflamed areas because the regenerative function of the stem cells is often hampered by certain substances released during inflammation. Moreover, inflammation can also interfere with calcium absorption. So, calcium absorption in the inflamed area is more difficult than in normal bone. These are reasons why cartilage and bone repair in osteoarthritis patients is so problematic.

Having too many fat cells in the body is not very good either. A lump of accumulated fat in the body is like a separate and independent organ that can produce hormones and substances like other human organs. If there is an excess of fat cells, these fat cells—mainly from the visceral fat cells—produce substances like cytokines and adipokines, which are released in response to inflammation and cause chronic inflammation throughout the body and your life. This makes the body's cells become less sensitive to the actions of insulin, which later leads to type 2 diabetes.[5] In addition, when the body releases substances during inflammation, it can make the inflammation and pain even worse. Inflammation also has a big role in hardening of the arteries, increasing the risk of heart problems. Moreover, inflammation over a long time can hurt DNA and increase growth of tumors. What's more, being overweight is bad because it puts too much stress on the immune system, causing it to attack itself, harm tissues, and even lead to cancer.

Apart from sugar, refined flour, white bread, ultra-processed foods, and alcoholic beverages, foods high in saturated fats can also cause inflammation, particularly in the brain, which is a contributing factor to dementia.[6] Foods high in saturated fats that should be avoided include red meat, beef, lamb, pork, bacon, ham, burgers, dairy products such as whole milk, cream, butter, cheese, cakes, cookies, fried foods, and palm oil. Additionally, consuming too much saturated fat can raise cholesterol levels, increasing the risk of narrowed or blocked coronary arteries. If the blockage occurs in an artery in the brain, it can cause a stroke, leading to paralysis. Furthermore, people who consume lots of processed foods made with trans fats face a 16% higher risk of coronary heart disease, and their eventual fate could be a heart attack.[7] Consuming trans fats can also result in inflexible and fragile cell membranes that hinder effective communication among cells, which would otherwise function optimally if composed of healthier fats. Therefore, consuming trans fats can interfere with the proper functioning of cells. In fact, how we eat is crucial to fight against inflammation and chronic diseases and to maintain our cellular and physical health.

Primeval age fat consumption

It's very true that fat can have a negative effect on the body. However, it doesn't mean that we should abstain from fat entirely, because fat is important for the production of hormones and the absorption of fat-soluble vitamins such as vitamins A, D, E, and K.

Instead, we should consume good fats rather than bad fats. Good fats, especially unsaturated fats and omega-3 fatty acids found in fish, nuts, extra virgin olive oil, and avocado, are healthy ones.

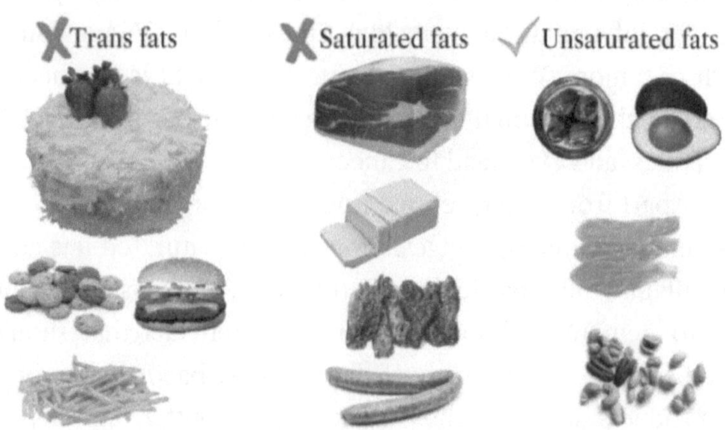

Both trans and saturated fats can cause inflammation, which is linked to long-term health problems like heart disease, stroke, type 2 diabetes, and memory loss. Saturated fats can raise bad cholesterol, increasing the risk of blockage in the arteries of the heart. Trans fats can become part of the walls of your cells, messing up how cells communicate to each other and potentially leading to health issues.

Omega-6 and omega-3 fatty acids are types of fats that our body can't produce them on its own. Studies of prehistoric human ancestors revealed that early humans consumed omega-6 and omega-3 fatty acids in a 1:1 ratio.[8] In the past, omega-3 fatty acids were found in almost all natural foods, especially meats, fish, nuts, berries, and wild plants. These foods contain a balanced ratio of omega-6 to omega-3 fatty acids. However, the dramatic shift in human dietary habits, which has been primarily driven by the widespread use of vegetable oils, such as soybean, corn, and sunflower oil, over the past few centuries starkly contrasts with the evolutionary patterns of our species. As a result, the human consumption ratio of omega-6 to omega-3 has changed from 1:1 a century ago to 16-25:1 these days.[9]

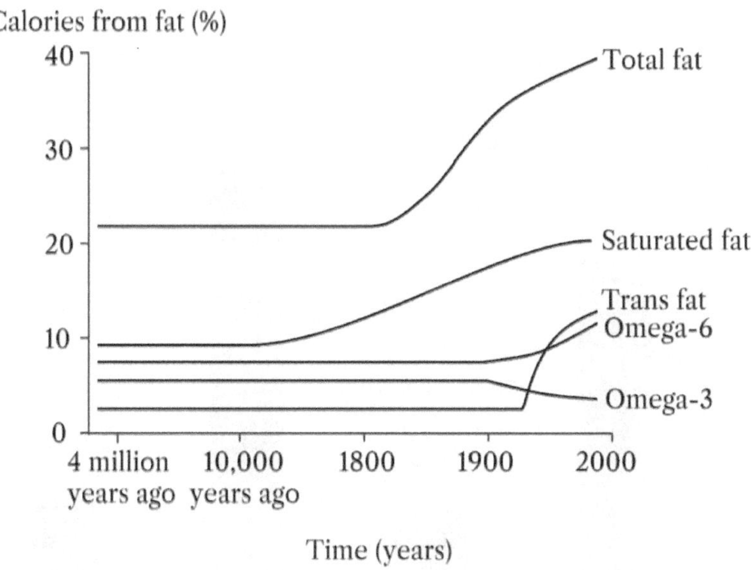

Human ancestors consumed omega-6 and omega-3 fatty acids in a 1:1 ratio, but this balance changed from the 1800s onwards.[9]

Diets high in omega-6 fatty acids increase inflammation due to their pro-inflammatory nature. Omega-6 fatty acids, like linoleic and arachidonic acids, contribute to inflammation and blood platelet clumping. Consuming too much omega-6 fatty acids is linked to diseases like obesity, type 2 diabetes, and cardiovascular disease. To lower inflammation, you should consume less omega-6 fatty acids and increase your intake of anti-inflammatory omega-3 fatty acids, like EPA and DHA. Since omega-3 fatty acids can counteract the pro-inflammatory effects of omega-6 fatty acids, a diet high in omega-3s and low in omega-6s will help reduce inflammation.

However, if your diet consists of more omega-6 fatty acids

than omega-3 fatty acids, the anti-inflammatory benefits of omega-3 fatty acids may be entirely negated. In fact, research has shown that if you have an unfavorable ratio of omega-6 to omega-3 fatty acids in your bloodstream, you can improve it by taking 2-3 g of omega-3 fatty acid supplements.[11]

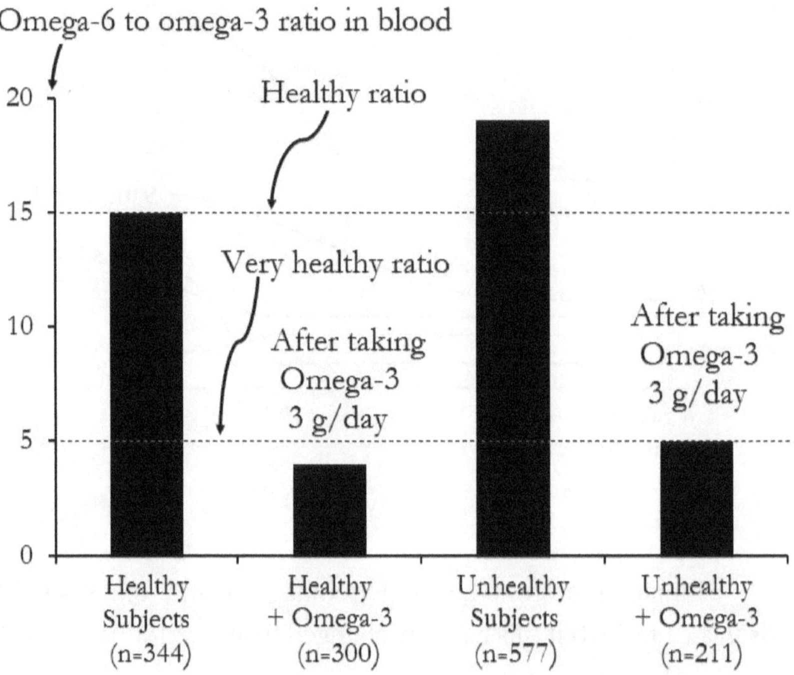

It's important to maintain a healthy ratio of omega-6 to omega-3 fatty acids for better health. People with diseases typically have higher omega-6 to omega-3 ratios, but taking omega-3 supplements (2-3 g/day of EPA and DHA) can help bring those ratios back to healthier levels.[11]

You need to consume a balanced diet of omega-6 and omega-3 fatty acids in a ratio of about 1:1, similar to our ancestors.[8] To do it, eat more omega-3 foods like fish and seeds, and consider supplements if needed. Focus on whole foods like fruits, vegetables, lean proteins, and whole grains. Opt for grass-fed meats and dairy, and eggs and poultry from free-range birds. Check food labels to avoid products with high omega-6 oils, and use olive or avocado oil instead of vegetable oils. Today, it's known that sacha inchi oil has the closest omega-6 to omega-3 fatty acid ratio, at 1.4:1, making it an ideal source for maintaining a balanced intake.[13]

Ratio of omega-6 to omega-3 fatty acids in some popular foods.[12]

Food	Serving Size	Omega-6 (g)	Omega-6: Omega-3 ratio
Corn oil	1 Tbsp (14 g)	7.2	46 : 1
Soybean oil	1 Tbsp	6.8	7 : 1
Sunflower oil	1 Tbsp	3.2	311 : 1
Beef	100 g	3	10 : 1
Canola oil	1 Tbsp	2.6	2 : 1
Palm oil	1 Tbsp	1.2	45 : 1
Olive oil	1 Tbsp	1.4	12.8 : 1
Butter	1 Tbsp	0.38	8 : 1
Rainbow smelt	4 oz (113 g)	0.2	1 : 2.5
Sacha inchi oil	1 oz (28 g)	8	1.4 : 1

***

Cut back on omega-6 fatty acids to lower your risk of chronic disease

The evidence supporting the idea of cutting back on omega-6 fatty acids to lower your risk of chronic disease can be traced back to the 1990s. During that time, people in Eastern Europe frequently consumed foods high in omega-6 fatty acids, such as beef and refined cooking oils. However, when the consumption of these foods decreased, it led to a decline in death rates from coronary heart disease in Eastern European countries.[14] For example, in Poland between 1989 and 2008, when the consumption of foods high in omega-6 fatty acids, such as butter, decreased from 7 kg to 3.8 kg per person per year, beef consumption decreased by 75%, and there was a significant increase in fruit consumption.[15] As a result, the Polish death rates from coronary heart disease decreased by 3% per year.[16]

For those who consume a Western-style diet, the intake of omega-6 fatty acids is often too high relative to omega-3 fatty acids. It's important to remember that if your diet contains more omega-6 fatty acids than omega-3 fatty acids, it can trigger inflammation and pain.

To achieve a balanced diet of omega-6 and omega-3 fatty acids, consider these steps: First, avoid processed and packaged foods, which often have unhealthy fats and high omega-6 to omega-3 ratios. Next, cook at home, allowing you to control ingredients and choose healthier fats. Finally, include more omega-3-rich foods in your diet, such as fatty fish (salmon, mackerel, sardines, and herring), flaxseeds, chia seeds, and walnuts. Following these steps can help reduce your risk of chronic diseases associated with high omega-6 consumption.

Begin walking to alleviate inflammation and pain

Another reason why chronic pain can persist and flare up even when the injury has healed or symptoms have subsided is that cells can still remember the previous pain and injury.[17] Individuals who experience chronic pain also possess a distinct nervous system in comparison to those who don't suffer from this condition. Currently, there is no way to erase the pain memory recorded in cells. Moreover, those who rely on ibuprofen to alleviate their pain may experience a recurrence of chronic pain after a span of 2 to 10 years.

We all need to realize that chronic pain and inflammation will eventually come back. If you have persistent pain or inflammation, you need to learn how to reduce chronic pain and inflammation in your body. For those who rely on modern medicine, oral treatments for inflammation pain can potentially lead to more adverse effects. The use of one drug can create far more problems than it would solve. Generally, the safest inflammation pain treatment is to medicate topically where the pain is most perceived. This may also benefit the elderly, who are more prone to adverse drug events from medicines taken orally.

However, to alleviate inflammation-related pain inside your body, you can start by engaging in moderate exercise, such as aerobic exercise or brisk walking, for 15-30 minutes every day, 5 days a week. The benefits of regular exercise include improved communication between cells, reduced levels of inflammatory cytokines, and increased production of anti-inflammatory substances in your body. For older individuals, consistent exercise helps maintain a healthy weight, decrease senescent white blood cells, and, of course, reduce inflammation-promoting substances.[18,19] Don't forget to also incorporate a variety of anti-inflammatory foods rich in lutein and zeaxanthin to further decrease widespread inflammation throughout the body.

The potential of fasting as a remedy for inflammation

Fasting can reduce the body inflammation that typically develops as we get older. How can fasting reduce inflammation? Fasting causes the body to produce beta-hydroxybutyrate, a substance generated by the liver in response to fasting.[20] Beta-hydroxybutyrate can help decrease inflammation in the body, similar to the effects of exercise or avoiding starchy carbs.

In humans, beta-hydroxybutyrate in blood circulation is usually scarce, but after 12-16 hours of fasting, its levels can be 10 times higher than normal.[21] Beta-hydroxybutyrate can even reach higher levels in people who consume a low-carb diet and exercise vigorously by cycling for 120 minutes.[22] When the body has an ample amount of beta-hydroxybutyrate, it suppresses the activity of inflammasomes, complexes of proteins that trigger an inflammatory and immune response.[20]

Moreover, like many previous studies, a 2019 study shows that, in humans, fasting for 19 hours can reduce the number of monocytes, which are a type of white blood cell that plays key roles in the inflammation response, in the blood.[23] Fasting also reduces the number of white blood cells in the affected area.[24] The job of white blood cells is to consume and destroy invading pathogens or foreign substances that enter the body. For those with chronic inflammation in their bodies, such as people with high body fat content, people who are overweight or obese, people with cardiovascular disease, diabetes or cancer, and even older people who have a higher number of senescent white blood cells and pro-inflammatory cytokines than younger people, intermittent fasting can reduce inflammation and maintain a well-balanced immune system. Importantly, fasting encourages autophagy, the body's natural process of self-digestion. This not only helps eliminate aged and dysfunctional cells but also supports the rejuvenation of the body.

However, fasting can have adverse outcomes when you fast for 24 hours and then refeed yourself, as it can stimulate inflammasomes again.[25] To solve this problem, you need to engage in aerobic exercise 3 days a week, for 40 minutes a day, with a heartbeat of 70-80% of your maximum heart rate, but not high-intensity exercise, to further suppress inflammasome activity during refeeding.[26] Alternatively, you may consider eating bitter melon, which in mouse models, has been shown to increase Sirt3 protein levels, thereby suppressing inflammasome activity.[27,28]

In the future, fasting could become a form of medicine. Doctors may prescribe intermittent fasting for patients with obesity, type 2 diabetes, cardiovascular disease, or cancer to balance their immune system and fight the disease.

In patients with arthritis, an arthritis flare can be caused by a diet high in carbohydrates, starchy, and sugary foods, which can increase inflammation as well. Therefore, to reduce inflammation in arthritis sufferers, it's necessary to cut back on foods high in carbohydrates such as candy, sugary drinks, white bread, cookies, and potato chips, as well as foods high in fat and cholesterol, like fast food, French fries, beef, pork, lamb, chicken, ham, sausage, bacon, cake, and ice cream. Moreover, arthritis is directly related to elevated blood cholesterol levels.[29] You have to manage arthritis and maintain healthy cholesterol levels by focusing on maintaining a healthy weight, eating a balanced diet rich in anti-inflammatory foods, limiting saturated and trans fats, and increasing fiber intake.

Ginger and turmeric are as effective as ibuprofen to reduce inflammation and relieve pain

Natural substances with anti-inflammatory properties can be taken instead of ibuprofen for inflammation. One such substance is gingerol, a constituent of ginger that gives it a pungent, spicy smell. Gingerol is present in ginger (*Zingiber officinale*), and its content is higher in ginger rhizomes aged 12-14 months. A clinical trial showed that when volunteers who underwent wisdom teeth removal took 500 mg of ginger rhizome powder, it elicited pain relief equivalent to 400 mg of ibuprofen.[30] However, it's recommended that people consume no more than 4 g of ginger a day, as taking more may cause heartburn.

For arthritis or osteoarthritis, curcumin is also as effective as ibuprofen in reducing pain and inflammation. A 2014 clinical study revealed that 171 patients with knee osteoarthritis who took 1,500 mg of curcumin extract daily for four weeks experienced inflammation reduction equivalent to a daily dosage of 1,200 mg ibuprofen.[31] In another study, curcumin can be used in a lower dose, 1,000 mg, to alleviate arthritis-related inflammation without causing significant adverse effects.[32] It suggests that curcumin may serve as an alternative to ibuprofen for reducing inflammation and pain.

Combining curcumin with piperine can boost curcumin

absorption by 2,000%. When taking 2,000 mg of curcumin alongside piperine, blood curcumin levels can rise from 0.006 to 0.18 mcg/ml within an hour.[33] Consuming fresh turmeric root with healthy fats, like extra virgin olive oil and avocado, can also help boost curcumin absorption by 7-8 times, as curcumin is a fat-soluble molecule. Pairing curcumin with good fats aids its absorption from the digestive tract into the bloodstream through the lymphatic system without passing through the liver.

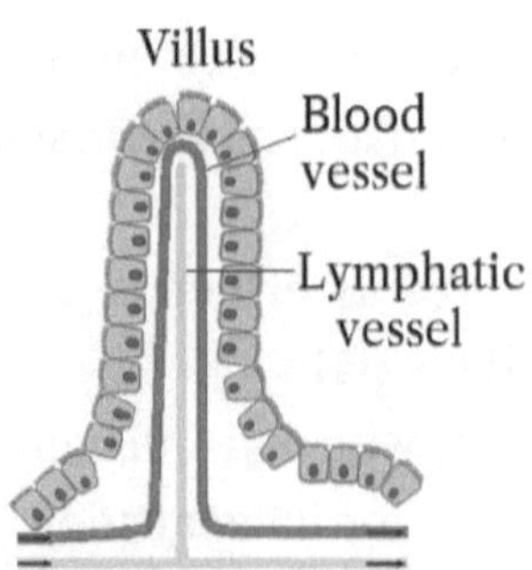

The villi are small, finger-like projections found in the small intestine.[34] Curcumin, a fat-soluble compound, can be absorbed from the digestive tract into the bloodstream through the lymphatic system within the villi, bypassing the liver.

Besides, extra virgin olive oil contains oleocanthal, which has an ibuprofen-like activity that helps inhibit pain. The stronger the stinging sensation in the throat, the more potent the oleocanthal content in the oil. Consuming four tablespoons of extra virgin olive oil a day provides about 10% of the recommended ibuprofen dose for adult pain relief.[35] This approach may offer some of the long-term effects of low-dose ibuprofen use (120 mg), making extra virgin olive oil a potentially safe way to reduce inflammation.

However, the effectiveness of ginger and turmeric as alternatives to ibuprofen may vary for each individual and condition. Personally, I consume 15 g of fresh turmeric root with a tablespoon of extra virgin olive oil. If fresh turmeric root is unavailable, I take about 1,400 mg of turmeric powder (equivalent to 125 mg curcumin) with a tablespoon of extra virgin olive oil. This approach has successfully kept arthritis flare-ups in my knees at bay for months or even years, all without the use of medication.

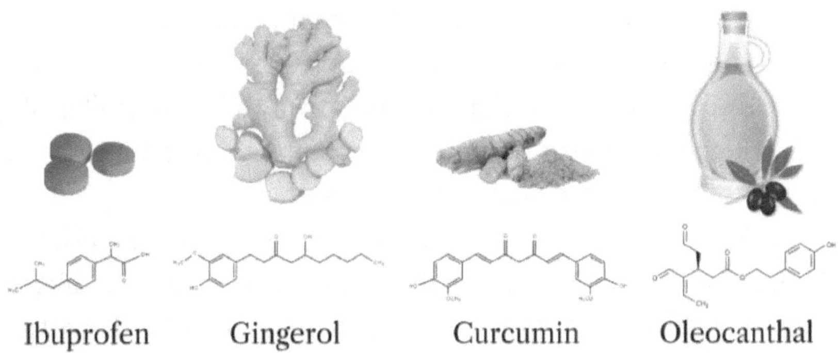

The natural anti-inflammatory properties of ginger, turmeric, and extra virgin olive oil, which are known to help relieve pain and inflammation in the body, similar to the effects of ibuprofen.

Importantly, the ideal time to consume anti-inflammatory foods like ginger, turmeric, and extra virgin olive oil is in the morning and at noon, which aligns with the active phase of the body's biological clock. Administering anti-inflammatory substances during these times can enhance their effectiveness in promoting healing.[36] The body has a rhythm that regulates activity during the day and inactivity at night, even switching genes on and off accordingly. Inflammation and tissue breakdown occur during the daytime, while wound healing and tissue regeneration take place during sleep. As such, it's crucial to synchronize the use of anti-inflammatories with the body's biological clock; using them during the rest phase could have adverse effects. For instance, taking non-steroidal anti-inflammatory drugs at night may exacerbate bone and cartilage damage in people with arthritis.[37] Proper timing is essential when using anti-inflammatories.

As you may know, inflammation is the body's response to harmful stimuli, but when the immune reaction is inappropriate, it can result in chronic inflammation. Chronic inflammation can impede stem cells' regenerative ability and is a significant factor preventing longevity. Excessive inflammation can damage healthy tissues, contribute to autoimmune disorders, increase the risk of chronic diseases, impair healing, and negatively affect overall quality of life. Hence, removing chronic inflammation is prioritized as the first step for the body to heal and mend itself.

At some point in our lives, everyone experiences inflammation in some parts of the body, such as the circulatory system, digestive tract, brain, liver, pancreas, or skin. Therefore, incorporating everyday anti-inflammatory measures is essential; otherwise, dependence on painkillers may become a lifelong necessity, benefiting pharmaceutical companies at the expense of one's health.

CHAPTER 11

You have to have the right bacteria to live a longer life

Humans are composed of 30 trillion cells, accompanied by 37 trillion microbes, including bacteria, viruses, yeasts, and molds. These microorganisms collectively weigh about 2 kg, equivalent to the weight of the human brain. They inhabit our bodies and derive energy from the food we eat. After obtaining necessary nutrients, these microbes produce substances that can regulate our immune system, affect our body and brain, or influence our hunger and emotions.

Scientific studies highlight the importance of tiny organisms, especially bacteria, in the first 1,000 days of life. Babies born vaginally acquire *Lactobacillus* bacteria from their mother's birth canal, while C-section-born babies often lack this type of bacteria. Instead, they have skin bacteria like staph and strep in their guts. This trend continues for about 2-3 years. In addition, the guts of babies who are breastfed are full of good bacteria like *Bifidobacterium* and *Lactobacillus*. The introduction of solid foods also brings new types of bacteria. By the age of 3, a kid's gut will have three times more types of bacteria, which continues to increase with age and stays pretty much the same during middle age.[1,2]

However, the diversity of the microbial population declines again in old age. Each person also has varying numbers, diversity, and types of bacteria. For example, Japanese people who regularly eat nori—a traditional ingredient in Japanese cuisine—have bacteria that can digest seaweed in their guts, while Americans typically don't have this type of bacteria in their intestines.[3] This connection between our diet and gut microbiome, all of the microbes that live in your intestines, has led to growing interest in the concept of personalized nutrition. By understanding the unique composition of an individual's microbiome, it may be possible to create tailored dietary recommendations that optimize their gut health, ultimately leading to better overall health.

You should know that our intestines are home to two key types of bacteria: Firmicutes and Bacteroidetes. Combined, these two types form 90% of our gut bacteria. Firmicutes often have a bad reputation because they can negatively affect how our bodies use glucose and fat. In contrast, Bacteroidetes are seen as good bacteria because they produce beneficial metabolites. The intestines of lean individuals generally contain a large population of good bacteria, whereas those of people with obesity are often populated with bad bacteria. The balance of these bacteria is essential for good health, as they interact with the intestinal epithelial cells that line the gut. Your overall health thus depends on how these bacteria interact with your gut cells. When good bacteria dominate, the gut epithelium is well-lined and thick, without any inflammation. On the other hand, when bad bacteria dominate, the epithelium becomes thin, inflamed, and may even leak, making it vulnerable to pathogenic invasion.

In addition to diet, lifestyle factors such as stress and antibiotics use can also disrupt the balance of gut bacteria. Chronic stress has been shown to reduce the diversity of gut bacteria, while the use of antibiotics can kill off both good and bad bacteria in the gut, leading to an imbalance.

Importantly, you need promote the good bacteria to rule your gut, and you can do this by eating healthy foods. Consuming lots of vegetables, fruits, nuts, and grains is one way to promote healthy microbes in your gut. This plant-based eating approach; however, takes time to develop and requires continuous reinforcement.

Sometimes, it takes about a year for people to alter and balance their gut microbiome. For others, changing gut microbiome may take up to 5 years. Adopting a healthy diet can encourage the growth of beneficial bacteria in your gut, which is critical since 80% of your immune cells reside there. In centenarians who have unique gut microbiome, their immune systems function at a high level, resembling the robustness typically found in younger individuals. Thus, having the right gut bacteria can improve your immune health too.

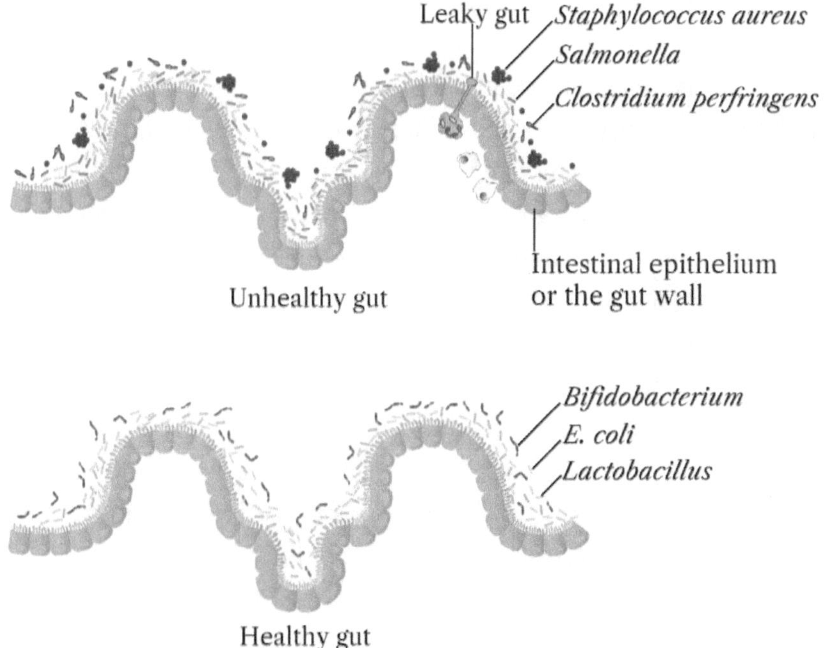

A healthy gut contains good gut microbes such as *Bifidobacterium, Lactobacillus* and *E. coli*, while an unhealthy gut contains disease-causing microbes such as *Staphylococcus, Salmonella* and *Clostridium perfringens*.

***

Probiotics

A shortcut for promoting good bacteria in your gut can be achieved by consuming "probiotics." Probiotics are beneficial, non-pathogenic bacteria that contribute to our health by helping to balance the bacteria in our gut and aiding in resolving digestive issues like diarrhea, constipation, and inflammatory bowel disease.

However, not everyone may benefit equally from consuming probiotic bacteria. It depends on the types of microbes already present in your gut. For some people, when someone eat foods with probiotics such as fermented milk, yogurt, kimchi, natto, and miso, the probiotics may not survive stomach acid or may be excreted in feces the next day. Building a healthy gut microbiota takes time and effort.

Consuming either animal products like eggs, bacon, pork, and cooked meats, or plant-based diets consisting of rice, vegetables, fruits, and beans for days can result in changes in the composition and metabolic activity of our gut microbiome.[4] However, eating a diet focused on vegetables and fruits for weeks can create an environment suitable for good bacteria to thrive.

A study in which participants reduced their fatty food or carbohydrate intake, or both, and instead consumed 43 g of walnuts a day for 6 weeks found a significant increase in the population of good bacteria like *Bifidobacterium*. Intake of a handful of walnuts daily also significantly decreased the population of bad bacteria, *Chloridium*.[5] In contrast, another study found that eating whole grains like brown rice, wheat, oats, beans, and sesame seeds, 75 g per day for 8 weeks, had no effect on the population of trillions of bacteria in our gut.[6] This highlights the importance of starting with a handful of walnuts a day for at least 6 weeks if you want to increase the good gut bacteria.

It's important to note that not all probiotics are created equal. Different strains of bacteria have different effects on the gut, and some may be more effective than others in promoting good health. Additionally, the amount of probiotics in the food or supplement you consume is also important. Some probiotic products may not contain enough live bacteria to have a significant impact on the gut microbiota. When choosing a probiotic supplement, it's essential to look for products that contain high levels of viable bacteria and to follow the manufacturer's recommended dosage.

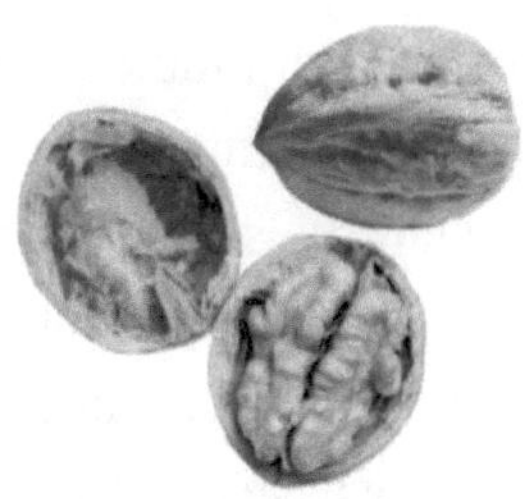

Walnuts help boost the number of beneficial bacteria called *Bifidobacterium* in your gut while decreasing the population of harmful bacteria known as *Chloridium*.

You can take prebiotics to foster the right bacteria

The term "prebiotics" refers to dietary fibers and sugars that the human digestive system can't digest. However, they can be digested by good gut bacteria. Prebiotics, food for good gut bacteria, are such as resistant starch, oligosaccharides, oligofructose, pectin, cellulose, and inulin.

Considering that your body is inhabited by 37 trillion microbes, which is 1.3 times greater than the number of cells making up the entire human body, these microbes act like another organ to us. Interestingly, both humans and microbes are also interdependent.

If we eat a low-fiber diet, the number of good bacteria living in the gut will decrease, while the number of bad bacteria will increase. Some bad gut bacteria like to eat mucus, a slimy secretion that covers the intestinal epithelium. Every time these bad gut bacteria eat mucus, they move closer to the colon's wall that protects against infection. If they eat the colon's lining, the body will produce an immune response to counteract these invasive bacteria. This causes the gut to become inflamed. If this continues to happen, it will lead to chronic inflammation in the intestines, resulting in complications like diarrhea and bowel disorders. Therefore, for those with a thick layer of mucus in their intestines are considered to have a healthier intestinal tract than individuals with a thinner layer of mucus.

Given that 80% of our immune cells reside in our gut, which makes our gut bacteria vital for managing our body's defenses. If you eat fewer fibers or prefer starchy, sugary, or fatty foods, you're more likely to stir up inflammation in your gut. This inflammation can spread throughout your body and may become a long-lasting issue, raising the risk of chronic diseases. Chronic inflammation is a big factor in cancer development, including colon cancer among others. It can promote cancer by damaging tissues, causing scarring, and prompting gene changes that support cancer growth. Additionally, as we get older, our immune system becomes weaker, increasing the chance of getting cancer, especially when there's ongoing inflammation.

Did you know that gut bacteria can regulate serotonin production too? In fact, 90% of the total body's serotonin is made in your gut.[8] Serotonin is a neurotransmitter that plays a key role in regulating mood, hunger, anger, and happiness. This may help explain why many young Americans are now suffering from depression. Part of this may be due to inflamed intestines caused by consuming Western, sugary, or low-fiber diets. However, if you want to rebalance the intestinal microbiota for better gut health and a good mood, you can feed the good bacteria in your gut with prebiotics.

You can gradually increase prebiotic intake: If you're not used to eating a lot of prebiotic-rich foods, start by gradually increasing your intake. Adding too much fiber to your diet too quickly can cause digestive discomfort. Beginning by incorporating a small amount of prebiotic-rich foods to your meals and slowly increase the amount over time.

FOS and inulin together fertilize good gut bacteria

A type of carbohydrate such as FOS (fructo-oligosaccharide), sometimes called oligofructose, and inulin are the best-studied prebiotics. They can only be digested by our gut bacteria. They have a low energy value or just 0-2 calories per gram but are only 30% as sweet as granulated sugar. According to scientists, we should consume 4-8 g of FOS every day.

Natural foods high in FOS, such as chicory, asparagus, scallion, onion, watermelon, Jerusalem artichoke (*Helianthus tuberosus*), and yacon, contain FOS ranging from 2 to 13 g per 100 g fresh weight.[9,10,11] Remember that whole foods are better than dietary supplements for the health of your intestines. That is because they provide easily absorbed nutrients, contain fiber for healthy digestion, promote a diverse gut microbiome, and offer a synergistic effect of nutrients. Additionally, whole foods are generally safer, more satisfying, and help with weight management.

Inulin is also a favorite food for good gut bacteria like *Lactobacillus* and *Bifidobacterium*. These bacteria are often taken as a supplement to improve gut health and strengthen the body's immune system. Actually, you don't need to spend your money on such probiotic products. All you need is to eat more prebiotic inulin in whole foods to nourish *Lactobacillus* and *Bifidobacterium* bacteria in your gut. Natural foods highest in inulin are chicory (15 g of inulin per 100 g), Jerusalem artichoke (3 g of inulin per 100 g), and pomegranate (1 g of inulin per 100 g).

However, approximately 1 in 3 people in Europe have fructose malabsorption. Because FOS and inulin are polymers of fructose molecules, those with fructose malabsorption who consume too many inulin-rich foods may experience abdominal discomfort, tummy bloating, and decreased bowel movements. But these symptoms can be minor. Europeans with fructose malabsorption may need to eat apples instead. Eating just one apple provides you with 100 million microbes.[12] These bacteria living in the core of an apple can also promote the growth of good bacteria, *Lactobacillus* and

Bifidobacterium, while inhibiting the growth of pathogenic bacteria in your gut.[13]

FOS and inulin content in natural foods.

Fresh food	Serving size (g)	FOS (g)	Inulin (g)
Chicory, chicory root	100	13, 22.5	15
Jerusalem artichoke	100	13	3
Asparagus	200	5	2
Scallion	100	4	-
Watermelon	400	3	-
Onion	100	2-2.5	-
Yacon root	100	0.7 - 13	-
Pomegranate	100	-	1

- ; no data

Ursolic acid can prevent the gut wall damage

Consuming foods rich in ursolic acid may help protect the intestinal wall from damage or even assist in repairing the damaged intestinal lining, as ursolic acid can help balance the gut microbiota. In a mouse model, ursolic acid enabled good gut bacteria like *Lactobacillus* and *Bifidobacterium* to grow and multiply in the mouse gut.[14] By supporting the growth of beneficial bacteria, ursolic acid may contribute to a stronger immune system, as a significant portion of the immune system is located within the gut. Nevertheless, it's possible that ursolic acid may improve intestinal health by inhibiting the growth of pathogenic bacteria that produce toxins and trigger immune responses, which can damage the gut lining.[15] Although studies have shown promising results in animals, its effectiveness in humans has not yet been demonstrated.

Ursolic acid can be found in several foods, but pomegranate has the highest content of ursolic acid, containing 450 mg per 100 g.

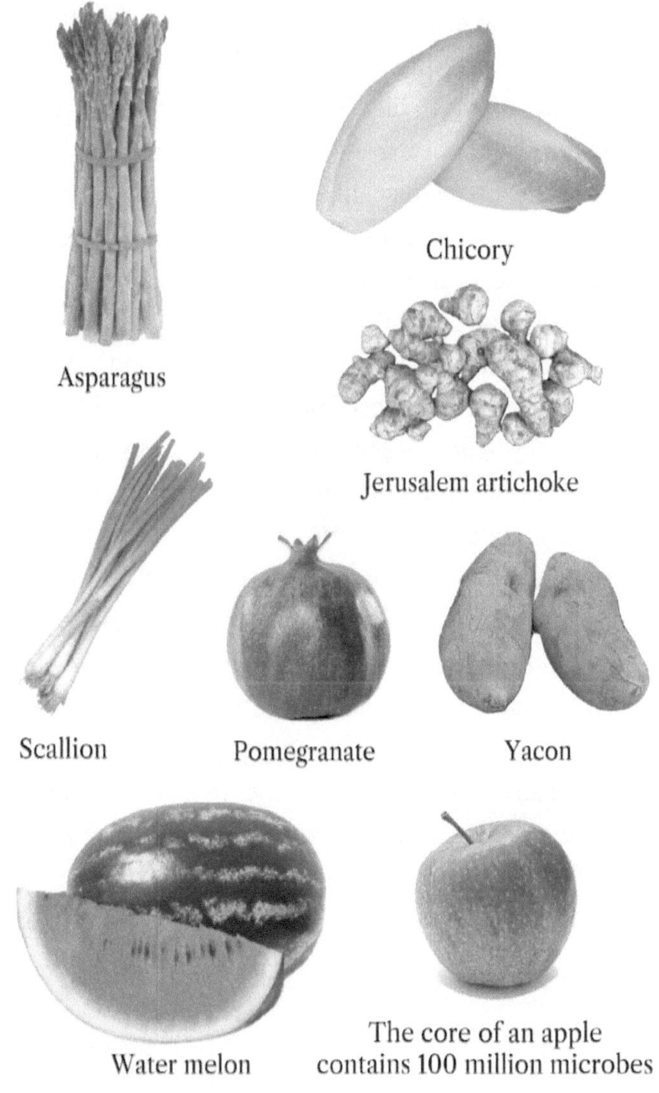

Food sources highest in FOS and inulin

In today's world, people tend to focus on material possessions. Most of us don't know that our body is composed of 30 trillion cells and is home to 37 trillion tiny microbes. These microbes are partners that we should look after. This interdependence makes humans and microbes rely on one another. The brain that governs systems in the body is not the only important part; the gut-brain axis also plays a crucial role. In fact, the brain-gut connection can even function automatically without the brain's command. If you don't take enough care of your digestive system, your gut may start to dictate your brain's actions. As a result, you could experience digestive system problems like constipation, celiac disease, inflammatory bowel disease, or even colon cancer. A poor brain-gut connection may also contribute to mental health problems such as anxiety, depression, stress and mood disorders.

Poor food and drink choices can kill off good gut bacteria and disrupt the balance of gut bacterial populations. The right gut bacteria play an important role in gut health and help nurture a good relationship between the gut and brain, which in turn helps prevent illnesses and prolong the life of the human host. Your gut and your gut bacteria are also the sources of substances such as propionate and butyrate that can keep your immune system working properly. The presence of good gut bacteria can enhance your body's defenses, helping fight major diseases such as heart disease, cancer, and autoimmune disorders. When your gut is healthy, your bowel movement typically occurs once a day, with a gut transit time of around 24 hours. Ultimately, caring for your gut bacteria can help maintain the right balance, leading to a healthier, happier, and longer life.

CHAPTER 12

Bone loss is a significant global health concern

The human body holds 1.2-1.4 kg of bone, with peak strength and density typically at age 30. Yet, in later years, bone density can drop by up to 10% annually. As you reach adulthood, only a small portion, around 10% or less, of bone can renew itself. This happens because, with age, the bone renewal process gradually slows down. After the bone renewal rate declines, your bones will gradually wear away at about 0.3% per year. However, some people experience bone loss at a rate of 1-10% per year. When bones begin to erode, the surrounding bone's structures, including calcium, break down, causing bone loss to become more severe. This can lead to bones becoming brittle and spinal bones shrinking and bending forward.

In India, women in their 40s, on average, lose 10 g of their bones every year, resulting in a third of them having osteopenia—lower bone density than normal.[2] In China, one-third of the population aged 50 and over has osteoporosis.[3,4]

One of the most common bone diseases is osteoarthritis, which is a form of degenerative joint condition caused by the deterioration of joint cartilage and the bone beneath it. Survey data collected in the US in 2006 revealed that 1 in 10 Americans have osteoarthritis. Osteoarthritis is the most common diagnosis made in older Americans—more than 4 million of them affected by this condition. According to a 2009 study, the economic cost of osteoarthritis in America was more than $185 billion a year.[5]

In some Asian countries, such as China, Japan, and Korea,

osteoarthritis affects around 30% of their elderly citizens. Indeed, bone loss and bone-related diseases are global health issues.

What causes bone erosion?

As we age, our bones undergo changes that can lead to bone erosion. Bone erosion refers to the loss of bone tissue, which can weaken bones and make them more susceptible to fractures. One of the primary reasons for bone erosion with age is the natural process of bone remodeling. This process involves the breakdown and replacement of old bone tissue with new bone tissue. Bone modeling is important because it helps our bones grow, stay strong, and heal from injuries. It also helps our bodies use calcium and adjust to different types of activities or pressures. However, as we age, the rate of bone breakdown can exceed the rate of new bone formation, leading to bone loss and erosion.

Other factors contribute to bone erosion as well. Hormonal changes that occur with aging, such as a decrease in estrogen levels in women, can contribute to bone erosion. Estrogen plays a key role in maintaining bone density, so its decline can lead to increased bone loss and erosion. Besides, in underweight women aged 50 to 84, gaining 3 kg of weight (1 BMI) after menopause puts them at greater risk of bone loss and osteoporosis. Another reason why women are more prone to osteoporosis is that they have smaller and thinner bones than men.[6] Therefore, if you are a woman aged 50 or older and want to avoid osteoporosis or bone fractures, it's important to maintain a healthy weight.

On average, drinking coffee results in a loss of about 4 mg of bone per cup.[7] This means that if you drink coffee every day, you could lose as much as 1,400 mg of bone each year. Moreover, in women aged 65-77, drinking 3 cups of coffee a day leads to approximately 2% loss of spinal bone per year. Some individuals with specific genetic traits can lose up to 8-10% of their spinal bone annually, amounting to about 120 g of bone loss per year.

Drinking coffee can cause even more bone loss if you add

sugar to it. Consuming sugar, including refined white flour, increases calcium excretion through urine by up to 36 mg per 100 ml of urine. Continual consumption of sugar and refined white flour every day may lead to a loss of around 13 g of calcium, which is equivalent to 1% of the total bone mass, each year.[8]

More importantly, avoid drinking coffee in the evening or before bed, as caffeine can cause sleeplessness. Lack of sleep can also contribute to a decrease in bone mass. For example, a 2019 study found that postmenopausal women who sleep less than five hours a night have lower bone density in their hips, thighs, and spine than women of the same age who sleep 7 hours a night.[9] Insufficient sleep disrupts the release of growth hormone, leading to reduced bone formation and increased bone breakdown. Furthermore, sleep deprivation can disrupt circadian rhythms, leading to alterations in bone formation and resorption.

You may not be aware that smoking stimulates the production of osteoclasts—specialized bone cells that break down bone in a process called bone resorption. Cigarette smoke contains a carcinogen called dioxin, which induces osteoclasts to multiply and cause bone breakdown at a rate 4 times higher than usual.[19] Smoking also interferes with the body's ability to absorb calcium and reduces blood flow to the bones.

In addition to cigarette smoke, certain medications, such as non-steroidal anti-inflammatory drugs and corticosteroid drugs used to reduce inflammation in the body, can also contribute to bone loss. Patients who received 2-5 mg of glucocorticoids, a class of corticosteroids, daily to reduce inflammation for over 6 months were 35% more likely to experience a spinal fracture.[11] The reason why steroid drugs cause bone loss is not well understood, but it may be related to back pain as well. Knowing this, would you still consider using these drugs?

Apart from smoking and certain medications, other factors can contribute to bone loss too. A sedentary lifestyle, for example, may lead to weaker bones over time. When you lead a sedentary lifestyle, your bones receive fewer mechanical stimuli, causing a decrease in bone formation and an increase in bone resorption. What's more, chronic inflammation can impair bone health by promoting bone resorption and suppressing bone formation. Besides, poor nutrition can play a significant role in bone health. A diet that lacks essential nutrients like calcium, vitamin D, and phosphorus can negatively impact bone density.

In addition, excessive alcohol consumption is another factor that can adversely affect bone health. Drinking alcohol in large amounts can interfere with the absorption of calcium and other nutrients necessary for bone formation.

When does the inevitable bone loss start?

In most people, around the age of 34, the rate of bone breakdown becomes higher than bone formation.[12] This leads to an inevitable gradual erosion of bones, around 0.3% per year. In fact, almost all men and women aged 70 and over suffer from osteopenia or osteoporosis. However, older women are more likely to experience more severe bone erosion. In other words, a 70-year-old woman's bone mass may be only half that of a 30-year-old.

Additionally, poor kidney function in the elderly is linked to greater bone loss. For example, a 2017 study revealed that older women aged 75 with normal kidney function experienced only 1.3% bone loss per year, but if kidney function declined, bone loss accelerated to 2.3% per year.[13,14] Kidney dysfunction can cause a buildup of acid in the body, known as metabolic acidosis. This condition can lead to the release of calcium from the bones to buffer the excess acid, which contributes to bone loss over time. Many people have chronic metabolic acidosis without realizing it. This can lead to an increase in bone resorption, which may result in a loss of 1-3% of bone mass per year. Also, when kidney function declines, the kidneys may not produce enough calcitriol, the active form of vitamin D. This can result in decreased calcium absorption. Interestingly, women who consumed more milk during the menopausal transition (the cessation of menstruation) did not see improvements in their bone strength.[15] So, it's better to take care of your kidneys to help prevent conditions like osteopenia and osteoporosis as you age.

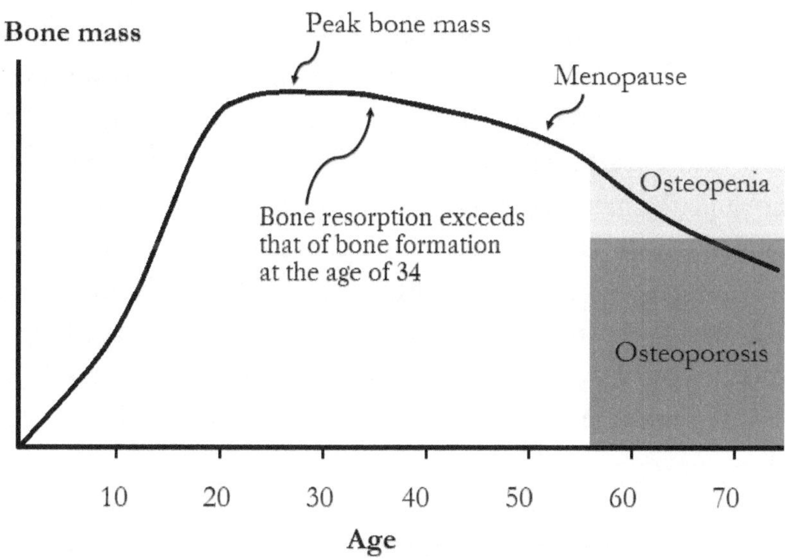

At around 34 years old, the rate of your bone resorption is higher than bone formation, which inevitably leads to bone loss.[16]

Bones can repair themselves and regrow

First, we now know that worn-out cartilage, the covering on bones' ends, in joints can repair itself, but the process takes 1-2 years before new cartilage can completely regrow. Cartilage healing takes so long because it doesn't have a blood supply, which limits its ability to repair itself. Regarding bones, experiments with mice have shown that if a mouse's fingertip is cut off, it can regrow. However, if the middle bone out of the three bones in a mouse's finger is cut off, it can't regrow. Similarly, if a child's fingertip is chopped off, it can regrow.[17] Scientists have also found that knee and ankle bones have a greater self-healing potential than the hip joint. This is why a hip fracture takes longer to heal than a fractured knee or ankle.[18] These findings provide scientific evidence that the body can heal itself, but bone regrowth just takes more time.

Moreover, it's possible that getting rid of senescent cells might speed up the process of cartilage formation. This is especially important as we know that, with age, old cells tend to build up in vital parts of the body, including the joints and cartilage. A 2017 study from Johns Hopkins University showed that clearing senescent cells from the articular cartilage (tissue covering the ends of bones) and synovium (the membrane surrounding the joints) is beneficial before rebuilding bone. Furthermore, clearing senescent cells can help arrest and even reverse osteoarthritis. More importantly, the removal of senescent cells from joints reduces inflammation and speeds up the formation of new cartilage.[19] So, before undergoing bone repair, consider removing senescent cells from your joints and cartilage as well.

Calcium is most essential mineral for bone regeneration

Calcium is the main mineral found in bones and makes up about 99% of all the calcium in your body. It helps create strong and rigid bones by combining with another mineral, phosphate, to form a substance called hydroxyapatite. Adults usually have blood calcium levels between 8.5 and 10.2 mg/dL. If there is not enough calcium in the blood, the body takes some from the bones, so important things like muscle movement and sending signals through nerves can keep happening.

The recommended daily calcium intake for adults is about 1,200 mg, and you shouldn't take more than 2,000 mg a day.[20] Exceeding this amount is not beneficial. Some studies have suggested that as excessive calcium intake can lead to health issues such as kidney stones and an increased risk of heart disease. However, if there is excess calcium, it will be excreted through urine, feces, and sweat instead. After your body gets the calcium it needs, any excess is excreted in sweat and urine, about 200 mg a day.

In calcium balance, it's assumed that the body can absorb 30% of calcium in foods. However, calcium absorption decreases to 15-20% as we age. For people who eat foods containing 1,000 mg of calcium a day, their body can absorb 300 mg of calcium. Thus, each day, the body will excrete 150 mg of calcium into the intestines. When the body absorbs 30% of calcium in foods (300 mg) and 45 mg of calcium via the intestines, the net calcium absorption is 195 mg a day (for foods containing 1,000 mg of calcium). In this calcium balance, we also lose 195 mg of calcium through the skin and urine a day.[21]

The fact is that postmenopausal women who take 500-1,200 mg of calcium a day still experience bone loss. Therefore, interventions for preventing bone erosion and restoring strong bones require something else.

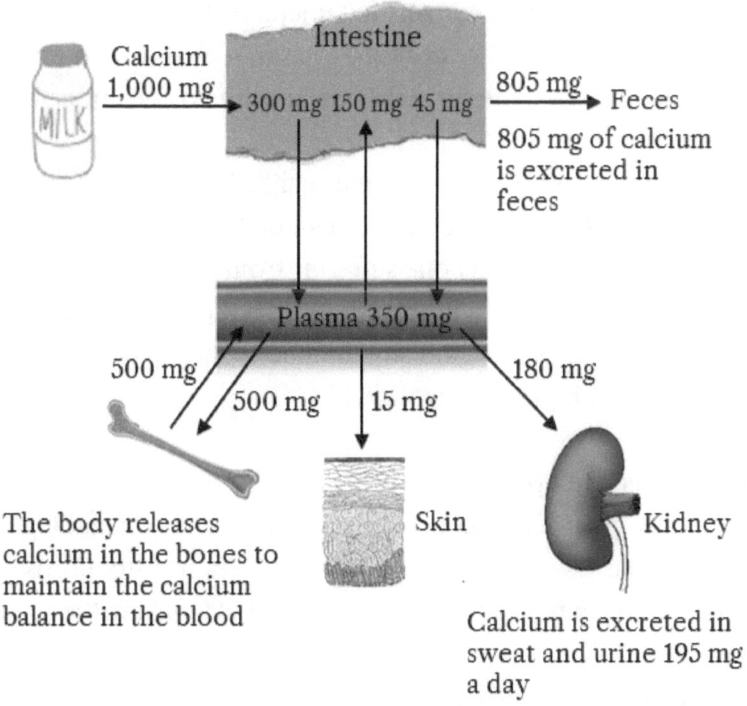

Calcium balance.[21,22]

Back pain is also a major concern across the globe

At the age of 45, I faced a significant problem in my life: being unable to find a job. Perhaps it's because the Thai context differs from the Western one, where workers can find employment regardless of their age. In Thailand, ageism exists. Here, job postings often set an applicant's age limit at 35 or 40 years old. As a result, many people over that age lose their opportunities or are implicitly excluded. Even though we don't always choose our jobs, many times jobs choose us. I was unemployed for 2 years, and apart from cooking, picking up and sending my children to school, doing laundry, and washing dishes, there were no other activities to do at home.

My back pain started in my 30s when I was working in a desk job at a government organization. When I switched to doing research, I still had to work at a lab bench for long periods, causing my back to continue hurting. Unemployment at the age of 45 and staying at home made my back pain even worse. I felt uncomfortable and emotionally frustrated. My back hurt every time I sat in a chair for an extended period. It felt like I was alone in the world, with no one understanding my feelings.

The past two years made me realize how harmful sedentary behavior and sitting for long periods can be harmful to my back. But the truth is, I'm not the only one suffering from back pain. In fact, 84% of people on this planet will experience back pain at some point in their lives.[23] This is a significant number. Back pain is indeed a widespread health problem worldwide.

What causes back pain?

Back pain can occur for several reasons, including poor posture, spinal issues, muscle or ligament strain, osteoporosis and obesity. Some people may even experience back pain without a clear cause.

In people with obesity, an increased mass of fat puts a burden on the spine, leading to its deterioration and, eventually, back pain.[24] Furthermore, there is strong evidence that a large stomach is linked to back pain. Excess fat can cause inflammation in the body, and when this occurs regularly, the body becomes chronically inflamed. This persistent inflammation changes the body's environment. The more fat tissue the body contains, the more inflamed it becomes. Over time, inflammation can cause even more back pain, eventually becoming a permanent problem. Moreover, back pain leads to physical inactivity, which in turn leads to obesity and more back pain—a vicious cycle. Did you know that back pain costs the United States around $80 billion per year?[25]

Back pain is most likely to affect people with sedentary behavior, such as couch potatoes or those who spend a lot of time sitting, or having poor posture. If you can change your behavior, you might be among the 16% of people who never experience back pain in their lives.

Bed rest or taking anti-inflammatory medications or painkillers can't cure your back pain. In fact, avoiding movement may make it worse. As mentioned earlier, taking non-steroidal anti-inflammatory drugs or corticosteroid drugs can increase bone loss and the risk of spinal fractures by up to 35%. However, weight loss and lifestyle changes can reduce back pain.[26] Nowadays, in the US and UK, doctors advise patients with back pain to self-medicate through activities like brisk walking and yoga.

After 2 years of being at home, frustrated and uncomfortable with back pain, I thought, "Never mind about all that," so I went on to work as a laborer in a waste-glass recycling plant. I spent most of my time lifting glass bottle sacks weighing 40-50 kg, totaling 3-4 tons a day, off clients' pickup trucks. But after working for about a year, my back pain improved. I was enlightened—this hard work has saved my life!

Let me explain this. Working hard is similar to exercising for me. It's true that each time we exercise, it causes tiny injuries to our muscles. This small injury activates cells in our body, and importantly, causes muscle cells to repair and rebuild new muscles. Moreover, muscles work together with bones. By giving muscles a workout, it also helps build strong bones. This is supported by evidence. A 2019 study found that exercise triggers the hormone irisin to be released from skeletal muscles, stimulating bone-building.[27,28] When we exercise, our muscles release a substance called irisin, which goes into our blood and travels to our bones. Once it reaches the bones, irisin encourages the development of new bone cells and can even help repair damaged bones. So, when we exercise, it not only benefits our muscles but also our bones, making them stronger and healthier.

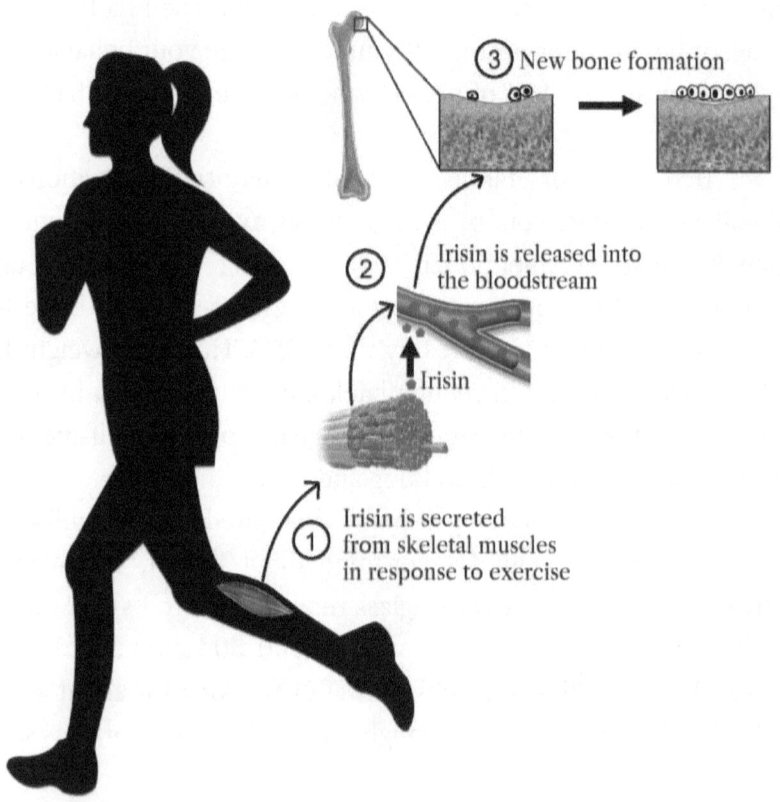

In humans, exercise can stimulate bone formation.[22,29,30] During exercise, the irisin hormone is released from skeletal muscles into the bloodstream and stimulates bone-building.

Additionally, exercise can help by strengthening muscles that support the back, improving flexibility, and increasing blood flow to the affected area, which can help to reduce inflammation and pain. Plus, exercise has been shown to promote the release of endorphins, which are natural painkillers that can help to reduce discomfort.

In combination with hard work, I also ate foods rich in calcium, vitamin D, and vitamin K2 in the form of MK-7, which can stimulate the body to build bone. All of this may be the reason I was able to fix my terrible back pain naturally. After all, don't live like an old man. "Be stronger than your excuses." Avoid sedentary behavior and adjust your life as if you were younger. The belief that older people shouldn't lift heavy objects is just a person's belief. The more muscles you use, the stronger your muscles and bones become.

However, this is only what I have experienced personally. To get the best help for your back pain, it's important to talk to a doctor who can give you a proper diagnosis and plan for treatment.

***

Prioritize removal of senescent cells for effective bone repair

If you have joint, knee, or back pain, taking calcium won't immediately help build up your bones. This is because inflamed joints contain senescent cells, which release inflammatory substances that interfere with bone repair and regeneration processes. Before restoring calcium in your bones, it's important to get rid of these senescent cells with senolytics. Some natural senolytics include fisetin, curcumin, and luteolin, which work in harmony with the human digestive and immune systems. Curcumin, in particular, can selectively destroy senescent cells and strengthen bones at the same time. It may also increase the activity of bone-building cells, leading to increased bone density. This is why curcumin may have helped me get rid of inflammation in my body and encourage bone healing. From my experience, without taking curcumin, I might not have been able to heal myself.

Curcumin induces bone formation

In a healthy body, there is a balance between bone formation by osteoblasts and bone resorption by osteoclasts, which break down bones and release minerals. However, if bone resorption exceeds bone formation, it decreases a person's bone density, which, over time, can lead to osteopenia and eventually osteoporosis. The mechanisms of bone formation and resorption are now better understood. One reason why bone formation occurs more slowly than bone resorption might be due to the buildup of senescent cells.

However, there is good news. Studies show that curcumin can do more than just remove aging cells in joints; it can also encourage the regrowth of bone.[31,32] For instance, in a 2017 clinical study, elderly volunteers took 1,000 mg of curcumin per day with vitamin D, vitamin C, and calcium, along with exercising by lifting light weights, jogging, or walking for 20 minutes, 4 days a week for 4 weeks. The results showed that, on average, the volunteers had a 5% increase in finger bone density and a 2% increase in upper jaw bone density.[29] As the study continued for six months, the volunteers' finger bone densities increased to 7%, and the upper jaw densities increased to 4%. Overall, the volunteers experienced 3-5 times more bone mass gain compared to those who followed the same routine but didn't take curcumin.[33] Curcumin's remarkable benefits for bone health make it a valuable supplement to consider for maintaining and improving bone density.

Emodin inhibits the bone cells that breaks down bones

Stimulating the stem cells in the body to build bone requires another factor: GDF2 (growth differentiation factor 2), a protein that can induce bone formation, which is produced in the liver. The blood of teenagers is high in GDF2, but this decreases as they age. Levels of GDF2 are even lower in people with type 2 diabetes. In addition to milk, which has long been known as a stimulator for bone growth, GDF2 is also known as a potent inducer of bone formation.

Emodin is a natural compound that can induce the production

of GDF2 and stimulate the cells to build bone.[34,35,36] In a mouse model, in which mice were fed emodin in a dose of 2 mg/kg a day for 2 weeks, it was shown that emodin can stimulate osteoblasts to produce bone matrix, yet inhibits osteoclasts from breaking down bone.

Emodin can be found in the Chinese herb Shou Wu Pian (*Polygonum multiflorum*). However, herbs are not always incorporated into culinary dishes, which is why I think vegetables are a more suitable option.

Rhubarb (*Rheum rhabarbarum*) is a vegetable with red stalks and green leaves. The red stalk of rhubarb is the edible part, and it has a sour taste. It's among the most popular vegetables found in Western markets. Rhubarb stalk is commonly used for making food and desserts such as cakes, pies, and jam. A hundred grams of dried rhubarb stalk contains 2.24 mg of emodin.[37] And 100 g of fresh rhubarb stalks may contain up to 0.2 mg of emodin. Research indicates that people shouldn't consume more than 2,000 mg of emodin.[38]

Excessive amounts of emodin that are greater than normal amounts of hormones or other substances in the bloodstream can have a negative impact on the functioning of various cells and organs in the body. However, in animal models, emodin is poorly absorbed because it's rapidly metabolized via glucuronidation and eliminated from the body through urine or feces. This results in less than 3% of emodin absorption. Fortunately, emodin is resistant to heat—cooking at high temperatures doesn't destroy emodin. Plus, cooking can also help get rid of oxalic acid in plant foods, including rhubarb.

However, the issue of poor emodin absorption can be addressed by taking emodin alongside piperine or black pepper. A study found that rats fed with piperine experienced an increase in emodin absorption by over 200%.[39] In fact, similar to low levels of calcium, low levels of emodin are sufficient to increase the number and activity of osteoblasts. Emodin should not be used at a concentration greater than 10 micromolar or equivalent to 13 mg of emodin in the body. Therefore, it's best to take small amounts of emodin. In addition, it's likely that taking repeated low doses of emodin could help stimulate osteoblasts to build bones, inhibit the bone cells that break down bones, and prevent bone loss.

A little bit of knowledge

Foods high in oxalic acid include spinach, cabbage, sweet potatoes, and rhubarb. Consuming large amounts of oxalic acid or oxalate over an extended period can lead to calcium deficiency. Oxalic acid binds to calcium and hinders calcium absorption. However, when foods high in oxalic acid are briefly cooked at 120°C, oxalic acid breaks down into carbon dioxide, carbon monoxide, and water.

Eat mangoes to promote bone building

If you want to have strong bones, mangoes might be able to help you. This is because mangiferin, a compound that gives the fruit its yellow color, has the ability to promote cartilage formation and repair. Cartilage a type of connective tissue that provides a cushioning and supportive layer between bones in joints. Experiments in animal models revealed that mangiferin can enhance cartilage formation in various joints.[40] Studies have suggested that mangiferin may stimulate the growth of chondrocytes, which are the cells that produce and maintain cartilage in the body.

Evidence also implies that mangiferin can promote bone building. Mice that received a daily dose of 10 mg/kg of mangiferin for 8 weeks had more new bone formation in their joints, which appeared thicker.[41,42] In a mouse model, researchers tested the potential of a 1% mango diet in improving bone density and found that mice fed 1% mango improved their bone density and strength, but not mice that received a 10% mango diet.[43] This is likely because mangoes are high in sugar, and too much sugar impairs bone formation.[44]

Mangoes are also abundant in essential vitamins and minerals, including vitamin C, which plays a key role in collagen synthesis; vitamin A, which is crucial for bone growth and development; and vitamin K, which is necessary for the activation of osteocalcin and proper bone metabolism.

While more research is needed to fully understand the potential benefits of mangiferin and mangoes for human bone health, there is no harm in enjoying this delicious fruit. Keep in mind to consume mangoes in moderation and aim not to eat more than 85 g of mango four times a week. Research shows that consuming more than 250 g of mango per day may cause accelerated aging.[45]

Which type of mango is best for you? The Kent mango from Peru and Azúcar mango cultivated in Colombia have the highest content of mangiferin, at 11 mg per 100 g, followed by the Pica and Tommy Atkins mangoes from Chile, which contain 3-4 mg of mangiferin per 100 g.[46]

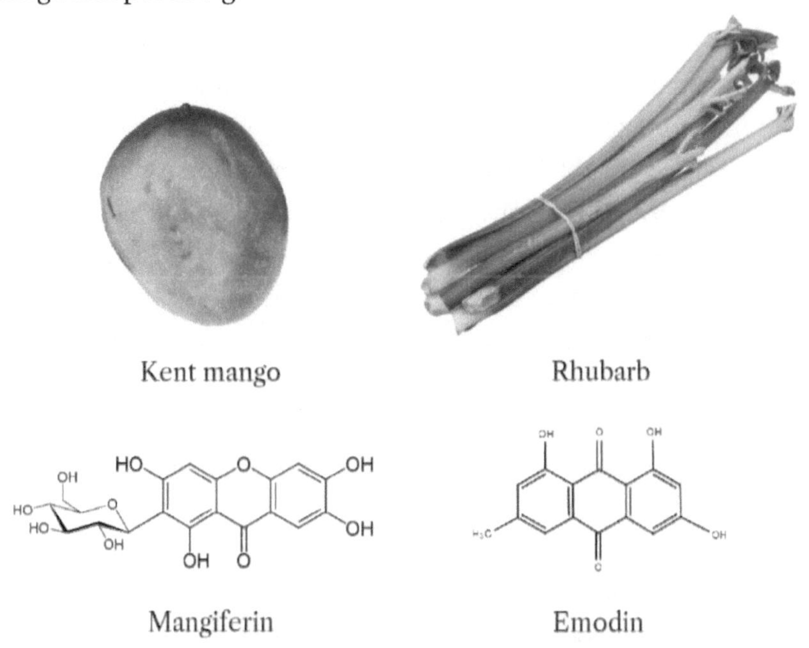

Kent mango   Rhubarb

Mangiferin   Emodin

Mangiferin in mango can stimulate cartilage and bone formation. Emodin, found in rhubarb, can promote bone building, inhibit the bone cell that breaks down bones, and prevent bone loss.

Strengthen weak bones with vitamin D

As mentioned before, consuming calcium alone is not enough to prevent osteoporosis in postmenopausal women. This is because the body needs vitamin D to absorb calcium and phosphate, essential minerals for new bone formation. Vitamin D is crucial, as it significantly impacts calcium absorption. Without sufficient vitamin D, only 15% of calcium is absorbed, while adequate vitamin D levels can increase absorption to over 30%. Vitamin D also plays a vital role in maintaining normal immune system function and helps fight infection. In children, a lack of vitamin D predisposes them to colds and flu. Additionally, vitamin D may aid in fighting off the COVID-19 virus.

There are two main types of vitamin D: vitamin D2 and vitamin D3, which are inactive forms until they are activated by enzymes from the liver and kidneys. While vitamin D2 is found in milk, yeast, and fungi, vitamin D3, the most important form for the human body, is found in animal sources. Actually, only 10% of vitamin D3 is obtained from our diet, while the other 90% is synthesized in the skin upon exposure to sunlight and stored in the liver.

However, not everyone gets the same amount of vitamin D3 from skin synthesis. As you age, your skin's ability to produce vitamin D3 decreases. In a 70-year-old person, their skin's capacity to produce vitamin D from sunlight is reduced to just 25%. For individuals with obesity, almost all of their vitamin D is stored in body fat. Therefore, only small amounts of vitamin D3 from the body's synthesis from sunlight can be drawn out.[47] That is why elderly and people with obesity are more likely to suffer from bone loss, flu, and infection.

In adults younger than 65, having low blood levels of vitamin D3 was associated with lower bone mass.[48] Active vitamin D3 levels in the blood are also related to muscle strength. People with higher active vitamin D3 levels in their blood tend to have stronger leg muscles.[49] For healthy people, a normal level of vitamin D in the blood is between 20-50 nanograms per milliliter (ng/ml). However, lower levels of vitamin D in the blood are found in patients with osteomalacia or rickets, which are mainly caused by vitamin D and calcium deficiencies, and osteoporosis.

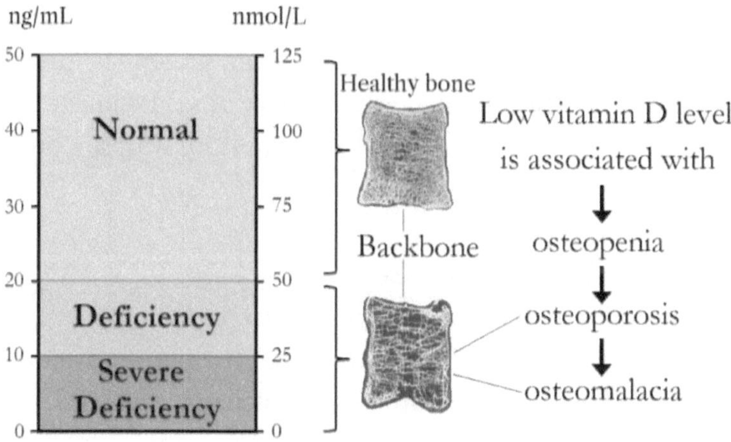

Vitamin D in the blood

The normal level of vitamin D in the blood is 20-50 ng/ml (or 50-125 nmol/L). Vitamin D levels falling below this normal range can cause clinical manifestations of vitamin D insufficiency, leading to a loss of bone density and bone diseases such as osteopenia, osteoporosis, and osteomalacia.[50,51,52]

Natural foods with the highest vitamin D3 content per 100 g include wild salmon fillet, containing 600-1000 IU of vitamin D3 (equal to 15-25 mcg), canned salmon, containing 300-600 IU of vitamin D3, and fortified milk, containing about 100 IU of vitamin D3.

It's challenging to get the recommended dose of 800 IU (20 mcg) of vitamin D3 every day unless you eat 150 g of wild salmon daily. The best way to get enough vitamin D3 without spending money is by getting sunlight. Generally, for fair-skinned individuals, approximately 15-20 minutes of sun exposure on the face, arms, and legs before 10 am or after 3 pm during the summer months may be enough to synthesize around 3,000 IU of vitamin D3.[53] And going out in the sun for 5-10 minutes daily will allow your skin to synthesize the recommended dose of vitamin D3 of 800 IU. This should be enough to give you strong and fracture-resistant bones. However, for darker-skinned individuals, it may take longer. Keep in mind that overexposure to the sun increases the risk of skin damage and skin cancer, so it's important to balance sun exposure with sun protection measures.

Vitamin K enhances bone strength

In addition to being an important factor in helping your blood clot in wounds, vitamin K is also required to activate osteocalcin, a calcium-building protein. After osteocalcin is activated, it binds calcium and incorporates it into the bone.[54]

It has been known that vitamin K deficiency can result in a higher risk of developing knee osteoarthritis.[55] However, if you are a postmenopausal woman, taking 45 mg of vitamin K2 daily for 3 years can significantly improve your bone density and strength.[56] Taking vitamin K2 as MK-7 also reduces the risk of developing osteoporosis and improves bone density in menopausal women.[57]

Vitamin K is found in high concentrations in green leafy vegetables, especially watercress. A hundred grams of watercress contains 250 mcg of vitamin K, representing 238% of the recommended daily intake. Vitamin K is also found in natto, a Japanese soybean food fermented by *Bacillus subtilis* natto strain. A 100 g serving of natto contains 1,034 mcg of Vitamin K2, of which 930 mcg is in the form of MK-7. Importantly, vitamin K2 as MK-7 in natto is well absorbed in humans, and it remains in the blood up to 2 days after consumption. Some other sources of vitamin K2 as MK7 are fermented vegetables such as sauerkraut and kimchi, which contain small amounts of MK-7.

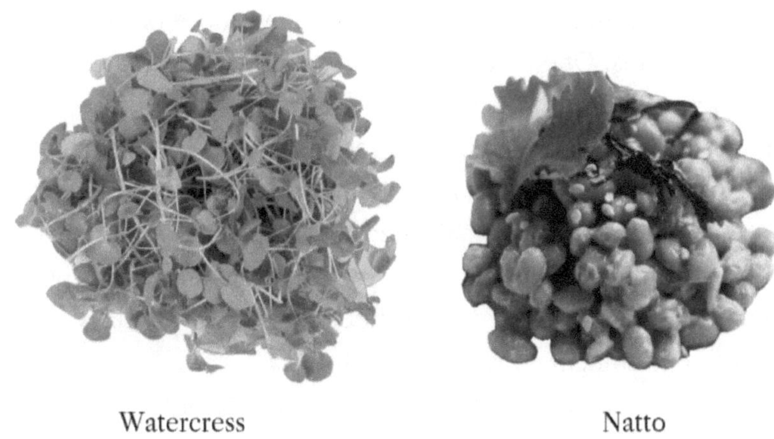

Watercress   Natto

Watercress contains 250 mcg of vitamin K. Natto has 930 mcg of vitamin K2 as MK-7. Eating either of them can improve your bone density.

Prebiotics help calcium absorption

A study shows that consuming prebiotics such as FOS (15 g a day) improves calcium absorption in adolescent boys by 10%.[58] In another study, after a year, teenagers who received 8 g of inulin a day added more new bone (35 g) to their bodies compared to the control group.[59] In older women, estrogen deficiency can lead to poor intestinal absorption of calcium. However, menopausal women who take 5 g of a mixture of FOS and inulin extracted from chicory for 6 weeks can increase their intestinal calcium absorption.[60] The FOS and inulin in this experiment are equivalent to 35 g of fresh chicory. Thus, cooking and eating chicory can help calcium absorption in the gut and improve your bone health.

Onions, containing 2-2.5 g of FOS per 100 g, are not only a flavorful addition to your meals but may have potential benefits for bone health. After being heat-treated, onions become slightly sweet due to their FOS content. Scientists at the University of Bern in Switzerland discovered that rats consuming a gram of dry onion per day for four weeks increased their bone mineral content by 17%.[61] This amount of onion would be the equivalent dose of 12 g of fresh onion in humans. One medium onion is about 100 g. However, this has been proven in animal models and has not yet been shown to be effective in humans. Further research is needed to determine the impact of onion consumption on human bone health. Meanwhile, adding an onion to a well-balanced diet offers valuable nutrients, such as vitamin C, vitamin B6, folate, potassium, phosphorus, calcium, magnesium, and dietary fiber (around 3-7% daily value), while also enriching the taste of your dishes.

Keep in mind that taking short-term prebiotics is unlikely to result in a significant change in bone density. If you want a noticeable increase in bone density, you have to take FOS and inulin for at least a year. Long-term intake of prebiotics could bring you closer to being free from bone disease. Food sources of prebiotics, such as affordable fruits and vegetables, can improve bone health when used properly, compared to medicines.

How exercise can reinforce bone health

A sedentary lifestyle can lead to weaker bones, as regular exercise is essential for maintaining bone strength and density. Studies have shown that exercise can stimulate the production and release of osteocalcin from the bones into the bloodstream. Osteocalcin is a protein hormone that is produced by bone-forming cells known as osteoblasts. Studies have shown that osteocalcin can promote the growth of new bone tissue and enhance bone mineral density, thus playing a role in preventing osteoporosis and bone fractures. Osteocalcin levels have been found to increase after both acute bouts of exercise and long-term exercise training. Plus, the increase in osteocalcin has been linked to several health benefits, including improved glucose metabolism, increased insulin sensitivity, and decreased fat mass.

In addition, exercise triggers the release of growth hormone from the pituitary gland. Growth hormone plays a vital role in bone growth, maintenance, and repair by directly stimulating bone formation and promoting the production of insulin-like growth factor-1 (IGF-1). IGF-1 is a hormone that promotes the activity of osteoblasts, leading to increased bone formation.

Moreover, engaging in regular physical activity has been demonstrated to balance the levels of sex hormones, including estrogen and testosterone, which are vital for maintaining bone health. Exercise also enhances blood circulation to the bones, delivering crucial nutrients, hormones, and growth factors required for bone development. Overall, exercise has been demonstrated to benefit bone health by influencing osteoblast activity, increasing osteocalcin production, promoting IGF-1 and sex hormone levels, and enhancing blood flow to the bones.

Finally, you may have heard stories of elderly individuals with fragile, brittle bones who became bedridden after a fall. If you want to avoid such a situation, there are numerous steps you can take now to maintain the health of your bones and joints.

CHAPTER 13

The very big problem of the aged: muscle loss

If you were to say that a human being is essentially walking flesh, it wouldn't be entirely wrong, since 40% of the human body is composed of muscle proteins. However, if you don't maintain your muscles by staying active, you may lose them more quickly.[1] This is because the body uses up to 40% of its total energy to keep muscles working, so when you don't engage your muscles, they shrink to conserve energy. Let's examine some evidence. For instance, astronauts in zero gravity who don't perform Earth-like exercises can lose about 20% of their muscle mass within two weeks.[2] Similarly, inactive individuals on Earth can lose muscle mass as well. Public health data from 1995 to 2013 revealed that half of the world's elderly population already experienced a loss of muscle function or mass.[3]

Loss of muscle

Thinking back to when I worked in a government office, I remember having lots of meetings and paperwork. In this kind of job, I sit for most of the day, about 80% of the time. I wondered if doing this for 30 more years, until I retired, might be bad for my body. Luckily, sitting at a desk is not as harmful as being in space; otherwise, I would have lost 20% of my muscle.

Sarcopenia, the gradual loss of muscle mass, is a condition that usually starts affecting people around the age of 40. As we get older, especially when we reach 70, this muscle loss speeds up. In fact, between 70 and 79 years old, we might lose up to 2% of our muscle mass every year. By the time people turns 80, they could have lost as much as 30% of their muscles. This decrease in muscle mass can lead to problems with mobility, balance, and overall strength, making it essential for older adults to find ways to maintain and improve their muscle health.

Sarcopenia occurs for a number of reasons, including inactive muscle cells, low testosterone levels in the body, chronic low-grade inflammation, and nutritional deficiencies. Sarcopenia is more common in the elderly, people with type 2 diabetes, and especially in menopausal women, affecting up to 20% of them.[5] Loss of muscle also makes internal organs less stretchy in older adults. Apart from an elevated risk of falls and fractures, sarcopenia affects heart muscles as well. It affects heart muscles by reducing their mass and function, leading to changes in the heart's structure. Thus, older adults with sarcopenia are likely to have a higher risk of heart failure and irregular heartbeat, especially if they already have underlying heart conditions.[6]

The bedridden and wheelchair-bound elderly are also at a greater risk of sarcopenia. Conversely, sarcopenia could make older adults become bedridden or wheelchair-bound due to muscle loss. This leads to weakness and inability to perform daily tasks. Moreover, as muscle mass decreases in older adults, tendons and bones will carry more weight. If this happens in the knee, it will carry more weight, increasing the risk of knee osteoarthritis. For patients, whether they are young or elderly, lying in bed for a long time can reduce their leg muscles by as much as 485 g. And if you happen to sit in a wheelchair all day for 2 weeks, you will lose about 250 g of your leg muscles.[7] Don't blame yourself. This is the body's way of adapting to the disuse of muscle.

In addition, sarcopenia may occur when calcium leaks in skeletal muscles, the muscles that attach to bones. It's believed that weakness in aging is related to calcium leak in muscles. When too much calcium leaks, it impairs the flexibility of muscle—the muscle's capability of contracting. If this happens in the heart, it may trigger an irregular heartbeat and heart failure.[9] Calcium leaked in muscles also produces free radicals that can damage cells and cell components, which, in turn, accelerate aging. Sarcopenia is a serious issue that can greatly impact an individual's quality of life, especially in older adults. While it's a common problem among older adults, it's not an inevitable part of aging.

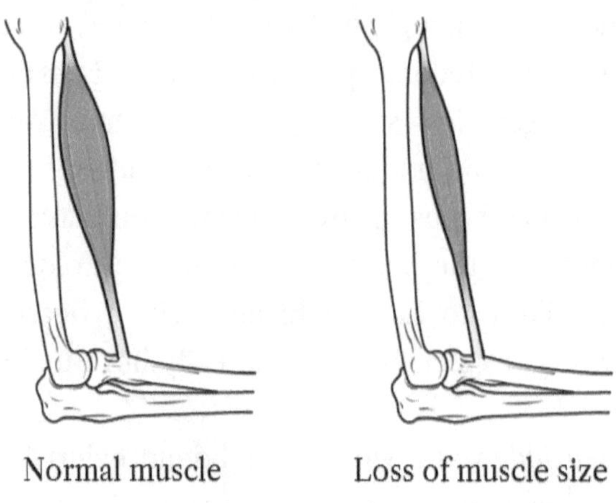

Normal muscle Loss of muscle size

Sarcopenia is the reduction of muscle size.[8]

With aging comes physical decline. In older people who are frail, physically weak, and lack exercise, their mitochondrial function in skeletal muscles has also been found to be impaired.[10] Scientists believe that impaired mitochondria in skeletal muscles are due to autophagy, a mechanism for cleaning up damaged proteins and organelles.[11] In the muscles of a healthy person, damaged cells or organelles from, for example, cellular metabolism, exposure to toxins, physical injury, or aging are degraded and immediately recycled. This helps conserve cellular energy by recycling cell components and makes space for new cells. But as we age, mitochondrial function declines, and injuries occur inside mitochondria. If damaged mitochondria aren't repaired and it causes permanent damage to the mitochondria, it become "zombie mitochondria," worsening other existing conditions or leading to disease such as Parkinson's and Alzheimer's.

The lack of certain nutrients such as calcium, magnesium, phosphate, and selenium, that play a role in muscle function, is also associated with sarcopenia.[12] Additionally, some medications, such as non-steroidal anti-inflammatory drugs, aspirin, and ibuprofen, if taken for extended periods, can lead to muscle mass loss.[13]

A little bit of knowledge

Statins, cholesterol-lowering drugs, may cause more harm than good. The clearest statin's adverse side effect during treatment is muscle problems. Statins can lower muscle coenzyme Q10, a compound that helps generate energy in your cells. As a result of this, the function of mitochondria are disrupted and thus cause the muscles to break down. If you take a statin, you may develop muscle pain and feel tired. Statins are also likely to cause insomnia and loss of libido. It happens quite often that people who have used a statin tend to quit it within a short period of time.[15]

With age, people also develop low-grade inflammation, a mild inflammation caused by an imbalance of cytokines, which mediate communication between immune cells. This is particularly true if you have a health condition such as arthritis, osteoporosis, cardiovascular disease, diabetes, obesity, or dementia, where inflammation is a problem. As you age, elevated cytokines also interfere with communication within cells, resulting in abnormal rates of protein synthesis and breakdown. Over time, even a small decrease in protein synthesis or increase in protein breakdown can lead to muscle loss.[14] As low-grade inflammation becomes more prevalent with age, it's crucial to take steps to reduce its impact on your muscle health.

With age comes sarcopenia. Currently, there is no medication available for treating sarcopenia. Non-drug treatments such as exercise, lifestyle changes, and a healthy diet are considered the most effective ways to manage sarcopenia. Compared to medications, these alternative therapies are generally safer and have fewer potential side effects. Sarcopenia can gradually happen in your body. Be aware of it.

***

Superfoods that can help build muscle mass

As we age, muscle health declines due to the loss of muscle mass and poor mitochondrial function; however, natural muscle recovery can help strengthen weak muscles in older people with sarcopenia. A clinical study was done on 60 elderly people (men and women) who didn't exercise regularly. They took either 500 mg or 1,000 mg of urolithin A every day for four weeks. The study showed that urolithin A can increase the activity of mitochondria in skeletal muscles. This helps their muscles use fat more efficiently, just like when they exercise.[16] The study suggests that urolithin A may be helpful in treating these issues in humans.

Pomegranates are rich in urolithin A and ellagic acid. In fact, our gut bacteria transform the ellagic acid from pomegranates into urolithin A. Urolithin A is an active ingredient that stimulates mitochondrial activities. It boosts mitophagy, which removes damaged mitochondria and supports healthy ones. This leads to better energy production and cell function. It also helps create new mitochondria in cells, improving energy output and overall cell health. In addition, urolithin A may improve muscle protein synthesis, which is essential for maintaining and increasing muscle mass and strength.

After it's consumed, urolithin A is absorbed through the intestines and into the bloodstream, where it's distributed to tissues throughout the body. However, everyone's gut has a different microbial population. The production of urolithin A is dependent on the presence of certain bacteria.[17] As a result, the amount of urolithin A that each person receives from eating a pomegranate can vary, and the effects of urolithin A may also vary from person to person.

Pomegranate is a superfood. One hundred grams of fresh pomegranate contain 9 mg of ellagic acid and 269 mg of urolithin A.[18] Plus, you can obtain ellagic acid from raspberries, which contain up to 37 mg of ellagic acid per 100 g.[19]

What's more, one hundred grams of pomegranate contain up to 450 mg of ursolic acid. The research revealed that ursolic acid can increase in the volume of muscles of lab mice, which is similar to an increase in muscular mass achieved through exercise.[20] However after being considered successful in animal tests, ursolic acid failed to show clinical effect in a human trial. Taking 50 mg of ursolic acid daily for 3 months had no effect on the male participants' muscle strength. However, it did help the female participants have significantly higher hand grip strength and muscle strength measure than the female subjects in the placebo group.[21] In this clinical trial, subjects may have been exposed to low amounts of ursolic acid. It's worth noting that the participants in the study had an average age of 40, which may not be old enough to experience the effects of sarcopenia. A study conducted on older adults with sarcopenia could potentially yield more conclusive results.

Eating superfoods like pomegranate could provide potential benefits of the three bioactive ingredients. They are ellagic acid, during ingestion, the bacteria in the gut convert it to urolithin A; urolithin A that can improve mitochondrial function and activity in muscle cells; and ursolic acid that may increase your muscle mass and strength.

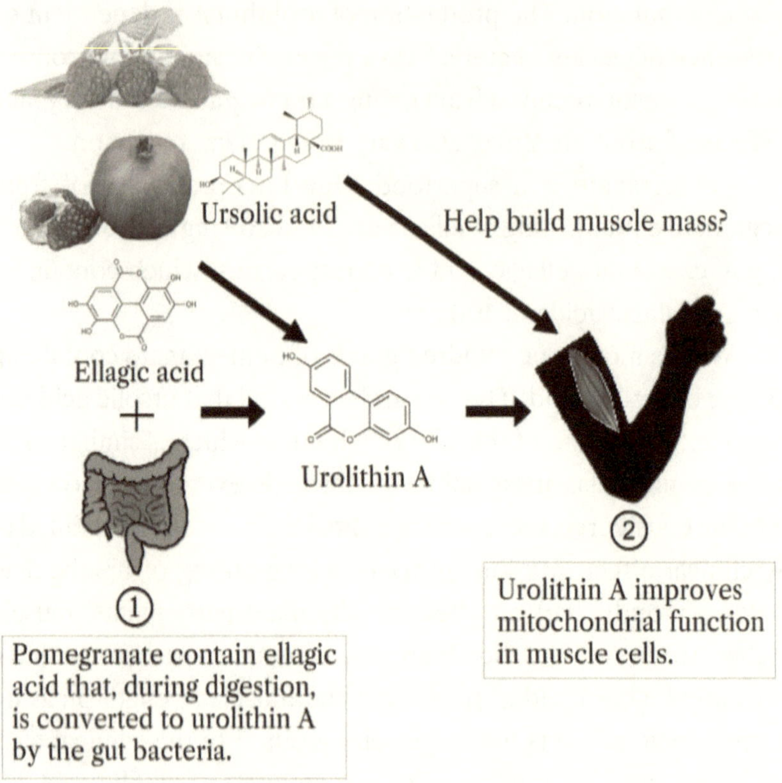

Urolithin A, ellagic acid and ursolic acid from pomegranate and raspberry can improve mitochondria function and build muscle mass.

Your gut bacteria can strengthen the muscles

In animal models, mice that had no gut bacteria had weaker muscles and less energy. However, when gut bacteria were transplanted back into mice without gut bacteria, their muscle mass and strength increased.[22]

Studying the human gut microbes has led experts to know that human gut microbial populations influence muscle strength. Experts have an easy way to assess the relationship between our gut bacteria and muscle strength: by having the elderly take prebiotics and measuring their hand grip strength.[23] Older adults (between 66-90 years old) who took 3.4 g of FOS and inulin daily after breakfast for 13 weeks experienced a significant increase in hand grip strength, meaning their muscles became stronger. However, this study only tested 22 volunteers. To determine its true effectiveness, a larger group of subjects may be needed.

In my opinion, consuming 3.4 g of FOS and inulin is very easy. Eating 30 g of chicory or 100 g of asparagus a day provides the same amount of FOS and inulin.[24] Additionally, two pomegranates contain about 3 g of inulin. You can modify your meals according to your preferences. However, it's important to note that some people in Europe may experience minor symptoms, such as abdominal pain and bloating, due to fructose malabsorption.

It's important to note that prebiotics are not a quick fix and take time to work. Studies have shown that it can take several weeks or even months of consistent consumption to see significant improvements in gut health and muscle function.

Overall, maintaining a healthy gut through the consumption of prebiotics and probiotics can lead to improved muscle function and strength in older adults. The evidence so far suggests that a healthy gut is an important factor in maintaining overall physical health and well-being.

You couldn't live without gut bacteria because they and the substances they make are important in helping you maintain muscle mass. Eating foods that can increase good gut bacteria and help maintain muscle strength and mass would be great. However, the best way right now to preserve our muscles is to exercise regularly because exercise is truly beneficial. Also, it's possible to gain muscle throughout your life, so it's important to keep going.

CHAPTER 14

Exercise is the key to a healthier and longer life

Exercise is not only effective in healing bones and muscles but is also known as the elixir of life, opposing sedentary lifestyles. It has been shown to help prevent and treat various diseases by boosting the immune system and increasing strength as we age.

There are four types of exercise: aerobic or cardio exercise, strength training exercise, flexibility exercise, and balance exercise. Exercise is considered as a physical movement that requires more energy and muscular effort than normal daily activities. These physical movements can be categorized into three levels:

Low level: This involves little physical movement, such as standing, sitting, walking slowly, washing dishes and doing laundry.

Intermediate level: This requires more physical movement and involves larger muscles, such as doing household chores that require lifting or reaching, brisk walking, dancing, yoga, golfing, jogging, and cycling.

Vigorous level: This requires continuous physical movement that engages larger muscles of the body, with a higher heart rate, such as running, swimming, basketball, aerobics, calisthenics, weight lifting, and activities like farming and athletics training.

Tips for making your exercise more effective

Exercise is good for you as it helps build your body's strength and prevent illnesses. However, getting effective exercise requires following these tips:

1) The exercise should be moderate to vigorous physical activity, and should involve more than just sitting and standing.

2) Morning exercise before breakfast is ideal, as it helps burn fat more effectively than other times.[1]

3) Incorporating high-intensity intervals into your workout can help you burn more calories and improve your fitness level. Try adding short bursts of high-intensity activity such as sprinting or jumping to your routine.

4) Aim for at least 7-8 hours of sleep each night to help your muscles repair and grow after exercise.

5) You should also aim to exercise at least three times a week.

6) Try to exercise at the same time each day to develop a routine. Exercising at the same time every day can synchronize cellular processes with the external environment for optimal health and performance.

7) Keep exercising regularly, even as you age.

The recommended exercise for beginners and older adults is cardio exercise. Cardio (heart) exercise refers to any exercise that raises your heart rate. Cardio exercise helps stimulate the metabolic and circulatory systems, build muscle mass, maintain hormonal balance, and increase bone density. Unlike strength training, cardio exercise doesn't focus on intense muscle exercise. Instead, it focuses on how the body moves to get the heart beating faster. Examples of cardio exercises include aerobics, brisk walking, jogging, and swimming.

Strength training involves the ability to force against one's weight or overcome resistance. It's suitable for people who want to strengthen their muscles and stimulate bone growth. For those who have lost muscle from being bedridden or in a wheelchair for a long time, cardio exercise by cycling four times a week for six weeks will help restore muscle mass, but it won't regain 100% of your muscle strength that you had before.[2] To recover and build muscle back to its original strength, strength training is necessary.

Exercise science has shown that just 2 minutes of vigorous exercise will cause the body to burn some amino acids for energy. After 15 minutes, the body converts glucose into energy, and an hour after exercise, the body breaks down glycogen stored in the liver for energy.[3] The body typically doesn't burn fat while exercising but often burns fat after the workout is over. However, there is an exception for people who run long distances, such as marathon runners. When a marathon runner's body glycogen is completely metabolized, the body will immediately burn stored fat for use during the run. Interestingly, the body literally burns fat while sleeping.[4] During an eight-hour sleep cycle, a person who weighs 70 kg might burn roughly 4 to 7 g of fat.

Some say older people should not work hard or lift heavy objects anymore, but this is incorrect. In fact, even just by moving and doing physical activities or exercises, older people can increase muscle strength and flexibility, and prevent muscle cramps and joint pain. However, if you are quite old, it's important to consider exercising according to your age and physical abilities.

Older adults are more prone to falls and injuries. Flexibility and balance exercises can help prevent falls and serious injuries. Activities such as yoga and walking on rough trails and terrain can help older people develop better balance and flexibility.

Don't let your muscles forget how to stretch and balance. Exercise not only improves your physical health, but also your overall well-being. It can be as beneficial as eating an apple a day, helping keep the doctor away.

***

How exercise reverses biological aging in mice and its potential impact on humans

Exercise can decrease disease progression, rejuvenate skin, and even slow down aging. In old mice with a sedentary lifestyle, their

224

bodies and health deteriorate. Similar to older humans, hair loss, baldness, and disease are common in old mice. However, after old mice were allowed to exercise on running wheels, they were in good health again. They regained muscle strength, had a healthy heart and sexual reproduction ability, and even had black, long, and shiny fur— signs of the reversal of biological aging. Scientists believe that if exercise can slow down aging and have a rejuvenating effect on mice, it could also be true in humans.

Exercise rejuvenates the skin of the aged

Did you know that the average person sheds 500 million skin cells, or 0.7-2 g of skin cells,[5] every day? This ongoing renewal process is necessary for healthy skin. In addition to eating antioxidant-rich foods, regular exercise can also help keep your skin looking youthful.

In order to explore how regular exercise can promote youthful skin, scientists compared the skin of people who regularly engaged in moderate to vigorous exercise (such as jogging, swimming, or cycling for at least 3 hours per week) to those who were mostly sedentary. They found that the exercisers, aged 40-65, had a thinner outer skin layer (stratum corneum) and a thicker deeper layer (dermis), which is similar to the skin of teenagers, despite their older age. In contrast, sedentary people of the same age had a thick stratum corneum and thin dermis, resembling the skin of an older person.[6]

This means that exercise can help rejuvenate even older skin. Another study found that regular exercise, such as cycling, can also help older adults aged 55-79 maintain a younger, healthier body than their inactive peers.[7] These findings suggest that exercise promotes cell renewal and may even reverse some aspects of aging in humans.

One possible reason for this is that exercise helps to improve circulation and oxygenation throughout the body, including the skin. When blood flow increases, it brings more nutrients and oxygen to the skin, which can help promote healthy skin cells and collagen production. Collagen is a protein that helps keep the skin firm and elastic, and its production decreases as we age. However, regular exercise may help slow down this process and even stimulate new collagen production.

Another way exercise can benefit the skin is by reducing stress. Stress can have a negative impact on the skin, leading to inflammation, breakouts, and other skin issues. Exercise has been shown to reduce stress levels and promote relaxation, which can help improve skin health.

Overall, regular exercise is a great way to improve not just physical fitness, but also skin health and appearance. Incorporating a variety of exercises, such as cardio, strength training, and flexibility exercises, can help maximize the benefits for both the body and skin.

Exercise increases FGF21—a longevity hormone

Exercise has a variety of health benefits, including lowering levels of harmful fats like triglycerides and LDL cholesterol, which in turn can reduce the risk of atherosclerosis and heart disease. Vigorous exercise can provide even greater benefits by increasing levels of FGF21, a hormone with anti-diabetic properties that has been referred to as a "longevity hormone" due to its association with increased life expectancy in some animal studies.[8,9] As we age, FGF21 levels were significantly lower in healthy older adults compared to younger adults, with a decline of approximately 30-40%. Studies on mice have shown that higher levels of FGF21 are associated with a 40% increase in life expectancy[10] Although running 8 km in 30 minutes like Olympic runners can increase the level of FGF21 in the blood by 200%, more moderate exercise can also positively affect FGF21 levels and improve health outcomes.[11]

Many people spend the majority of their day sitting or lying down, which can have negative health effects like reduced blood flow and muscle atrophy. Recent research suggests that even 11 minutes of exercise can be enough to counteract some of these negative effects.[12] Additionally, increasing daily exercise to 15 minutes may further decrease the risk of chronic diseases and premature death by

10%, while exercising for 60 minutes a day may provide even greater benefits.[13]

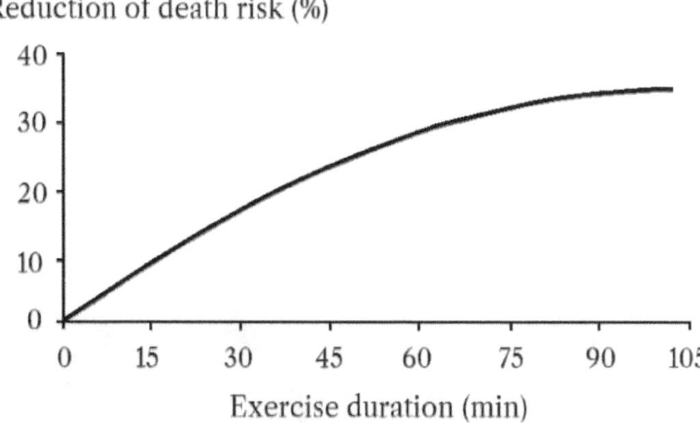

Just 15 minutes of daily exercise can reduce the risk of death by 10%. Even greater benefits can be achieved with longer exercise sessions: 30 minutes of exercise can reduce your risk of death by 20%, while 60 minutes can reduce the risk by 30%.[13]

Exercise does more than just make us stronger. It improves blood flow, reduces inflammation, and helps prevent cell damage. Regular workouts can also slow down the effects of illnesses and improve our bodies' ability to fix damaged cells. For example, being active often can help slow down type 2 diabetes. It can do this by improving how our bodies use insulin, helping to control blood sugar, and reducing belly fat.

The evidence is clear that exercise is an important part of a healthy lifestyle and has many benefits including improving cardiovascular and musculoskeletal health, rejuvenating skin, enhancing mental well-being, and extending lifespan. By making physical activity a regular part of our daily routines, you can enjoy these benefits and maintain good health and vitality throughout our lives.

Personally, if I can't go jogging or brisk walking, I often

perform burpees, a type of calisthenics exercise. I usually do around 20-30 repetitions at a time, which helps build my muscle strength and increases my heart rate to about 140 beats per minute, or about 85% of my maximum heart rate. I also include at least 20 rounds of 5 kg weight lifting in my daily routine.

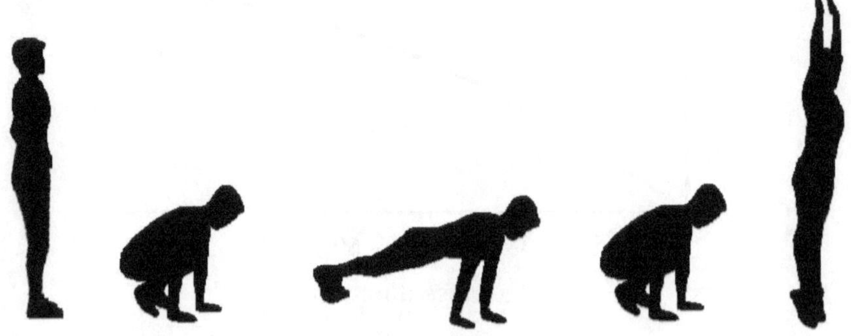

Burpee is a simple exercise that can help build muscle strength and improve cardiovascular fitness.

As we get older, our bodies find it harder to repair tissue, mostly due to a drop in stem cell function. However, adding regular exercise to our daily routine could boost the healing power of these cells, leading to better overall health and even slowing down the aging process. Exercise can help counteract to the natural decline in stem cell function. Plus, regular physical activity has been shown to increase blood flow through bone marrow and stimulate bone marrow stem cells into circulation and migrate to where they are needed. Once there, these stem cells can then transform into specific types of cells as required. Exercise can also help our brains to make new cells. This means that being active not only helps prevent illness but can also foster a healthier, younger-looking brain, as seen in people who consistently workout. Lastly, it's essential to choose age-appropriate activities that strengthen your heart, muscles, and bones. When done correctly, exercise can indeed be one of the best medicines for a person.

CHAPTER 15

Under stress, depression and lack of sleep

How much are you craving this food right now?[1]

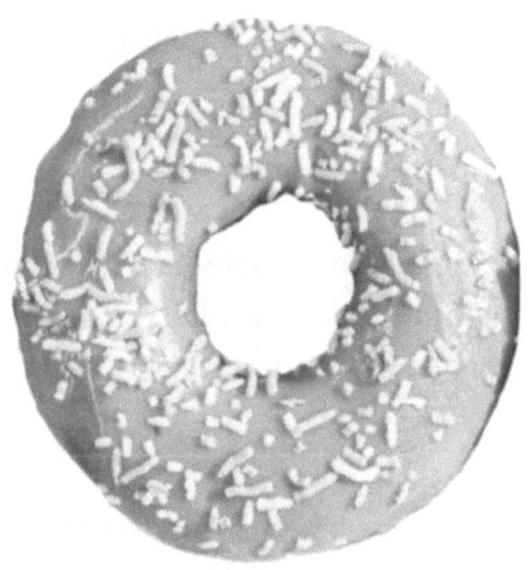

☐ Strongly do not want

☐ Somewhat do not want

☐ Somewhat want

☐ Strongly want

Scientists have known for a while that the less you sleep the better chance you say yes to fatty-starchy food. Why is this so? The reason is: lack of sleep increases hunger and appetite.

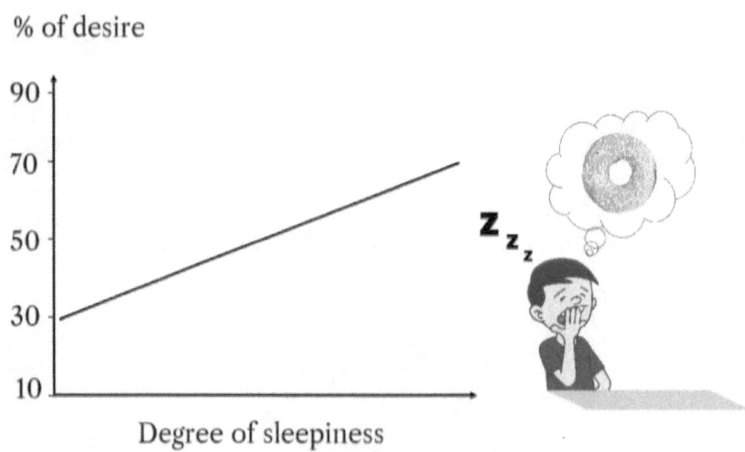

Lack of sleep causes people to crave high-calorie diets.[1] Surprisingly, your brain even values fatty-starchy foods more than foods containing only fat or starch.[2]

Usually, occasional lack of sleep may not cause much harm. But if you sleep lightly, awakening frequently throughout the night for days, weeks, months, or even years, then you may already be experiencing sleep deprivation. For adults, the optimal amount of sleep needed for good health is 7-8 hours a night.

There are several reasons why people don't get enough sleep. One of them is aging. As we grow older, sleep deprivation becomes a more significant problem. Falling asleep at the age of 65 is more challenging than it was at 20. As we age, our bodies undergo various changes that affect our sleep patterns. These changes include a reduction in the production of certain hormones, changes in our circadian rhythm, and an increase in chronic health conditions that can interfere with sleep. Additionally, as we age, our bodies may require less sleep, but many older adults have trouble falling and staying asleep, leading to sleep deprivation. Older adults may also have lifestyle factors such as medications, caffeine, and alcohol consumption that can interfere with sleep. Moreover, sleep disorders such as sleep apnea and restless leg syndrome become more common as we age, contributing to sleep deprivation.

Regarding the hormones that cause sleep deprivation, one of them is melatonin, which plays a crucial role in regulating our sleep-wake cycles. This hormone is released in response to darkness and helps promote sleep. However, as we age, our body's production of melatonin decreases, leading to difficulty falling asleep and staying asleep. Also, cortisol and adrenaline are hormones that can significantly contribute to sleep deprivation. Cortisol is the hormone responsible for regulating the body's response to stress, and its levels naturally fluctuate throughout the day, with higher levels in the morning and lower levels at night. However, if cortisol levels remain elevated at night due to chronic stress, it can interfere with the body's natural sleep-wake cycle, making it harder to fall asleep and stay asleep.

What's more, stress is a common cause of sleep problems. Whether it's stress from work, money, family, or health, everyone experiences stress. Stress is not easy to deal with, as it can have both physical and mental effects. We all have to face stress; thus, we should, at least, understand how our bodies respond to stress.

How the stress takes a toll on your body?

First of all, when the body is stressed, cortisol, a stress hormone, in the body increases even more than when exercising. Cortisol causes an increase in your heart rate, blood pressure, and levels of glucose in the bloodstream. It's part of your natural fight or flight response that prepares your larger muscles to fight a threat or to run away.

However, when the glucose in the blood has not been used when the body is stressed, the body tends to store excess sugar in the form of fat. It's even worse after the stress hormone is released, as it triggers the brain into high alert.[3] At bedtime, cortisol levels continue to rise, making it hard to fall asleep and leading to a restless night, which, the following day, results in a 28% increase of ghrelin, a hunger hormone. Ghrelin makes us feel hungry and directs us to eat more. But it's not over yet, because the stress hormone also reduces leptin, sometimes called a satiety hormone, by 18%, so instead of feeling more satiated after eating, you will feel hungrier. In addition, sleep deprivation causes some mechanical changes in the brain that regulate appetite and hunger. It makes you crave more high energy-dense foods. And over time, the stress hormone also triggers some cells to convert to fat cells and leads to obesity.[4,5,6,7] Both stress and lack of sleep are major contributors to the current obesity epidemic.

When stress strikes, we can't stop it. After the brain has already perceived a danger, it can't be undone. Therefore, you may overeat when you feel stressed. However, for some people, stress can make them lose their appetite and refrain from eating. Everyone reacts differently to stress. But if you have to live with stress for days or even months, your stress can become chronic. This is going to increase the levels of the hunger hormone in your body for years to come, even after the stressful event is over. It's for this reason that some people are unable to control their appetite and have to overeat for years after experiencing a traumatic event. And it's this chronic stress that causes fat cells to build up over time and leads to weight gain.

Chronic stress can also lead to long-term changes in the body. For example, high levels of cortisol over time can impair the immune system and increase the risk of developing heart disease. Apart from negatively impacting the quality of sleep, leading to tiredness and trouble focusing, stress can also raise the chance of accidents and injuries. Besides, too much stress can spark or make anxiety issues worse, causing symptoms like constant worry, restlessness, and moodiness. Elevated cortisol levels during stress can also decrease the production of serotonin and dopamine. This can cause feelings of deep sadness, lack of interest, tiredness, and low self-worth. To deal with stress, some people may use alcohol, nicotine, or drugs, which can lead to addiction and exacerbate mental health issues further.

It's essential to recognize the signs of excessive stress and take steps to manage it effectively. In some cases, professional help may be necessary to address the underlying causes of stress and provide support for managing mental health concerns. By reducing stress and getting enough sleep, you can mitigate its negative effects on our body and mind, and improve our overall quality of life.

A little bit of knowledge

Apart from DNA damage and hair loss, stress also causes collagen in the skin to reduce.[8] This is because high levels of cortisol in the body can break down the skin's collagen to make amino acids for energy, causing more wrinkles. The more wrinkles you have, the faster you age. Furthermore, upon consumption, sugars enter your body and can react with amino acids found in collagen and elastin, which help support the skin's deeper layer called the dermis. As you know, this creates advanced glycation end products, or AGEs. When sugar levels in the body are high, this process happens faster, and exposure to ultraviolet light from the sun makes this damage even more visible. Over time, the formation and buildup of AGEs in the skin lead to the appearance of wrinkles and less stretchy skin. People start to have AGEs in their skin when they're around 20 years old, but wrinkles become noticeable when they're about 35. Aging is a gradual process, and often, changes may not be noticeable until it's too late. In fact, the amount of AGEs increases by around 3 % each year, resulting in an increase of up to 50% by the time a person reaches 80 years old. If you notice fine lines and wrinkles, mainly around the eyes, mouth, and forehead, and age spots on your face and body, these tell-tale signs may indicate the presence of AGEs in your skin.

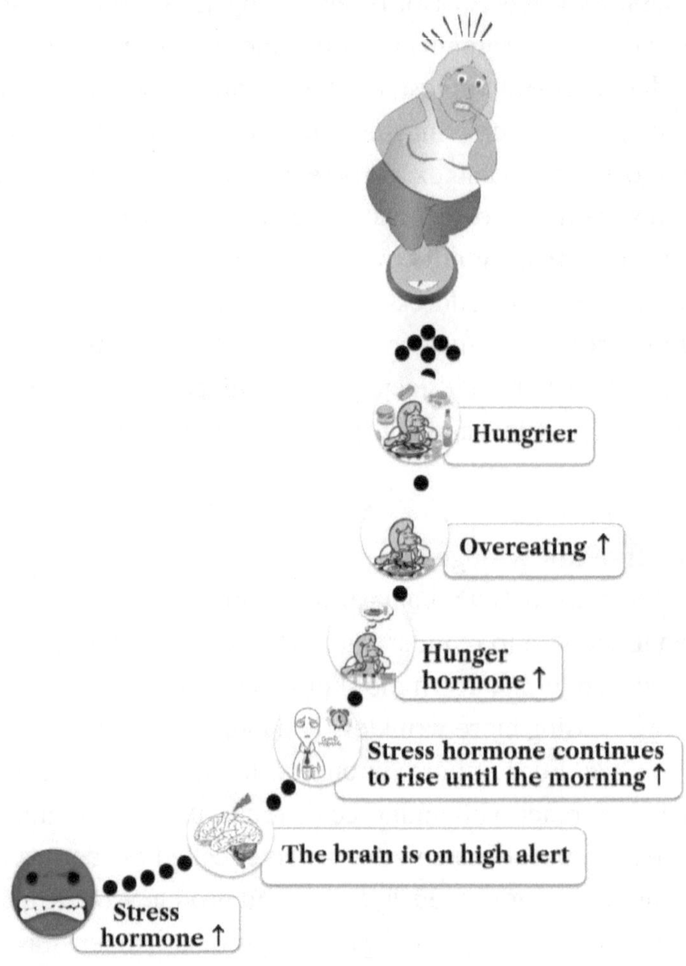

Stress takes a toll on your body.

Understanding sleep cycle

In general, sleep can be broadly divided into 4 stages:[9]

1. Lightest sleep is the first stage of the sleep cycle, lasting approximately 10-15 minutes. This stage is a transition between being awake and falling asleep.

2. Light sleep occurs when eye movements slow down, and muscles relax to enter deeper sleep. This stage lasts no more than 1 hour.

3. Deep sleep is the stage where eye movements and muscle activity cease, while breathing and heartbeat slow down. During this stage, growth hormone is released, promoting cell repair, regeneration, muscle growth, and bone building. Immune proteins are also released to fight infections if necessary. Deep sleep helps clear toxins from the brain and typically lasts about 2-4 hours per night.

4. REM (rapid eye movement) sleep, also called "dream sleep," is characterized by rapid eye movements and dreams lasting 5-35 minutes. REM sleep occurs in cycles, with the first cycle lasting about 10 minutes and subsequent cycles increasing in length, potentially up to an hour. In this stage, the brain is active, but the body is paralyzed. REM sleep is crucial for memory formation, learning, and stress recovery. The longer the REM stage, the better the recovery from stress. REM sleep may last 2-3 hours per night, but it tends to be shorter for elderly individuals.

Your sleep and body clock

The deep sleep is the most important sleep phase for repairing any tissues and cells of your body. That is between 11 PM to 3 AM, if you can sleep before midnight. During this time, the body regenerates, repairs itself, and builds muscles and bones. During deep sleep, the immune system also works to fight infection. Besides, in this sleep phase, there is less blood in the brain. It means that the liquid around your brain and spinal cord can flow in to fill the space and helps to carry away toxins trapped in your brain. This allows you to clear your mind and wake up with a clear head in the morning. Deep sleep typically lasts around 4-5 hours for younger individuals, but decreases as one ages. This is why achieving 4-5 hours of deep sleep for older people could have anti-aging effects.

REM sleep is associated with brain development, especially in infants and young children, who spend a lot of their sleeping time in this phase. This stage is crucial for the growth and maturation of the central nervous system. Moreover, REM sleep is thought to help with creativity, as it lets the brain make new connections between different ideas, leading to unique and inventive thoughts. While in REM sleep, our brains refill important chemicals like serotonin and dopamine, which are vital for mood regulation, motivation, and overall cognitive function. REM sleep also helps us get better at physical skills and coordination by strengthening muscle memory. REM sleep diminishes with age and could be associated with frailty in the elderly. By maintaining 2 hours of REM sleep per night as you age, you may be able to lead a healthier life.

The sleep-wake mechanism and the functioning of cellular processes in humans and other organisms are governed by cycles known as "biological clocks" or "circadian rhythms." These daily cycles control nearly 80% of the genes in the human body, playing a vital role in maintaining our overall well-being.

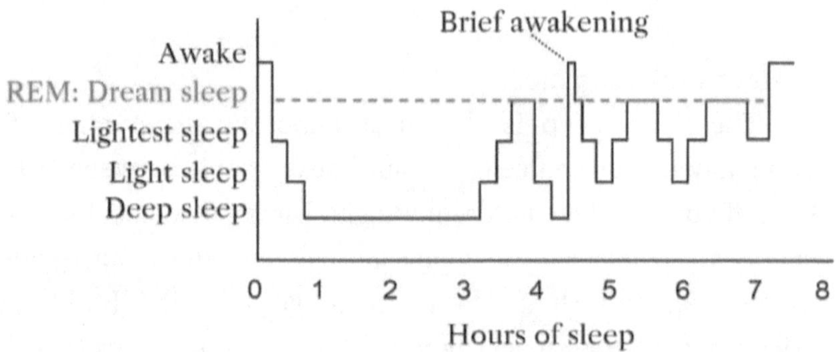

There are 4 stages in the sleep cycle: 3 stages of non-REM sleep and an REM stage. Stage 1 is the lightest sleep, the period just before actually falling asleep. In Stage 2, light sleep, the heartbeat and breathing gradually slow down, and eye movement stops. Stage 3 is the deepest state of sleep, during which growth hormone is released and works to restore and rebuild the body. The rapid eye movement (REM) stage, also known as dream sleep, is important for stress recovery and the development of cognitive abilities.

Tuning in to your circadian symphony

Circadian rhythms regulate various physiological processes, such as metabolism, hormone secretion, body temperature, and cognitive function. These rhythms are influenced by external factors like social cues and light exposure, as well as internal factors such as hormonal fluctuations.

For instance, at night, light—especially blue light—can suppress the body's production of melatonin. This disrupts the biological clock, either slowing it down or speeding it up, and increases the risk for health implications.[10] It's possible that light might trick your body into thinking it's daytime. Therefore, while sleeping, you should avoid having the light on, and try to prevent light from entering your room.

There is a pile of evidence showing that blue light can also disrupt the biological clock. One study, investigating iPad use before sleep, found that the blue light from the device reduces melatonin and delays the body clock by 1.5 hours.[11] Consequently, this can cause insomnia when going to bed. Insomnia is common in the older population, with up to 50% of older adults experiencing poor sleep.[12]

Why is the human body so sensitive to blue light? The answer lies in the presence of cryptochromes—a blue-light sensitive pigment in our bodies. Cryptochromes control the circadian clock ticking in your body in a light-dependent manner. So, if you're looking at a tablet or phone screen with blue light before bedtime for a long time, your body thinks it's daytime. That's why it's tough for you to sleep. This evidence should be enough to discourage you from using your tablet or mobile phone at least an hour before bed.

Hormones like melatonin, cortisol, and insulin are closely linked to the body's internal clock and crucial in maintaining its rhythm. Melatonin production increases when it gets dark, signaling the body to prepare for sleep. As daylight approaches, melatonin levels decrease, promoting wakefulness. Cortisol helps maintain alertness and energy levels during the day, while its decline in the evening allows the body to relax and prepare for sleep. Disruptions in cortisol secretion can lead to sleep disturbances and affect the biological clock. Insulin is a hormone that regulates blood sugar levels and plays a role in the circadian rhythm. Insulin sensitivity and secretion follow a daily pattern, with increased sensitivity in the morning and decreased sensitivity at night. This pattern helps maintain stable blood sugar levels throughout the day and night.

At the end of the day, you might feel exhausted because your body is preparing for rest and repair during sleep. Around 9 pm is the average time our bodies produce melatonin, a hormone that makes us feel sleepy. However, your body can release melatonin before or after that, depending on your age. For men and women aged 18-32, melatonin usually secretes around 11 pm and drops around 8:30 am. The timing of melatonin release may also be influenced by your sleeping habits. For older people aged 59-75, melatonin is secreted around 10 pm and decreases around 7:30 am.[15,16] This is why older individuals tend to go to bed earlier and have shorter sleep periods and longer wake periods.

Our cortisol levels follow a diurnal rhythm, peaking in the morning around 8-9 am and gradually decreasing throughout the day, reaching their lowest point at midnight.[9] This pattern is important for maintaining a healthy sleep-wake cycle and ensuring that we have enough energy during the day.

Testosterone is a hormone mainly produced in the testicles in men and ovaries in women. It plays a crucial role in developing and maintaining muscle mass, bone density, and sex drive. Additionally, testosterone levels follow a diurnal rhythm, with the highest levels occurring in the morning and gradually decreasing throughout the day. Like cortisol, testosterone levels are also affected by sleep, with sleep deprivation leading to decreased testosterone levels. In fact, if you had insufficient sleep last night, your testosterone levels could drop to the same level as someone 15 years older than you.

Around 2 am, the leptin hormone made by fat cells peaks. High leptin levels make you feel full, while low levels make you feel hungry. Leptin levels typically follow a circadian rhythm. Lack of sleep or poor sleep can disrupt leptin levels, leading to more hunger and cravings, which may cause weight gain or trouble losing weight. High leptin levels, often seen in obesity, are associated with insulin resistance, which can contribute to the development of type 2 diabetes.

The biological clock also affects physical and mental performance. For instance, muscle strength follows a 24-hour cycle, with the best performance often seen in late afternoon or early evening. This matches the natural rise in body heat and hormones like cortisol and testosterone, which boost muscle function. Alertness and thinking ability also have a rhythm, with high levels usually during daytime, especially in late morning and early afternoon. Motor skills often peak in the late afternoon or early evening, as higher body temperature and hormone levels help nerve signals and muscle work.

What's more, the body's biological clock influences other physiological parameters, such as blood pressure, which follows a diurnal rhythm. During daytime, our blood pressure is typically higher because our bodies are more active, demanding greater blood flow to muscles and organs. As we get ready for sleep, our blood pressure starts to decrease, reaching its lowest point during the night. Normally, blood pressure falls by about 10-20% during sleep. This pattern, known as the "dipping" phenomenon, signifies a healthy circadian rhythm.[9]

However, disruptions in our sleep-wake cycle, like irregular sleep patterns or sleep deprivation, can result in abnormal blood pressure patterns. For instance, people who work night shifts or have inconsistent sleep schedules might experience a "reversed dipping" pattern. In this case, their blood pressure stays high at night, which increases their risk of serious diseases such as atherosclerosis, heart disease, stroke, and kidney disease. Maintaining a regular sleep schedule and prioritizing good sleep hygiene can help prevent these disruptions and promote a healthier circadian rhythm, ultimately reducing the risk of adverse health outcomes.

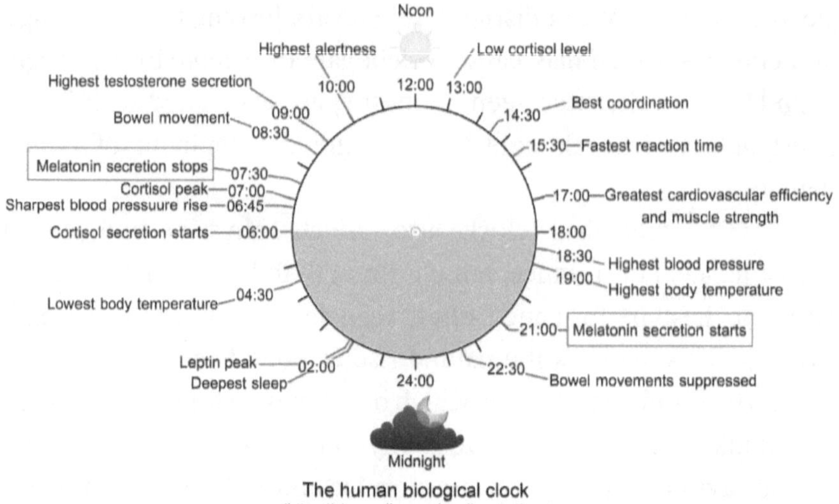

The human biological clock
(https://nigms.nih.gov.circadian-rhythms)

As adults, you need 7-8 hours of sleep per night for a healthy lifespan.[13] If you sleep less or more than 7-8 hours, you can increase your risk of death. That is because it may involve impaired immune function, hormonal imbalances, cardiovascular health, metabolic health, and mental health. Additionally, you should aim to sleep and wake up at the same time every day. This will help improve sleep quality, regulate your circadian rhythm, and ensure you go through each day feeling energized.

Death by sleep deprivation

If you don't get enough quality sleep at night, you are more likely to get sick than those who do. Lack of sleep can also make you more forgetful and impair brain functions.

Insufficient sleep disrupts the blood-brain barrier, a protective barrier that determines which substances can and can't enter or exit the brain. It shields the brain from bacterial and viral infections. The blood-brain barrier permits small molecules like oxygen, carbon dioxide, hormones, glucose, amino acids, and alcohol to cross from the bloodstream into the brain. However, when the blood-brain barrier becomes disrupted, the transport of substances into and out of the brain is also affected. This disruption can even damage the blood-brain barrier and cause neurodegenerative diseases involving the death of certain brain regions.[17,18]

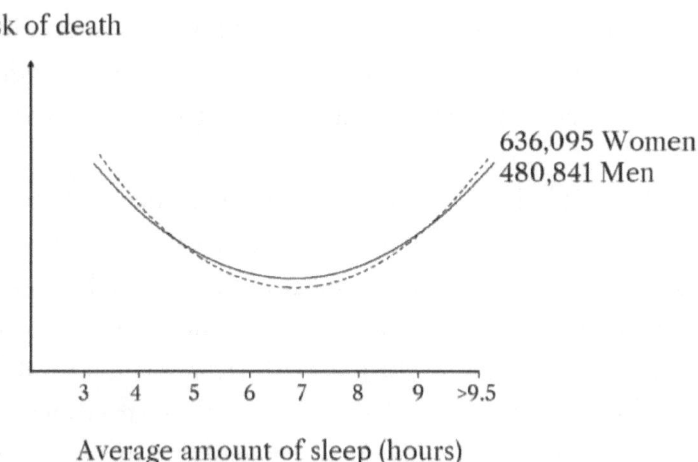

In this U-shaped curve, people who sleep less than 7 hours or more than 8 hours have an increased risk of death compared to those who sleep 7-8 hours per day.[13,14]

Moreover, lack of sleep increases the accumulation of proteins called "beta-amyloid" in the brain. When beta-amyloid accumulates and clumps together, it damages the brain, leading to dementia and Alzheimer's disease. Just one sleepless night can increase beta-amyloid levels in your brain by 30%, which is comparable to levels seen in people at very high risk for dementia and Alzheimer's disease.[19,20]

Some people think that if they had a bad night's sleep the night before, they can catch up on the sleep they lost the next night. However, science doesn't support this idea. If you sleep less than 7 hours one night and then sleep 10 hours two nights later, you can't fully recover from the damage done to memory performance and some brain connectivity.[22] Frequent sleep deprivation slowly damages your brain, and it may take more than 2 nights to eliminate the buildup of beta-amyloid in the brain and for the brain to recover completely.

Sleep affects your muscles too. On one hand, lack of sleep can cause you to lose muscle mass instead of body fat when dieting; on the other hand, sleeping too much can lower serotonin production, a mood-boosting chemical, and cause you to gain 1.5 kg of weight per year.[23]

Lack of sleep can also cause or worsen atherosclerosis. Insufficient sleep increases the number of white blood cells in the blood, leading to inflammation similar to that caused by an infection. Although inflammation typically lasts a few hours or days, prolonged inflammation can become chronic. This inflammation resulting from lack of sleep can cause large lesions or cracks on artery walls.[24]

In some cases, sleeplessness can lead to death. A famous study in 1989 showed that, at least in animals, a total lack of sleep for 11 days could result in death.[25] But what happens if humans don't sleep for 11 days? In 1965, a 17-year-old boy named Randy Gardner managed to stay awake for that long.[26] However, I found mixed answers when researching this topic. In 2012, a 26-year-old Chinese man reportedly died from sleep deprivation after staying awake for 11 days to watch every football game in the European Championship.[27] The difference between these two cases may be related to the fact that the Chinese man was not physically fit, drank alcohol, and smoked, unlike Randy Gardner.

As mentioned above, health problems such as Alzheimer's, dementia, atherosclerosis, and obesity can partly result from a misaligned sleep-wake cycle with the day-night cycle. Thus, you need to synchronize your sleep-wake cycle with your environment to maintain a healthy, disease-free life.

***

How to reset your biological clock

Your body is designed to sleep at night and be awake during the day. However, in today's era of globalization, many people work night shifts, consequently disrupting their biological clocks. People working at night are likely to have poorer health than those who work during regular hours. Night shift work can also lead to an increased risk of developing chronic diseases such as breast cancer, heart disease, obesity, and Alzheimer's.[28]

Examples of those who work the night shift include doctors, nurses, security guards, 24-hour convenience store workers, and factory workers. This also applies to people with jet lag; traveling across time zones can make them sick. Jet lag can cause daytime fatigue, anxiety, loss of focus, and problems in the digestive and cardiovascular systems. Typically, if you travel 12 hours across time zones, you would need at least 12 days to adjust to the new time zone because you can only bring the biological clock back to its ideal state a little bit each day.

In fact, the human biological clock is constantly adjusting to changing social and work activities. For example, on workdays, you go to bed early to get a head start on the next day's tasks, but on weekends, you might go to bed and wake up late. Your body's circadian clock often adjusts on a daily basis. A 2018 study revealed that, on average, Americans experience about 75 minutes of social jet lag every day.[29] Frequent changes in daily bedtime and wake-up time due to social jet lag cause confusion in the biological clock. This leads the body to continuously adjust its circadian rhythm. Inconsistent bedtimes and wake-up times also negatively affect overall health.

If your biological clock falls out of sync, here are some tips that may help you realign your biological rhythms faster and improve your sleep:

A promising 2008 study done on mice found that the sleep-wake cycle could be reset by fasting. While the study has only been applied to mice thus far, researchers suggest that the implications for travelers are promising. The author, Clifford Saper at Harvard

Medical School, advised that fasting for about 16 hours may help adjust your body clock to the new time zone more quickly.[30] Plus, this 16-hour fasting can be done easily by, for instance, eating your dinner around 4 pm and then breakfast at 8 am the next day. Another equally important fact is meal timing play a vital role in synchronizing your circadian rhythms as well.[31] That is because food can turn on the body clock. Especially, eating late can shift your internal clock and change sleep patterns. You should be aware of this too.

Another way to reset your biological clock may involve medicinal mushrooms. A new study in 2020 revealed that the circadian rhythm can be reset with cordycepin, a substance found in fungi called *Cordyceps sinensis* and *C. militaris*. Mice with jet lag were fed cordycepin (15 or 45 mg per kg of body weight), allowing them to regain their circadian rhythms within 4 days. In contrast, it took 8 days for the mice that didn't eat cordycepin to readjust their circadian rhythms. This study shows that cordycepin shortens the time needed to readjust the circadian rhythm by half and enables subjects to recover faster. How does cordycepin molecularly affect the circadian rhythm? The answer is that cordycepin can regulate the switching on and off of genes that govern the circadian rhythm, helping to bring it back to an ideal state.[32]

The dose of 15 mg cordycepin used in mice would be the equivalent dose of 85 mg in humans. Cordycepin is currently readily available from cultivated *C. militaris*. A gram of *C. militaris* contains about 2.6 mg of cordycepin.[33] Thus, if 85 mg of cordycepin were needed, approximately 33 g of *C. militaris* would have to be consumed. However, this amount of *C. militaris* is excessive. It would be prudent to wait for outcomes from human research. If you hasten to consume this fungus now, it may enhance male sexual function[34] instead of resetting your biological clock.

In fact, the best way to reset your biological clock is by getting more sunshine and exercising in the morning. This is because sunlight signals the brain to reduce melatonin production, which can stimulate changes in the body's biological clock.[35] Exposure to sunlight in the morning causes your biological clock to shift to an earlier time.

Can turmeric help treat depression?

Everyone experiences stress from time to time, but if you aren't coping with stress well, chronic stress could lead to anxiety and depression.

Several studies indicate that curcumin can help treat depression. In humans, studies show that taking 1,000-1,500 mg of curcumin a day for 3-4 months reduces symptoms of anxiety and depression.[36,37,38] What's more, one study found that taking 1,000 mg of curcumin for 6 weeks is as effective as 20 mg of Prozac in treating depression.[39] Especially for male volunteers, taking curcumin significantly reduced symptoms of anxiety and depression.

As the above studies demonstrate, curcumin can be used to reduce symptoms of anxiety and depression. However, don't forget that curcumin is poorly absorbed and mostly degraded in the liver. This problem can be solved by taking curcumin together with 20 mg of piperine, which can increase curcumin's bioavailability and lengthen its lifespan by 1 hour.[40] Turmeric varieties from the south of Thailand contain almost 10% curcumin.[41] Intake of 1,000-2,000 mg of turmeric powder together with 5-7 black peppercorns and good fat may be equivalent to the amount of curcumin used in clinical trials.

Art of natural remedy

Have you ever pondered why being in nature brings us so much joy? In Japan, there is a concept called "Shinrin-yoku," which translates to "forest bathing." The Japanese term "shinrin" means "forest," while "yoku" refers to "bath." Together, they describe immersing oneself in the calming atmosphere of a forest.

Spending just 2 hours immersed in nature has been scientifically proven to significantly lower blood pressure and improve people's mood.[42] The reason forest bathing can enhance your mood is that it substantially reduces levels of the stress hormone cortisol.[43] Moreover, spending at least 2 hours per week walking or jogging in a park can help you maintain physical and mental fitness.[44] I believe that we, as human beings, need to connect with nature for these beneficial reasons. Therefore, when you have free time to spend with your loved ones, consider immersing yourselves in nature and trees. The healing power of the forest can alleviate stress, anxiety, and depression.

Now, let's consider people with depression. What do they think is the best stress reliever for them? A survey of 11,443 people worldwide by the health information website, CureTogether, reveals that exercise is the most effective way to treat depression, followed by spending time with a pet, playing outside, and getting a good night's sleep. In other words, participants in this online community found these treatments more effective than vitamins, dietary supplements, and even antidepressant medications.[45]

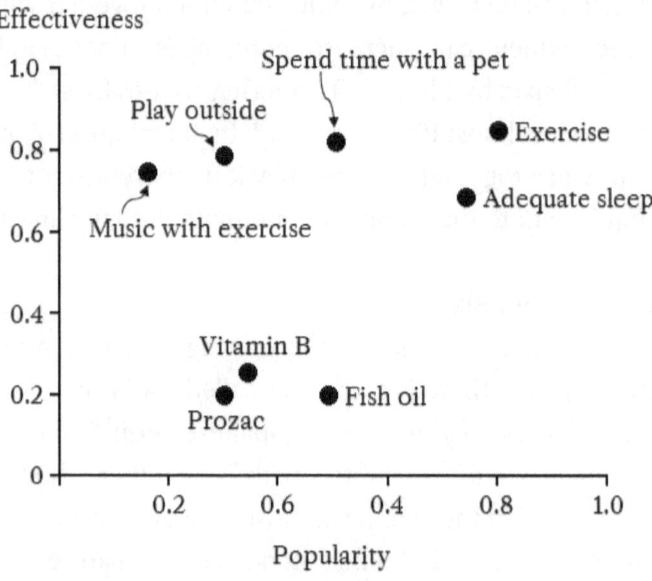

Top treatments for depression according to 11,443 patients at an online community called CureTogether.[45]

This comes as positive news for older adults, as antidepressants may not always be the best choice. Most commonly prescribed antidepressants are associated with adverse outcomes such as stroke, falls, fractures, and can even increase the risk of suicide.

In fact, people's intuition about exercise is accurate, as it can genuinely reduce stress, particularly in older adults. Cardio exercises like aerobics, brisk walking, jogging, cycling, and swimming, 150 minutes per week, can indeed lower stress hormone levels.[46] Why do people feel good after exercising? Not only does exercise increase endorphin levels, but it also boosts serotonin production. Both endorphins and serotonin are well-known as "happy hormones" that promote joy and happiness.

Besides, good news for people already engaging in cardio exercise: if you are under stress, you will cope with it more effectively and recover from stressful events more quickly than those who don't exercise.[47] This is because regular exercise acts like a stress immunization, reducing levels of stress hormones and protecting you from mental ailments. Thus, exercise can help both in treating depression and preventing stress. Cardio exercise is especially beneficial for depression. Some experts recommend engaging in 20 to 30 minutes of cardio exercise, three or more days a week. The more you exercise, the better you can manage your depression and stress. A healthy long life begins in nature or at the gym. Some experts also suggest that joining a group fitness class can be a great way to start.

How *Lactobacillus* and *Bifidobacterium* probiotics help improve depression

Depression is a major public health problem and is linked to the burden of disease. About 1 in 5 Americans aged 65 or older is affected by depression. Depression is also a potential adverse effect of the use of prescription drugs, such as anti-allergy drugs, medications for chest pain, and antihypertensive drugs. One in three

Americans uses these drugs on a daily basis.[48] This might be another reason why young Americans' health begins to decline at the age of 27. In 2020, the WHO reported that globally, more than 264 million people of all ages suffer from depression.[49] Studies also confirm that depression can shorten life.

However, scientific evidence indicates that not only could probiotics help you live longer, but they may also help with depression. Every study on the effect of probiotics on depression suggests that *Lactobacillus* and *Bifidobacterium* may help reduce depression.[50] One study in 2016, like several earlier studies, indicates that the intake of 100 g of probiotic yogurt per day or one probiotic capsule containing *Lactobacillus* can reduce depression.[51] Furthermore, people have reported feeling happier after consuming products like *Lactobacillus*-fermented milk, milk containing *Lactobacillus*, and supplements with *Lactobacillus* and/or *Bifidobacterium*.[52] Scientists believe that depression can be reversed by *Lactobacillus* and *Bifidobacterium*. If you aren't depressed, you will be happy. Happiness leads to a healthier life.

Melatonin, tryptophan and bell pepper for sleep

Melatonin is a hormone that promotes good sleep. Your melatonin level is related to your happiness level as well. Melatonin even plays a role in anxiety and depression. This is where antidepressants come into play, as they are used to help increase melatonin levels in the blood.

Did you know that teenagers with depression often have lower melatonin levels during sleep compared to their healthy counterparts?[53] In our body, it has a system that helps handle stress, and when someone is depressed, this system might not work as it should. This can lead to changes in the production of melatonin. Depression also often goes hand in hand with sleep problems, like having trouble falling asleep or not having a regular sleep schedule. These issues can cause the release of melatonin to become uneven and lead to lower amounts of melatonin during sleep.

Even though research on melatonin and emotional problems is ongoing, studies have suggested a connection between low melatonin levels and conditions like cancer and type 2 diabetes.[54,55] Both cancer and type 2 diabetes can lead to sleep disturbances, which may disrupt the normal production of melatonin. Pain, discomfort, and anxiety associated with cancer, as well as sleep apnea and restless leg syndrome, which are common in people with type 2 diabetes, can contribute to disrupted sleep patterns. Type 2 diabetes involves insulin resistance, which can influence the way the body processes tryptophan, a vital amino acid needed for making melatonin. This may potentially alter melatonin production.

In fact, reduced melatonin secretion during sleep may be linked to a lack of the amino acid tryptophan.[56] Our bodies can produce melatonin using tryptophan as a starting material. So, could taking tryptophan supplements help increase melatonin secretion during sleep?

Melatonin (pg/mL)

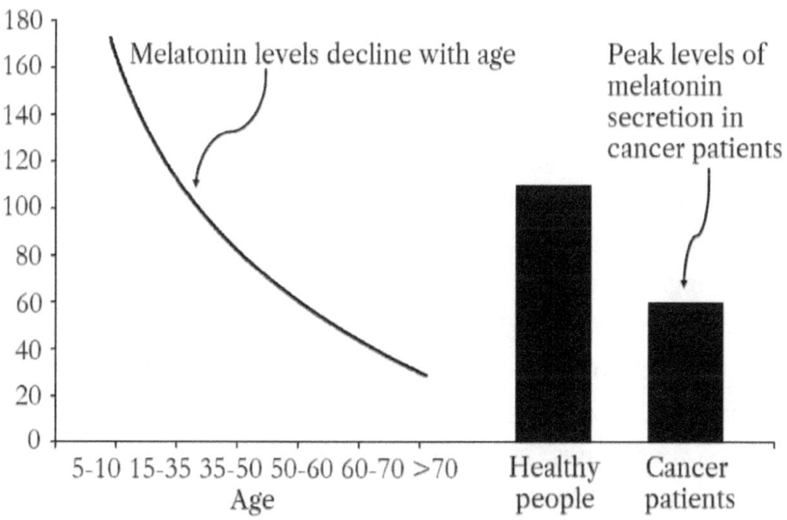

Melatonin levels naturally decline as a person ages. Some chronic diseases, such as cancer and type 2 diabetes, are associated with low melatonin levels at night.[54,55,]

The body produces melatonin from tryptophan, and once it's made, melatonin is immediately released into the bloodstream. In animal models, melatonin levels in the blood are elevated after feeding tryptophan. In humans, taking a tryptophan supplement can't increase melatonin secretion at night, but eating natural foods rich in tryptophan, such as soybeans, eggs, and bananas can. [57,58,59,60]

Among natural foods, red bell pepper has the highest tryptophan content, containing up to 7,000 mg of tryptophan per 100 g. In my experience, red bell pepper is more effective than bananas at improving sleep quality. For me, consuming a 1/4 of a red bell pepper an hour before bed works like a sleeping pill.

How melatonin and cherries can help you get a good night's rest

As mentioned before, as you grow older, your body produces 50% less melatonin, which may contribute to sleeplessness in older people. In individuals with cancer and type 2 diabetes, their bodies also produce 50% less melatonin.[54,55] People who work night shifts produce 33% less melatonin as well.[61]

When people experience insomnia, many of them turn to melatonin to achieve better-quality sleep. Some individuals with jet lag and those who work rotating shifts also take melatonin, which can help reset the biological clock and induce deep sleep.[62]

Recommended oral doses of melatonin range from 0.5 to 5 mg. In fact, a dose of 0.5 mg melatonin is nearly as effective as a dose of 5.0 mg. A bedtime dose of 0.5 mg melatonin may help you stay asleep longer at night.[63] However, if you take more than 3 mg of melatonin, it could cause adverse reactions, such as headaches and dizziness after waking up. In your body, excessive melatonin can affect other genes, as melatonin interacts with different cellular processes. What's worse, if you consume too much melatonin, it may even prevent your body from making it on its own. Therefore, you should use melatonin occasionally and consult your doctor before taking melatonin at a dosage of 3 mg or more.

On average, about 33% of melatonin is absorbed in the intestines, and it takes effect within the first 45 minutes. Melatonin is best taken no more than 30 minutes before bedtime. It's important to note that melatonin acts as an antagonist to the hormone cortisol. Normally, the body releases the most cortisol in the morning to provide energy for the day ahead. Taking melatonin at other times of the day will suppress cortisol's activity.

Melatonin can also be found in natural foods. It's found in the highest concentrations in cherry fruits and leaves. In nature, melatonin may protect cherries from the damaging effects of free radicals caused by UV rays. The highest melatonin amounts are found in Montmorency or tart cherries, a cherry cultivar commonly grown in Europe, the United States, and Canada. One hundred grams of Montmorency tart cherries contain 1.3 mg of melatonin.[64] One clinical study found that consuming 30 ml, or an ounce, of tart cherry juice concentrate twice daily can significantly increase melatonin in people's blood.[65] In this study, an ounce of tart cherry juice concentrate, equivalent to about 100 cherries, contains only about 42 mcg of melatonin. The reduced melatonin in this cherry juice concentrate may be due to food processing during its production.

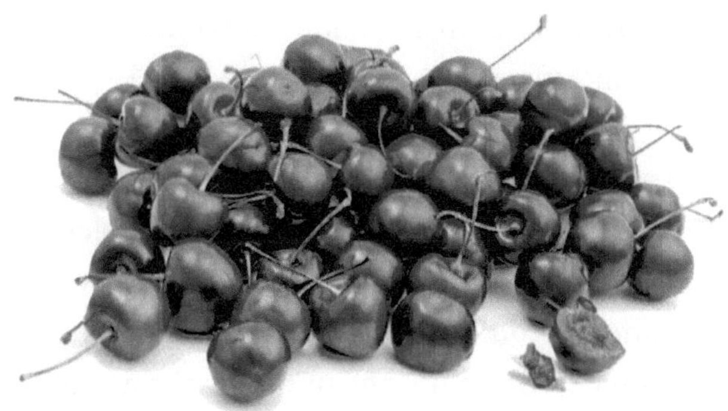

One hundred grams of Montmorency tart cherries contain 1.3 mg of melatonin, which can increase circulating melatonin levels and may help you achieve a good night's sleep.[64,65]

Due to their demonstrated advantages, I propose consuming around 200 g of Montmorency tart cherries, which boast a higher melatonin concentration. When eaten fresh, this serving size is equivalent to roughly 2.6 mg of melatonin. Keep in mind that whole foods are generally superior to supplements.

There is 400 times more melatonin in the intestines than in the brain

Believe it or not, your gut is the most important source of melatonin production; moreover, over 90% of serotonin is also formed in your gut.

In the human gut, enteroendocrine cells—specialized epithelial cells found within the digestive tract—are responsible for producing most of the melatonin in the body. The amount of melatonin in the intestines is 400 times higher than that in the brain and 100 times higher than that in the bloodstream.[66]

However, melatonin secreted from the gut is controlled by the food you eat—not by the biological clock, as is the case for melatonin produced by the pineal gland in the brain. Melatonin can also regulate gut bacteria, and vice versa. Over time, consuming melatonin-rich foods may contribute to a balanced gut microbiome, foster improved communication between the gut and brain, and promote better overall health and bodily functions, while also helping to regulate your internal body clock.

How exercise can boost dopamine and improve your Zzz's

Have you ever wondered why your REM sleep shortens as you get closer to your 50s? As people age, factors such as brain changes, modified brain chemicals, changes in neurotransmitter levels like dopamine, serotonin, and norepinephrine, disrupted sleep, and shifts in sleep cycles can shorten REM sleep.

Did you know that exercise can enhance your sleep? Studies show that exercise can improve the quality and duration of REM sleep. This improvement is due not only to increased levels of serotonin and norepinephrine but also to the increase in dopamine in the brain. Dopamine is an important chemical that helps start REM sleep. When you sleep, your brain moves from non-REM to REM sleep, and during this change, dopamine levels temporarily go up. This increase in dopamine is believed to help initiate the REM sleep stage. This stage is essential, as it plays a major role in a restorative sleep experience, crucial for keeping our well-being and everyday function in check. Thus, incorporating exercise to boost REM sleep as you age is important. Engaging in regular physical activities, such as walking, running, swimming, or cycling, can't only increase your dopamine levels but also promote longer REM sleep.

Additionally, other essential methods to boost dopamine levels and enhance REM sleep include sunlight exposure and moderating alcohol and caffeine intake. Regular exposure to natural sunlight is crucial for regulating dopamine levels and maintaining a healthy sleep-wake cycle. Aim for at least 15 minutes of sunlight exposure daily to support dopamine production and improve sleep quality.

Excessive consumption of alcohol or caffeine can disrupt dopamine production and negatively impact sleep quality. Limit your intake, especially in the evening hours.

To sum up, I believe that the suggestions in this chapter will contribute to your restful night's sleep, enabling you to lead a life unburdened by stress, anxiety, and depression, and ultimately promoting a longer lifespan. Sleep plays a crucial role in your overall health and well-being. It's important to remember that while younger individuals may need 9 or more hours of sleep, adults should aim for a minimum of 7-8 hours of sleep each night. The ideal sleep duration for a longer lifespan tends to align with these numbers.

Part 4

Cell Regeneration, Slowing Down Aging and Healthy Eating Forever

Chapter 16 Biohacking your body to rejuvenate old cells and slow down aging

Chapter 17 Eat less and live longer

Chapter 18 Design your own healthy plates

CHAPTER 16

Biohacking your body to rejuvenate old cells and slow down aging

One day, I found out that my LG top load washer was not working properly. I searched for the error code on Google and learned that "OE" indicated a problem with the drain pump. Later that morning, I visited the nearest electrical appliance store and bought a new drain motor to replace the faulty one.

When a washer's drain motor is broken, we can disassemble it and find a new one for replacement. However, when it comes to human organs, obtaining a replacement is not as simple. In the medical field, the process of replacing body parts is known as "organ transplant." This procedure is more complex than replacing machinery parts, as organs are usually transplanted to patients in critical need, and the donor's organs must be compatible with the recipient's blood and tissue types. Nevertheless, there are a couple of components in the human body that can be easily replaced or transferred with minimal adverse effects or immune system rejection, such as bone marrow and blood.

As scientific advancements continue, researchers believe that it's possible to slow down aging. Various treatments for extending life are already available. One such treatment involves using young blood plasma—the liquid portion separated from whole blood—to combat aging. Another way is biohacking, where you make changes to your body to improve how it works, boost your health, and maybe live longer. The idea of life extension is gaining popularity these days, with high-profile billionaires such as Jeff Bezos of Amazon and Larry Page, co-founder of Google, putting money into new medical companies that want to find ways to extend life. Their obsession with longevity may stem from the idea that in the future, time will become a more valuable asset than money. However, as we see today, the desire to lead a healthier and longer life is not limited to billionaires but is shared by an increasing number of people.

Nourishing your way to a longer and healthier life

Upon discussing the path to a long, disease-free life, it's fascinating to ponder whether nature might also intend for us to live beyond an average lifespan, much like Jeanne Calment. Otherwise, it could seem unfair for creatures like the immortal jellyfish to enjoy eternal life while we humans barely reach a century. Some scientists and futurists even suggest that human immortality may be attainable within the next decade of the 21st century. If not, why would body's cells, tissues, and organs continuously work together to maintain a favorable internal environment, prolonging our lives? Our bodies possess remarkable abilities to repair damage and prevent cells from aging, but we can't yet fully harness these capabilities. At some point in our lives, these abilities cease, and the aging process begins as growth comes to a halt.

Throughout this book, you have learned about various aspects of aging, age-related diseases, anti-aging foods, and the use of senolytics to delay illnesses and slow down aging. As numerous studies indicate, we can reduce the risk of developing diseases, enhance the body's ability to repair itself, improve health, decelerate aging, and extend lifespan. To achieve a healthy and long life, one must rely on scientific advancements. In this chapter, you'll discover research-backed biohacking techniques to delay illnesses and nutritionally slow down the aging process.

***

Step 1: Get rid of the senescent cells

The foremost principle in rejuvenating old cells and decelerating aging is to first eliminate inflammation that causes your body to overreact. This is crucial because any chronic inflammation present in your body can interfere with the activity of senolytics and the cellular rejuvenation process.

Scientific research on aged animal models has proven that when old or aging cells are removed, the aging process can be reversed. In animal studies, eliminating senescent cells has been shown to extend lifespan by 25%. Otherwise, if senescent cells are allowed to accumulate in vital organs such as the heart, liver, and kidneys during adulthood, these organs will deteriorate, leading to a shorter lifespan.[1]

Furthermore, senescent cells are easier to eliminate at a young age compared to older individuals. In animal models, senescent cells had a half-life of 5 days in young mice, which increased to 25 days in older mice.[2] Some studies have also shown that it takes 40-50 days to rejuvenate old cells into young ones. Based on this information, you can consume a senolytic in accordance with the turnover rate of senescent cells, that is, every 5 days, depending on your age. And continuous rejuvenation nutritionally may last for up to a few months. Here are the key natural senolytics presented in this book that can be used to enhance your body's ability to repair itself, help delay illnesses, and slow down aging.

Fisetin The recommended dosage for fisetin is 20 mg/kg of body weight. For instance, a person weighing 70 kg should not take more than 1,400 mg per day for over two consecutive days and should only take it once a month. Consuming foods rich in fisetin, such as strawberries, may enhance absorption compared to taking fisetin supplements. One hundred grams of fresh strawberries contain 16 mg of fisetin.

Curcumin To increase the bioavailability of curcumin, one can consume 1,400 mg of turmeric powder (equivalent to 125 mg of curcumin) along with 5-7 black peppercorns and a source of healthy fat. This method may raise the concentration of curcumin in the bloodstream to micromolar levels. Alternatively, eating 15-20 g of fresh turmeric root with 5-7 black peppercorns and a good fat can also boost curcumin absorption by 7-8 times. Consuming curcumin with good fats such as 150 g of avocado, extra virgin olive oil, or sacha inchi oil allows curcumin to be absorbed through the lymphatic system. Lymphatic vessels are found throughout the body, except in areas that lack blood vessels, allowing curcumin to enter the bloodstream without passing through the liver.

Resveratrol This natural compound is primarily found in grape skins. The human body can absorb 70% of resveratrol. Within our bodies, a concentration of 0.1-1 micromolar resveratrol is a dose that is not larger than that of other hormones or substances normally present. A 0.1 micromolar dose is equivalent to consuming 1.25 mg of resveratrol or eating 1,000 g of red Merlot grapes from Japan.[3] If you prefer to avoid consuming too much sugar, you can eat 1,000 g of mulberry instead.[4]

Quercetin Red onions have the highest concentration of quercetin, with 2,405 mg per 100 g. The outer skins of yellow onions contain 22-51 mg of quercetin per 100 g. After consuming 43 g of fried yellow onions, a plasma quercetin concentration of 22 mcg/L can be obtained. Quercetin can inhibit specific cellular pathways that promote the survival of senescent cells. By blocking these pathways, quercetin helps to promote the natural death of senescent cells.

Luteolin Celery and onion leaves contain up to 17 and 39 mg of luteolin per 100 g, respectively. A person consuming this amount of luteolin was found to have about 0.2 micromolar concentration of luteolin in their plasma.[5] Apart from its antioxidant actions, luteolin might block pathways that support the survival of old cells, leading to their death. Moreover, luteolin shows senolytic traits by reducing inflammation and halting the production of chemicals tied to cell aging. It also promotes autophagy, a process that cleans up and recycles damaged cell parts, potentially preventing aged cell buildup.

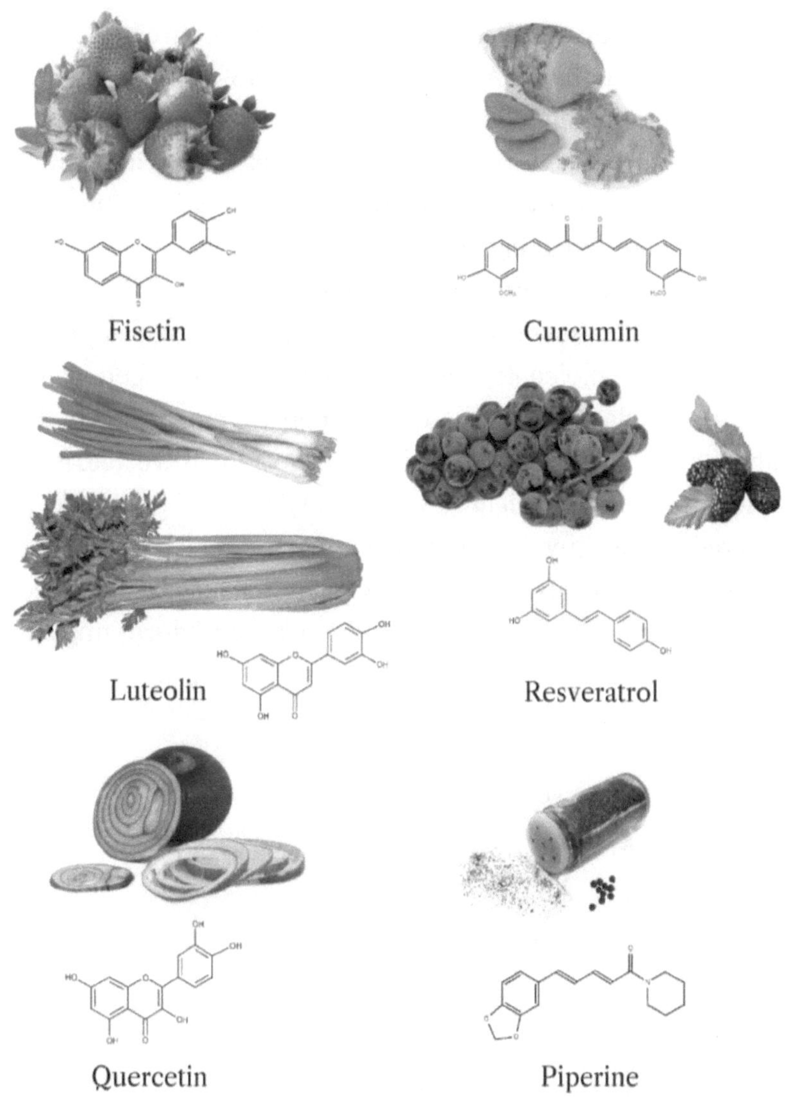

The key natural senolytics.

Step 2: To raise NAD+ and re-energize your body

NAD+ (nicotinamide adenine dinucleotide) is an essential substance in our body that helps produce energy. As you get older, the amount of NAD+ in your body decreases, leading to various health problems like inflammation, weaker muscles, memory issues, and a higher chance of getting cancer. People between 40 and 60 years old may see their NAD+ levels drop by 40-50%.

Scientists think that senescent cells contribute to this decrease in NAD+ as we age. These older cells cause inflammation, which increases the levels of an enzyme called CD38.[6] This enzyme is responsible for breaking down NAD+.

When there's more inflammation and higher CD38 levels, NAD+ gets broken down faster. CD38 uses up 100 molecules of NAD+ to make just one molecule of another substance. Senescent cells also cause other cells in our body to use up NAD+ more quickly than it can be made.[7] That's why NAD+ levels drop a lot as we age. Besides, people who are overweight have less NAD+ available in their body compared to healthy individuals. Eating too much and having a chronic disease can also lower NAD+ levels in young, healthy people, as these factors contribute to metabolic stress and disrupting energy balance.[8]

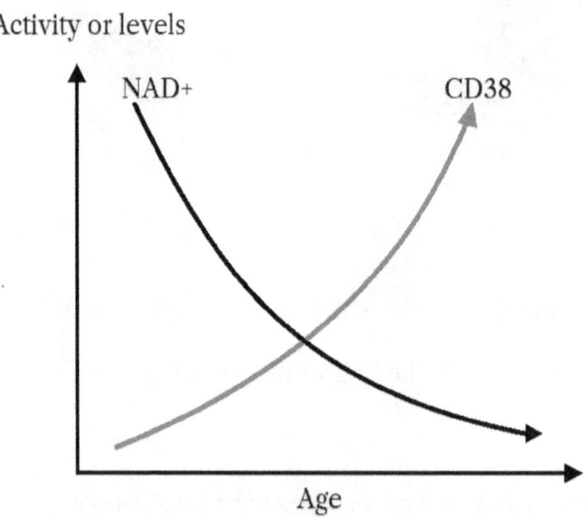

As we age, NAD+ levels decrease, while CD38, also known as an NAD+ degrader found in immune cells, increases.[9]

Moreover, when NAD+ levels decline, the capacity of cells to repair DNA damage and maintain cellular functions may decrease. Keeping NAD+ levels up can help with cell repair, DNA damage recovery, and support overall health for a longer and healthier life.

Besides taking NAD+ boosting supplements, another natural way to increase NAD+ production in your body is by consuming enough vitamin B3 and tryptophan in your diet. Both vitamin B3 and tryptophan help create NAD+.

In fact, consuming just 15 mg of vitamin B3 daily is enough to improve your body's NAD+ levels. Vitamin B3 is found in high amounts in various fish, such as American shad, Atlantic salmon, garfish, anchovy, mackerel, and Bluefin tuna, as well as in milk and ginkgo nuts. Foods rich in tryptophan include red bell pepper, pistachio nut, cashew nut, egg, and milk. However, without stopping CD38 activity, eating NAD+ boosting foods and supplements might not effectively increase NAD+ production and rejuvenate your body. So, it's important that when you reach middle age, you have to learn how to inhibit the NAD+ degrader CD38.

Interestingly, both luteolin and apigenin are natural substances that can enhance NAD+ levels in the body by blocking CD38 activity. In animal studies, mice treated with apigenin experienced a 50% increase in NAD+ production.[10]

Celery leaves are rich in luteolin and apigenin, with 100 g packing in 17 mg of luteolin and 56 mg of apigenin. Yet, not much attention has been given to testing the NAD+ enhancing compounds in celery. We'll need to await the outcome of human studies. If such a study were to be carried out, the findings could benefit the public rather than being a proprietary product.

In my opinion, employing a slightly enhanced strategy for managing a specific health issue, especially one without adverse side effects, could enhance your prospects for a healthier life. Even though the immediate impact might be minor, over a span of 5 to 10 years, it could culminate into a substantial health benefit.

Step 3: Nutrition can repair telomeres

Shortened telomeres are associated with the consumption of red meat, processed meat, and alcohol.[11] Shorter telomeres can accelerate the aging process. Men who adopt lifestyle changes such as healthy eating, increased exercise, sufficient sleep, and improved mental health can protect and lengthen their telomeres, compared to those who don't.[12] However, even with these lifestyle changes, it may take at least five years to lengthen your telomeres. So, it's better to start now.

There are natural substances that may help increase telomere length. In fact, it might only take 5 days to activate the enzyme responsible for lengthening telomeres. A recent human study conducted by scientists from the University of Freiburg in Germany involved participants consuming 15 g of dry Ethiopian kale powder (*Brassica carinata*), equivalent to 150 g of fresh Ethiopian kale leaves, per day for 5 days. The study found that only cooked Ethiopian kale, which had been boiled to remove the pungent odor and bitter taste of allyl isothiocyanate, could activate the enzyme telomerase by 25%.[13]

Telomerase is an enzyme that lengthens telomeres by adding DNA to their ends. Telomerase is not usually active in body cells but is active in stem cells. Thus, increasing telomerase activity slightly could bring youth to cells, similar to how stem cells use telomerase to maintain their telomere length.

It's believed that sinigrin in kale is likely the active ingredient that activates telomerase activity. In addition to Ethiopian kale, sinigrin is also found in Brussels sprouts (55 mg per 100 g), cauliflower (5-30 mg per 100 g), and cabbage (20 mg per 100 g).[14] Steaming these vegetables at lower temperatures could help preserve more sinigrin, as opposed to boiling or frying them. Moreover, there is an Indian pennywort, called gotu kola (*Centella asiatica*), which triggered an 8.8-fold increase in telomerase activity, but this is in test-tube experiments.[15,16]

Furthermore, in humans, a daily intake of 50 mcg of vitamin

D3, or 2,000 IU, for four months can induce a 19% increase in telomerase activity.[17] In fact, vitamin D3 is synthesized in our skin upon exposure to sunlight. If you expose your arms and legs to sunlight for 15 minutes, it's equivalent to taking 3,000 IU (75 mcg) of vitamin D3 through an oral supplement. However, strong sunlight can be harmful to your skin, so you should be in the sun before 9 am or after 3 pm. If your arms and legs are exposed to sunlight during this time for slightly longer, say, 15-20 minutes, your skin should produce enough vitamin D3 for you. In milk fortified with vitamin D, there is about 1-3 mcg of vitamin D3 per 100 ml. The natural food with the highest vitamin D3 content is salmon; it contains exactly 50 mcg of vitamin D3 per 100 g.

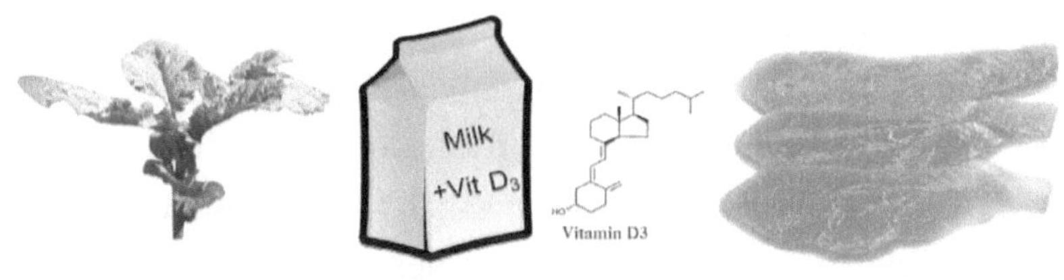

Ethiopian kale   Vitamin D3 fortified milk   Salmon fillet

Ethiopian kale can increase telomerase activity by 25%; and taking 50 mcg of vitamin D3 for four months can also increase telomerase activity by 19%. Wild salmon has 50 mcg of vitamin D3 per 100 g.

A little bit of knowledge

When eating fruits and vegetables, it's important to be mindful of pesticides. Ingesting foods with pesticide residues can be harmful to your body, accelerating the aging process and causing cells to become old. It's nearly impossible to entirely avoid pesticides in food, and even organic foods might not be completely free from them. However, using a baking soda or sodium bicarbonate wash is suggested as an effective method for removing pesticide residues.

Step 4: Strategies to boost regenerative potential of stem cells

Firstly, if you want stem cells to flourish in your body, consider reducing sugar intake, as sugar can decrease the ability of stem cells to grow and multiply.

In fact, cells can transition between stemness states when they are competent. Laboratory experiments have also shown that any cell in the body can be transformed into a pluripotent stem cell—a self-renewing cell—by introducing cMyc, Sox2, Oct4, and Klf4 factor, known as Yamanaka factors, into the cell.[18] These factors work together by tricking the cell into believing it's in an embryonic environment, causing it to become a stem cell. Exercise, though it doesn't boost all Yamanaka factors, has been shown to increase the expression of the Oct4 factor, which is important in the early development of stem cells.

Another method for generating stem cells involves using substances that can activate or deactivate genes, which has proven to be as effective as Yamanaka factors.[19] Such substances include fisetin, curcumin, and resveratrol, which can help revert cells in the body into stem cells.[20,21,22] Thus, not only do fisetin, curcumin, and resveratrol act as senolytics, they also act as "stemness rejuvenators." These compounds can revitalize cells, stem cells and enhance stem cell production in our bodies.

Although 100 g of strawberries contain 16 mg of fisetin, people who consumed 40 g of dry powdered strawberries, equivalent to about 400 g of fresh strawberries, had higher levels of pelargonidin, an anthocyanin pigment, which was more easily absorbed. It's believed that fisetin may be degraded or transformed, leaving only a small amount to be absorbed into the bloodstream.[23] Perhaps, for fisetin, less is more. As mentioned earlier, scientists recommend taking only 20 mg/kg of fisetin for no more than two consecutive days, and only once a month. That is because fisetin may interfere with the immune system and lead to a decrease in the number of white blood cells in our body.[24]

For curcumin, most studies have focused on its ability to

induce stem cells to regenerate bone and treat brain diseases. However, quercetin has been observed to help prevent aging of cells by influencing specific signaling pathways, allowing stem cells to maintain their regenerative capacity. And research suggests that curcumin concentrations should not exceed 10 micromolar. Similar findings have been also revealed for resveratrol.

In a mouse model, resveratrol has been shown to function similarly to Yamanaka factors, allowing for the creation of induced pluripotent stem cells.[25] What's more, a study successfully used resveratrol to boost stem cell production to repair and restore damaged hearts in mice with heart disease.[26] In humans, resveratrol also works by activating genes to increase stem cell production.[27]

Resveratrol in natural foods is found in smaller amounts and is poorly absorbed in the intestines. Attempts to increase resveratrol bioavailability have included feeding mice resveratrol with piperine, which increased resveratrol absorption by 1,544%.[28] A human study showed that taking 2,000 mg of resveratrol with breakfast resulted in very low blood concentrations of only 2-3 mcg/ml.[29] Unfortunately, neither piperine nor quercetin can significantly improve resveratrol absorption in human intestines. Additionally, a high-fat diet can decrease resveratrol absorption by 45%.[30,31]

Less is more

Let's discuss resveratrol in more detail. Scientists recommend the principle of "less resveratrol is more." A low dose of resveratrol is more beneficial than a high dose. A small amount of resveratrol can activate Sirtuin 1, an enzyme responsible for DNA repair, immune response regulation, cell protection from free radicals, mitochondrial function control, and slowing down aging. Sirtuin 1 activation is essential because its levels decline with age and decrease significantly in old age.

So how can a small amount of resveratrol boost Sirtuin 1 enzyme activity? The answer lies in resveratrol's estrogenic properties.[32] Resveratrol acts like estrogen to enhance the body's sirtuin 1 secretion. However, higher amounts of resveratrol have the opposite effect and reduce Sirtuin 1 secretion.[32,33] Since estrogen is produced in both men and women, consuming an appropriate amount of resveratrol benefits everyone. Menopausal women may benefit the most due to falling estrogen levels during menopause. In test-tube experiments, resveratrol concentrations of 1-10 micromolar or 0.2-2.5 mcg/ml blood are sufficient to stimulate Sirtuin 1 enzyme expression.[33]

Consuming red grapes may not achieve the desired blood resveratrol level (1-10 micromolar) because 100 g of red grapes contain approximately 9-160 mcg of resveratrol. Therefore, relying on resveratrol in dietary supplement form is necessary. In fact, scientists know that consuming just 40 mg of resveratrol daily can stimulate Sirtuin 1 production in the human body.[34] In another study, six participants who took a 25 mg resveratrol tablet and 50 mg of vitamin C had blood resveratrol and metabolite levels of 0.49 mcg/ml.[35] That's a good concentration of around 2 micromolar in human body. Another clinical study found that participants who took 250 mg of resveratrol had no more than 10 micromolar of resveratrol in their blood.[36]

Thus, taking around 12.5-250 mg of resveratrol can achieve the same 1-10 micromolar concentration of resveratrol in your blood as mentioned above. This blood concentration of resveratrol, 1-10 micromolar, is the right amount and sufficient to activate Sirtuin 1 to promote DNA repair and slow down aging. Excessive amounts may have the opposite effect.

A smaller dose of resveratrol is more effective in increasing stem cell proliferation and growth

A study in lab dish experiments, published in the journal PLOSONE, found that resveratrol concentrations of 0.1-1 micromolar are required for stem cells to divide and renew themselves.[37] However, long-term use of resveratrol at 1 micromolar or resveratrol at 5 micromolar or higher inhibited stem cell self-renewal and turned stem cells into senescent cells. Therefore, it's important to use a lower dose of resveratrol intermittently.

Now let's do the math on the dose. Resveratrol levels in the bloodstream at a concentration of 10 micromolar are likely equivalent to consuming no more than 125 mg of resveratrol.[38] Consuming 12.5 mg of resveratrol may be equivalent to resveratrol levels in the bloodstream at a concentration of 1 micromolar. Thus, resveratrol and its metabolite levels in the bloodstream at a concentration of 0.1 micromolar are probably equivalent to consuming 1.25 mg of resveratrol.[39]

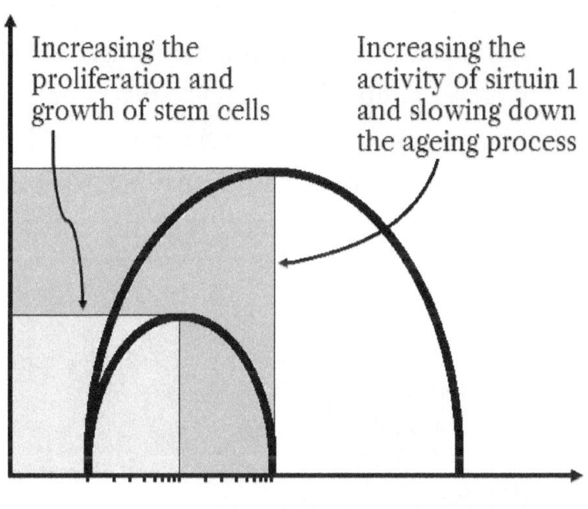

While resveratrol at concentrations of 1-10 micromolar enhances the secretion of Sirtuin 1, which is responsible for DNA repair and slowing down the aging process, at concentrations of 0.1-1 micromolar, it increases the proliferation and growth of stem cells.[33,37,44] When consuming approximately 12.5 mg of resveratrol in the form of dietary supplements, which corresponds to a 1 micromolar concentration, resveratrol is capable of both boosting the activity of the sirtuin 1 enzyme and promoting stem cell growth.

Incidentally, 1.25 mg of resveratrol can be found in a liter of fresh red grape juice,[40] or 1,000 g of red Merlot grapes from Japan.[41] Due to the high sugar content—about 15-25% of the grape is sugar—which may negate the benefits of resveratrol, it's advisable to choose mulberries over red grape juice or red grapes. A thousand grams of mulberries contain about 1.25 mg of resveratrol.[42]

Natural or whole foods are the ideal choices for our bodies, as they work in harmony with our bodily systems. The timing of resveratrol consumption is also crucial. Taking resveratrol with meals increases its bioavailability and helps it work in sync with the body's biological clock. For older individuals, the best time to take resveratrol is about the middle of the day. Moreover, the composition of gut microbiota has a significant impact on the bioavailability of resveratrol.[43] In some people, after taking resveratrol, their bodies may not absorb it effectively. If taking resveratrol for the first time, it can also alter some individuals' intestinal microbiota and cause diarrhea.

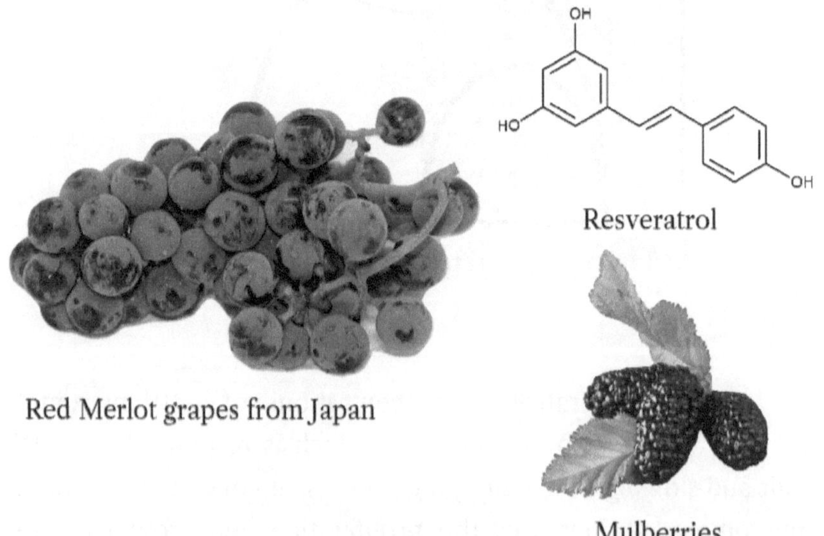

Resveratrol

Red Merlot grapes from Japan

Mulberries

Red grapes of Merlot from Japan and mulberries contain a resveratrol content of 1.25 mg per 1,000 g, which may be the about amount to encourage stem cells to divide and renew themselves.

Step 5: Decelerate facial aging

Inside the body, aging within the vital organs can't be noticed before symptoms manifest. However, aging on the skin that covers the body is noticeable, especially under the eyes and on your forehead where skin is thinnest.

Youthfulness makes the dermis thicker and skin cells more densely packed together. However, youthful skin disappears and turns into wrinkles in old age. The main causes of skin damage and wrinkling include AGEs, free radicals, chemicals, air pollution, and UV radiation from the sun. Consider this—AGEs, which are a result of sugar, harm skin cells. Additionally, free radicals generated by UV rays speed up the breakdown of collagen and elastin. This results in the formation of wrinkles and lines that appear as a cross-hatch pattern on the skin. Also, when free radicals and oxidants accumulate, they give rise to a state known as oxidative stress, which is harmful to DNA and cellular structures.

In spite of that, you can help protect cells from damage caused by free radicals and slow down your aging face. One option is eating anti-aging foods. Nature provides antioxidants that can increase your skin's ability to combat aging, such as vitamin A, E, C, carotene, and lycopene. Vegetables and fruits are full of antioxidants that can bring down the harmful effects of free radicals. You might already know about vitamins A, E, and C. Now, let's talk about another equally important antioxidant: lycopene

Lycopene is a carotenoid antioxidant that can scavenge free radicals, reduce oxidative stress, and act as a natural sunscreen. Lycopene is found abundantly in tomatoes, red guavas, and gac fruits (*Momordica cochinchinensis*). For example, 100 g of tomatoes contain 5-10 mg of lycopene, 100 g of red guavas contain 5 mg of lycopene, and 100 g of gac fruit has 222 mg of lycopene.

Scientists know that higher levels of lycopene in people's skin are due to the regular intake of these natural foods. Consuming a cup of tomato juice is equivalent to taking 10-20 mg of lycopene. It's important to know that lycopene can be presence in your facial skin.

It stimulates the production of collagen and elastin in your skin while strengthen the antioxidant defense of skin cells, which in turn help protect against UV rays.[45,46,47] Lycopene is a fat-soluble nutrient; thus, for the body to absorb it, you need to eat it with good fat or oil. Eating tomato salsa with a few teaspoons of extra virgin olive oil or 150 g of avocado will help your body absorb lycopene better.

Furthermore, it has been proven in a clinical trial that regular consumption of pomegranate juice, 240 ml a day, can help protect your skin from the sun.[67] In summary, tomatoes, red guavas, gac fruits, and pomegranates are anti-aging foods that are rich in antioxidants, which help fight free radicals and prevent them from causing the body's cells to age faster.

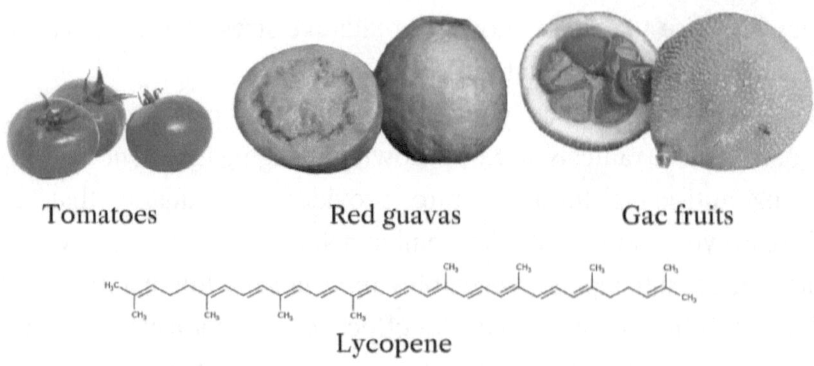

Tomatoes   Red guavas   Gac fruits

Lycopene

Lycopene is found in tomatoes 5-10 mg per 100 g; in red guavas 5 mg per 100 g; in gac fruits 222 mg per 100 g.

Some other anti-aging foods are often exotic and may be difficult to find. For instance, fingerroot (*Kaempferia pandurata*), a common ingredient in Southeast Asian cuisine, contains a substance called panduratin A, which can boost procollagen production. One hundred grams of fingerroot contains 900 mg of panduratin A.[48]

Research indicates that panduratin A has significant potential to prevent and reduce fine lines and wrinkles on the skin, as well as increase procollagen synthesis.[49,50,51] Studies show that panduratin A substantially enhances procollagen production to a greater extent than EGCG from green tea, a well-known anti-aging agent. In a cellular model, panduratin A at a very low concentration (0.1 micromolar—the part-per-million level) inhibits collagen degradation and, conversely, boosts skin's procollagen production by more than 200%. Skin cells produce collagen from procollagen. Failure to replace damaged collagen with newly made ones results in improperly repaired skin and the formation of wrinkles.

Importantly, panduratin A also helps regenerate skin cells by stimulating skin stem cells to divide and create more skin stem cells. By incorporating this anti-aging food into your diet, you could potentially preserve their youthful looks and extend their overall vitality for as long as possible.

Reduce facial wrinkles naturally by adding mangoes to your diet

Vitamin C is essential for the production of collagen, a protein that gives skin its elasticity and firmness. Long-term vitamin C deficiency can result in impaired collagen synthesis. Without adequate collagen production, the skin can become less resilient, leading to the development of fine lines and wrinkles.

Mango is one of the highest food sources of vitamin C and beta-carotene. One hundred grams of sliced mango provides 9-186 mg of vitamin C and 3-400 mcg of beta-carotene, depending on its ripeness and variety. Mangoes also contain mangiferin, which is thought to decrease wrinkles in women after menopause. In a randomized clinical pilot study, eating 85 g of mangoes four times a week for 2-4 months resulted in a 32% reduction in facial wrinkles for these women.[52] However, consuming 250 g of mangoes may actually increase wrinkles by almost 3%. One possible reason for this is the high sugar content in mangoes, which can cause the formation of AGEs and accelerate skin aging. The mangoes used in this study were Ataulfo mangoes, a cultivar from Mexico. Eating mangoes in moderation could be the key to reducing facial wrinkles.

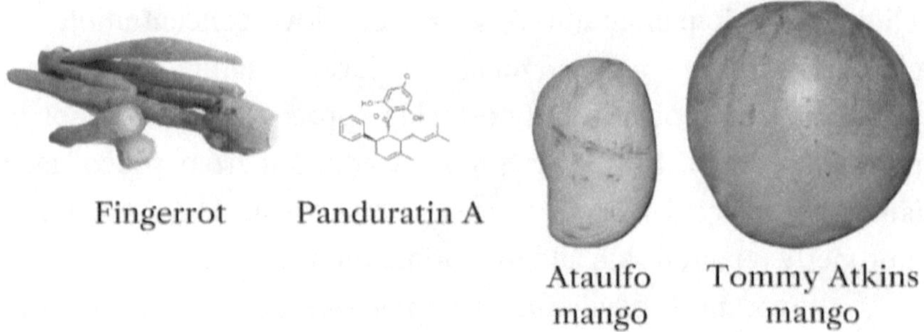

Fingerrot   Panduratin A   Ataulfo
mango   Tommy Atkins
mango

Fingerroot contains 900 mg of panduratin A per 100 g. Panduratin A has a higher potential to prevent and reduce wrinkles on the skin than EGCG from green tea. Ataulfo mangoes 85 g can also help reduce facial wrinkles in women after menopause.[52,53]

How do you know if aging has been slowed?

Externally, aging is visible on your face. Internally, when your tissues and organs start to decline or sustain damage, your body gives off alert signals. These might appear as creases in your earlobes, bags under your eyes, or deep wrinkles on your forehead.

In 2018, a study that followed 3,221 healthy French individuals with no history of cancer, heart disease, or liver or kidney diseases for 20 years suggested that forehead wrinkles might be an early indicator of atherosclerosis. Consequently, the more wrinkles on your forehead, the higher your risk of dying from cardiovascular disease.[54] While atherosclerosis occurs in other parts of the body, it can affect circulatory health in a way that manifest in the skin. Because blood vessels in the forehead are so small, they are susceptible to injuries and inflammation. When injuries and inflammation occur within these blood vessels, it becomes more noticeable. Additionally, due to the thin skin on the forehead, signs of blood vessel inflammation can be more clearly visible in this area.

It's not surprising when you look at pictures of the world's oldest men, there's one thing that almost all of them have in common: they don't have a warning sign of blood vessel inflammation in the middle of their foreheads. Instead, they have wrinkles appearing above their eyebrows. This could imply that the absence of mid-forehead wrinkles is a sign of healthy aging and longevity.

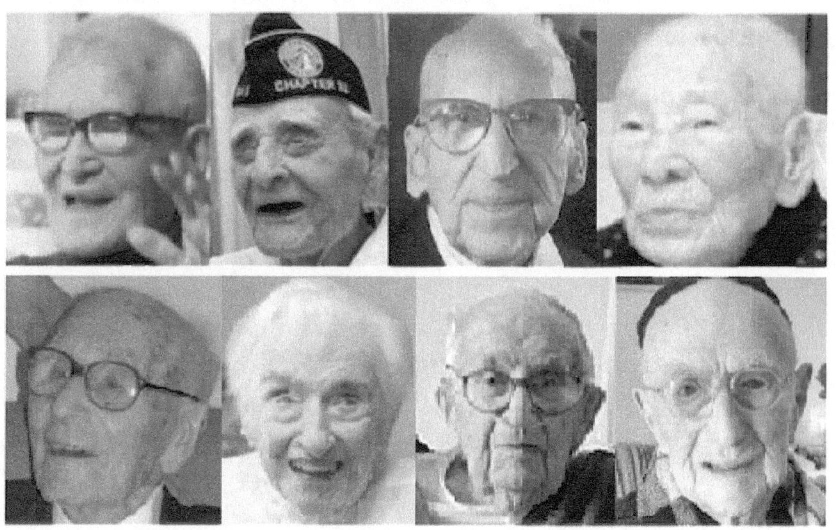

Oldest verified men ever: (left to right) top row: Jiroemon Kimura, Emiliano Mercado del Toro, Walter Breuning, Yukichi Chuganji; bottom row: Joan Riudavets, Gustav Gerneth, Fred H. Hale, and Yisrael Kristal.[66] Their forehead wrinkles seem less visible.

Visible changes on your face can serve as mirrors, reflecting a slowed aging process that's happening deep within your organ systems. But there's more to the story of decelerating aging. There are other signs, often subtle, that could suggest your body's aging process is slowing down.

Firstly, your physical abilities may seem to be improving or at least not declining as quickly. You might find that your movements are easier, your strength is maintained, and your balance is more stable. This reduces your chances of encountering accidents like falls, which can lead to fractures.

Secondly, your cognitive abilities could remain sharp. Your memory stays robust, you're able to concentrate better, and your problem-solving skills don't falter. As the years pass, you might notice you're not facing as many age-related health problems as your peers. This could translate to a reduced risk of developing conditions like heart disease, diabetes, or cognitive disorders.

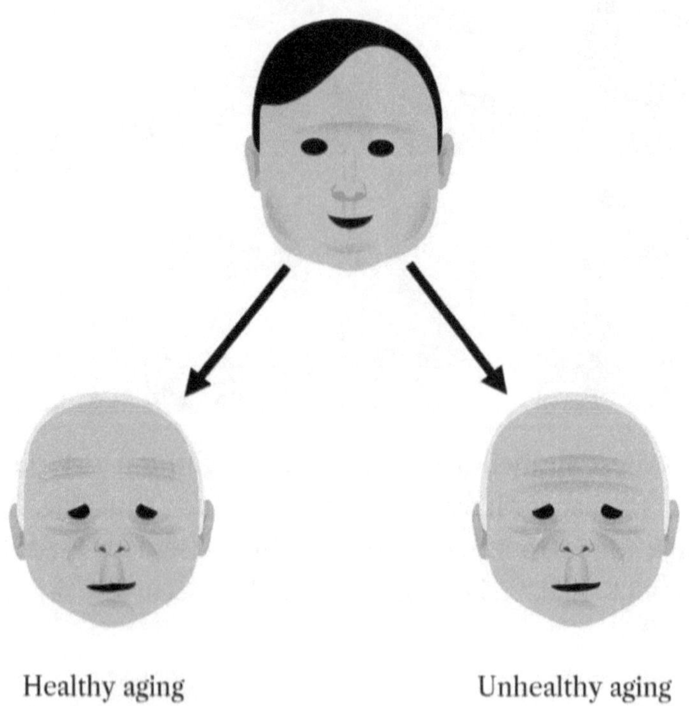

Common among supercentenarians, forehead wrinkles appear to form on the two sides of the forehead, rather than in the middle. This pattern of mid-forehead wrinkles seems to be indicative of atherosclerosis. This suggests that a person's mid-forehead wrinkles could serve as a warning sign of atherosclerosis and unhealthy aging.

Thirdly, your resilience to stress might be elevated. You're able to bounce back from challenging situations more easily, and your body can manage the harmful effects of stress, like inflammation or cellular damage.

Lastly, your emotional well-being could be thriving. You feel generally happier, you're able to form meaningful connections with others, and overall, you derive greater satisfaction from life. These signs all suggest that the aging process in you could be slowing down.

The right blend of elements for a longer life

Fascinatingly, researchers at McGill University conducted a study in which they fed fruit flies "Triphala", a traditional Ayurvedic herbal medicine from India, and a probiotic *Lactobacillus* similar to the one found in fermented milk drinks. The results demonstrated that the combination of Triphala and *Lactobacillus* increased the life expectancy of fruit flies by 60%.[55] This evidence indicates that Triphala and *Lactobacillus* can mitigate free radical damage, offer anti-inflammatory benefits, bolster the immune system, and help prevent illnesses in fruit flies.

Notably, in this study, the combination of Triphala and *Lactobacillus* proved to be more effective than either substance alone. This research exemplifies how the right blend of these elements can be crucial for achieving longevity. Triphala is rich in antioxidants, which help neutralize harmful free radicals, thereby reducing oxidative stress and cellular damage. This, in turn, can help slow down the aging process and improve overall health. It also underscores the importance of good gut bacteria for maintaining a healthy body and preventing or even treating chronic diseases.

So, enhancing longevity could be as simple as turning to natural foods and adjusting your gut's microbiota. The study suggests that a duo of Triphala and *Lactobacillus* may potentially aid in leading longer, healthier lives. The future might bring a time when increased longevity and improved health can be achieved just by including these three fruits and beneficial bacteria in our diet.

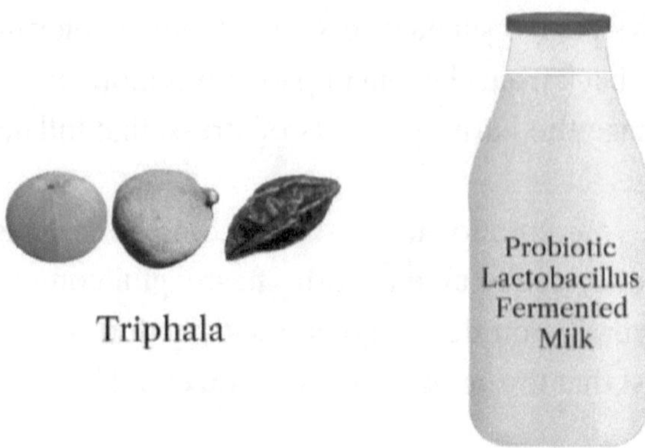

Triphala and probiotic *Lactobacillus* similar to the one found in fermented milk drinks can extend the lifespan of fruit flies by 60%. Triphala is made of three plum-like fruits: amla, bibhitaki and haritaki.

Step 6: To preserve the stemness of stem cells

After getting rid of old cells and boosting stem cell growth and ability, the next step involves preserving the youthfulness or regenerative capacity of stem cells as long as possible. This can be achieved by using, what I refer to "stemness preservers." Natural foods serve as important sources of stemness preservers, including melatonin and glutathione.[56]

Melatonin is an extremely effective stemness preserver due to its outstanding antioxidant and free radical scavenging properties. It protects stem cells from damage caused by free radicals, which in turn prevents stem cells from becoming senescent cells and allows them to continue dividing, multiplying, and maintaining their youthfulness. However, melatonin levels decrease with age. Healthy individuals aged 65-70 years typically have peak melatonin levels around 49 pg/ml, while those aged 75 and older have substantially lower peak melatonin levels, around 27 pg/ml.[57]

The depletion of melatonin and the accumulation of senescence can have negative consequences on the body. However, maintaining sufficient levels of melatonin can protect stem cells from self-destruction and potentially slow down the aging process. The recommended dosage of melatonin is 0.5 to 3 mg, and for melatonin to align with the body's biological clock, it's best to take it 30-60 minutes before bedtime. Plus, natural melatonin is found in cherries, with up to 1.3 mg per 100 g, and it's well absorbed at 33% in the intestines. Consuming 100-200 g of cherries should adequately boost your melatonin levels naturally.

Additionally, glutathione can also protect stem cells from free radicals and maintain their stemness. However, in experiments, human subjects needed to take 3,500 mg of glutathione to detect 1-2 micromoles of glutathione in blood or plasma. This indicates that only a relatively small amount of glutathione is absorbed, and its bioavailability is quite poor.[58] To increase your blood glutathione level by 30%, you would need to take 1,000 mg of a glutathione supplement daily for 6 months.[59]

In fact, glutathione is quickly broken down by stomach acid and has a mere 1.6-minute half-life in the body. Due to its short half-life, maintaining therapeutic levels of glutathione can be difficult, which is why glutathione drips are often employed. A glutathione drip is a type of intravenous (IV) therapy that delivers a high dose of glutathione directly into the bloodstream. This method is thought to provide higher bioavailability and faster absorption compared to oral glutathione supplements.

Although glutathione supplements and drips are available, purslane (*Portulaca oleracea*) is a natural food with the highest concentration of glutathione, containing up to 150 mg per 100 g. However, to match the amount used in clinical trials, you need to consume at least 700 g of purslane. While natural food glutathione may be absorbed better than glutathione in supplement form, it's not yet fully understood.

However, there are other ways to boost glutathione production in our body, such as consuming foods that are high in precursors to glutathione production. Examples of these foods are sulfur-containing foods like garlic, onions, and cruciferous vegetables. Another way is taking supplements that contain N-acetylcysteine (NAC), a precursor to glutathione. Furthermore, consuming 500 mg of vitamin C for 13 weeks can increase glutathione levels in white and red blood cells by 18%.[66] These increased levels in blood cells may suggest a systemic boost, as it indicates that the body is producing more glutathione. Increasing consumption of foods that are high in selenium, an important mineral for glutathione production, can also be helpful.

What's more, regular exercise and physical activity have been shown to increase glutathione levels in the body. Reducing stress is also important since chronic stress can deplete glutathione levels in the body. Besides, getting adequate sleep is important since sleep deprivation has been shown to decrease glutathione levels. Therefore, all of these factors help maintain the stemness of stem cells, contributing to overall health and longevity.

Get 7-8 hours of sleep a night to balance melatonin and growth hormone

Deep sleep, which is regulated by melatonin, plays a key role in the repair and regeneration of damaged cells, including stem cells. Without adequate melatonin levels and sleep, stem cells may not function optimally, leading to a decline in their regenerative potential. Some research suggests that melatonin can directly promote the proliferation and differentiation of certain types of stem cells, including mesenchymal stem cells and neural stem cells. To maintain proper melatonin levels and preserve the stemness of stem cells, you need a good night's sleep.

Various factors can negatively impact stem cell function, so it's crucial to regularly maintain and support them to ensure their continued effectiveness. Part of this maintenance could include establishing a beneficial bedtime routine, as proper rest can play a vital role in naturally rejuvenating your stem cells and overall body health. Getting good sleep can even help to maintain or increase telomere length.[60] However, if you are unable to sleep well for just one night, the negative effects can exceed your body's ability to repair damage, resulting in potential harm to your metabolism, brain, arteries, and stem cells. It may not harm them away, but over time the damage may accumulate and become irreversible and turn into a serious disease.

As you age, the levels of melatonin and growth hormone in your body decline. These hormones work together, and the body's growth hormone increases when melatonin levels rise. Conversely, if melatonin levels decrease, growth hormone levels also decrease.[61] Sleep is known to increase growth hormone levels, with peak levels occurring about an hour after the onset of sleep. Therefore, it's crucial to achieve deep sleep during the first few hours of a good night's sleep to ensure proper levels of both hormones.

If an increase of body's melatonin is associated with an increase of growth hormone, can melatonin supplements stimulate growth hormone secretion? Unfortunately, taking 2 mg of melatonin has no effect on the level of growth hormone in the body due to its low dosage. However, a higher dosage of 5 mg can double the growth hormone levels in men, increasing it from 3 to 6 ng/ml.[62,63]

There are other ways to stimulate growth hormone production. For men, taking 0.5 mg of melatonin and exercising at 85% of their heart rate can result in a 2-fold increase.[64] However, women's bodies have low responses to melatonin, and exercise alone may not be enough for older adults and people with obesity. To increase growth hormone naturally in these groups, they need to lose more than 10% of their body weight by cutting calories and exercise at least 5 days a week to stimulate growth hormone secretion.[65]

As humans, you aren't perfect. By acknowledging and addressing conditions such as melatonin and growth hormone deficiency, you can improve our physical health and overall wellness. In doing so, you can also enhance our body's regenerative abilities and increase your longevity. Then, when a person resides in an environment that fosters prolonged life, they will evolve their body's abilities to sustain this longevity. These adaptations can even be passed down as traits to future generations.

To sum up, in this chapter, you have learned how to biohack your body to rejuvenate old cells and slow down aging. By applying these techniques to your life, you can create your ability to bounce back from aging. Embracing these habits not only promotes a longer life but also supports overall well-being, allowing you to live a more vibrant, disease-free life. As you continue to implement these strategies, you'll be better equipped to maintain optimal health and enjoy a higher quality of life as you age gracefully.

CHAPTER 17

Eat less and live longer

Did you know there are three waves of aging? The first one arrives when you are 34 years old,[1] marking a critical health turning point in your life. As the first wave of aging hits you, you might notice your face becoming more wrinkled, feeling tired more easily, and losing strength while experiencing ill health. This wave doesn't only affect your appearance but also impacts virtually all of your body's cells. Following that, the second and third waves of aging will occur at ages 60 and 78, causing further health deterioration or even putting your life at risk. So, how will you cope with these aging waves?

The waves of aging result from the accumulation of senescent cells in vital tissues and organs such as adipose tissue, arteries, heart, kidneys, eyes, liver, pancreas, and brain. These senescent cells can create a transformative effect, much like a perfect storm. They cause your body to break down at specific points in your life. This instance occurs when the detrimental impacts surpass your body's capacity for repair itself. If senescent cells continue to progress past the point of no return, which could happen years after the onset of senescence, reversing the process becomes difficult. Thus, eliminating these cells as soon as possible or intermittently is often the best way to address aging waves.

You're already aware of using senolytics to eliminate senescent cells and employing stemness rejuvenators and stemness preservers to encourage stem cell growth in your body. Here, approach to slow down aging and rejuvenate your body, potentially extending your lifespan, involves eating fewer calories—a strategy often referred to as "dietary restriction" or "calorie restriction." Ultimately, it all depends on one thing: the sooner you can change your lifestyle, the better. If you can do it, making these changes before the first wave of aging hits your life is even more beneficial. If possible, you should also help others make similar changes. The ideal time to modify your eating habits and lifestyle ranges from your adolescent years to your early 30s, as this period offers the highest chance of success.

When I visited a wealthy person's home, I saw them eating expensive, seemingly unexciting foods such as fish maw, shark fin, abalone, sea cucumber, and sea squirt, all in the name of health. What they may not know is that to truly benefit from the anti-aging properties of plasmalogens found in sea squirts, one would need to consume about 700 kg of the food to achieve an effective dosage.

In reality, healthy foods do not have to be costly, rare, or exclusive to royalty; they can be affordable and readily available. Certain cultures may already be consuming these nutritious foods as part of their daily diet, which is excellent. However, people from other cultures might need to adapt and make better food choices for improved health.

You have the power to choose a healthy lifestyle and strive to be the healthiest version of yourself. Eating natural foods that slow down the aging process, rejuvenate stem cells, and maintain their youthfulness can help you manage aging and improve your health.

Besides making a significant impact or pursuing meaningful goals, what are your health aspirations? If you are older, health concerns may be a priority, and you likely don't want to spend your days confined to bed due to illness. To achieve freedom from disease, it's essential to break free from habits that negatively affect your health. Many people feel weighed down by life's burdens, often neglecting self-care. To be courageous, explore new healthy diets, adopt a wholesome lifestyle, and prioritize your well-being before it's too late.

***

The Minnesota starvation experiment and longevity

Since the 1930s, researchers have known that eating fewer calories can lead to a longer and healthier life. Dr. Clive McCay first discovered this when he noticed that rats with a 40% reduction in calorie intake, while still receiving all essential nutrients, lived 40% longer and had fewer health problems related to aging compared to rats eating a normal diet. This discovery also inspired more studies on how limiting calories affects the lifespan and overall health of different animals.[2]

It might seem surprising that anyone would eat 40% less, but there have been groups of people who consumed a lot fewer calories. For example, in the early 20th century, people living in Okinawa, Japan, ate 17% fewer calories than those in mainland Japan and 40% less than American workers.[3,4] A lot of these Okinawans lived past 100 years old, earning them the title of "centenarians." Another example is the Cretans, who lived on the Greek island of Crete in the 1940s and 1950s. They consumed about 40% fewer calories than people in the United States at that time. The Cretans followed a traditional Mediterranean diet, which focused on plant-based foods, healthy fats, and lean protein sources. Their lower calorie consumption, along with their nutritious diet, is thought to have contributed to their exceptional longevity and low rates of chronic diseases.

Furthermore, during World War II in 1944, the University of Minnesota conducted the "Minnesota starvation experiment" to study the effects of starvation on 32 young male volunteers around the age of 24. These participants received two meals per day and experienced a 40% reduction in daily food intake, consuming roughly 1,800 calories a day. They were also required to walk an extra 5 kilometers daily to burn 3,000 calories. Over six months, they lost 25% of their body weight, resulting in an average BMI of 16. By 2005, half of these individuals had reached 80 years old, living eight years longer than their same-age peers.[5] This experiment really suggests that consuming fewer calories could extend human lifespan and delay health issues by at least eight years.

If the idea of cutting your calorie intake by 40% feels worrisome, don't worry! You can gradually reduce your food consumption over several months without causing malnutrition. However, it's essential to avoid crash diets that promise quick weight loss in a short period, such as shedding 3 kg in 7 days or 5 kg in 10 days. These types of diets can be harmful to your health.

Instead, slow and steady weight loss, such as cutting 500 calories per day, is more beneficial. This approach results in about 1% of body weight loss, with 75% coming from fat and 25% from a combination of water and muscle.[6] On the other hand, losing weight too quickly result in excessive muscle breakdown, as the body can only tolerate a diet limit of about 400 calories per day before it starts burning muscle.

Though quick weight loss can reduce abdominal and liver fat, it can harm the heart. When fat is released from the abdomen and liver, it enters the bloodstream and reaches the heart. After a week, the amount of fat in the heart may increase by 44%, impacting its pumping ability. While this effect can return to normal after eight weeks,[7] it's unknown if the fat accumulation around the heart could cause long-term damage. Rapid weight loss can also harm the liver. When a person loses weight too quickly, the liver may struggle to process the increased amount of fat released from the body's fat stores. This can lead to a buildup of fat in the liver, a condition known as fatty liver disease. In some cases, fatty liver disease can progress to more severe liver damage, including inflammation and scarring.

Actually, weight loss should be strategic so that it's both healthy and sustainable. By following a well-thought-out plan, you can reach your goals in a way that promotes better health. For those with heart and liver issues, consulting a doctor before starting a new weight loss program is highly recommended.

By utilizing the Pennington biomedical weight loss predictor calculator, we can make an estimation of the daily weight loss for a 46-year-old who weighs 75 kg and plans to reduce their weight by 10% through a daily calorie deficit of 500.[8] In this gradual and healthy approach, creating a daily caloric deficit of 500 calories would result in a 1 kg weight loss over a couple of months. The person could potentially lose 8 kg and reach a weight of 67 kg within 600 days, provided they remain consistent. Please refer to the following diagram.[8]

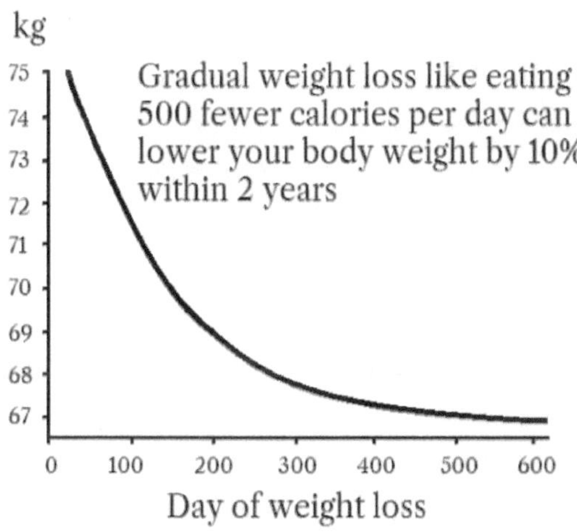

However, it's crucial initially to understand your daily caloric requirements, prior to setting a target of weight reduction percentage through a daily calorie deficit, which you can adjust further based on your specific weight loss goals.

To determine your daily caloric intake, you can use a Basal Metabolic Rate (BMR) calculator. BMR represents the number of calories needed when your body is at rest. The Mifflin-St Jeor formula is widely considered the most accurate method for calculating BMR. Numerous online BMR calculators utilize the Mifflin-St Jeor formula, such as the one found at this website: http://www.bmrcalculator.org. By inputting your age, gender, weight, and height, the online BMR calculator will estimate your daily caloric needs.

For example, if you are a 46-year-old male who currently weighs or aspires to weigh 75 kg, with a height of 172 cm, your calculated BMR would be 1,603 calories per day. This means that your body needs about 1,603 calories daily to maintain your current weight without any physical activity. Furthermore, to calculate your Total Daily Energy Expenditure (TDEE), you need to multiply your BMR by an activity factor that corresponds to your daily physical activity level. Here's a general guideline for activity factors:

1. Sedentary (little to no exercise): BMR x 1.2
2. Lightly active (light exercise/sports 1-3 days a week): BMR x 1.375
3. Moderately active (moderate exercise/sports 3-5 days a week): BMR x 1.55
4. Very active (hard exercise/sports 6-7 days a week): BMR x 1.725
5. Extra active (very hard exercise/sports and physical job): BMR x 1.9

In short, if your BMR is 1,603 calories and you're lightly active, your TDEE is 1,603 x 1.375, or around 2,204 calories per day. This is what you would need to eat to keep your weight steady.

Your BMR gives you a starting point to figure out your daily calorie needs. You can adjust this based on how active you are and your goals for cutting calories. Knowing your BMR lets you plan your diet and work out how to cut calories in a way that's healthy and sustainable for losing weight.

An improved strategy for reducing calories intake

As mentioned earlier, cutting down your daily calories by 40% can be concerning. However, as Les Brown said, "Shoot for the moon. Even if you miss it, you'll still be among the stars."

Consider this example: in 2005, exercise experts at

Washington University School of Medicine conducted a study on 48 overweight volunteers aged 50 to 60 (BMI 23.5-29.9) who were asked to reduce their daily calorie intake by 20%. After six months, the participants couldn't maintain their calorie-restricted diets, only managing to reduce their daily calories by 11%. Despite this, the results were surprisingly successful; although they fell short of the 20% calorie reduction goal, the volunteers still managed to reduce their belly fat by an average of 37%.[9] This demonstrates that even if you don't reach your target, you can still make significant progress.

Here are two more studies supporting the idea that cutting calories promotes health and longevity. In the first example, a 25% calorie-restricted diet regimen reduces food intake by 25% for an overweight person, or alternatively, they can eat 12.5% less and increase exercise by 12.5% through activities like walking, running, or cycling five days a week. Within 6 months, both approaches improve mitochondrial function by over 20% and result in a 10% weight loss and 24% fat loss.[10]

In the second example, a 15% calorie-restricted diet reduces food intake by 15% without causing malnutrition for two years. This 15% reduction can also decrease free radical buildup in the body, which, if left unchecked, can lead to oxidative stress and contribute to diseases like type 2 diabetes and cancer. This could also help slow aging and add years to your life. In fact, cutting your calories by 15% a day for two years could lead to about an 8 kg drop in weight and a 5% cut in body fat.[11]

It's key to note that cutting calories by 10-15% for two years is more doable and can be kept up, making it suitable for those who can't make big cuts in calorie intake. For adults who eat 2,000-2,500 calories daily, cutting 10-15% would mean eating 350-525 fewer calories each day. Foods that have 350-525 calories, like 100 g of fries, 10 pieces of nuggets, 100 g of potato chips, 100 g of chocolate chip cookies, 2 fizzy drinks, and 200 g of vanilla ice cream, should be avoided to achieve this reduction.

Older people with higher levels of hormone DHEA

In the human body, DHEA serves as a precursor for the production of sex hormones—estrogen and testosterone. Less estrogen leads to menopause signs, while low testosterone brings on andropause or male menopause signs like less sex drive, hair loss, bone loss, and depression. DHEA levels typically peak in people during their late 20s and then gradually decline by around 5% each year. As one gets older, their DHEA levels can drop significantly.

Interestingly, a distinct group of elderly people, known as the elderly Okinawans, don't display the same low DHEA levels as others in their age group. One possible reason is that being overweight has been tied to less DHEA, but the elderly Okinawans tend to consume fewer calories without consciously intending to, which may help maintain their DHEA levels.

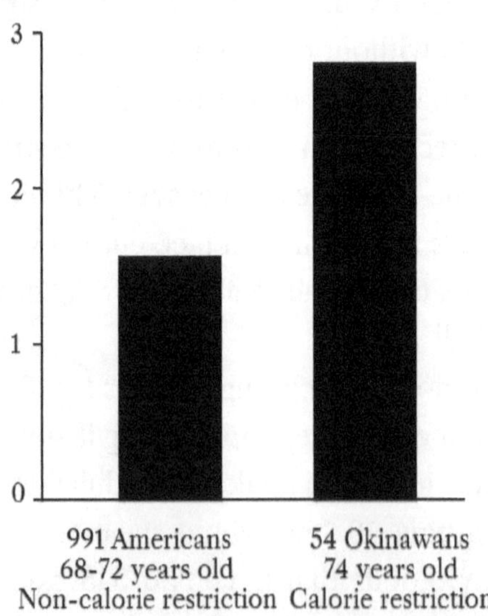

The difference in DHEA levels between elderly Okinawans and their American counterparts is significant, with the former having almost twice the amount of this hormone.[12]

You should know that long-term stress can also mess with hormone levels, including DHEA. Elderly people in Okinawa who manage stress well, often through social activities, tend to have better DHEA levels. This might be why they have nearly twice the DHEA levels of elderly Americans. So, it seems being active in your community and keeping up social ties might also help keep DHEA levels from dropping too fast as you age.

While eating less has shown good results for some groups, it's key to understand that it's not a fix-all for everyone. A more lasting way to manage weight would be to adopt a balanced diet, rich in whole foods, fruits, and veggies, paired with regular physical activity. For young people who are still growing and developing, calorie restriction may not be suitable. Adequate nutrition is vital during this stage of life to ensure proper growth, brain development, and overall well-being. Besides, long-term calorie restriction without malnutrition may have unintended effects, for healthy young adults. For instance, after practicing calorie restriction for an extended period of 3-7 years, some young people might experience lower testosterone and thyroid hormone levels compared to their peers who eat a regular diet. These hormonal imbalances can lead to issues such as fatigue, mood swings, decreased muscle mass, and impaired metabolism.

The 10:1 carbohydrate-to-protein ratio in the diets of centenarian Okinawans

The people of Japan's Okinawa Island are often regarded as some of the world's longest-lived people. When experts sought to understand why Okinawa has the highest number of centenarians globally, they traveled there for research. One such expert is Dr. Bradley Willcox, an expert in healthy aging, visited Okinawa in 1994 to study the island's longevity. He was particularly interested in the health differences between Okinawans and other Japanese people.

Upon arriving in Okinawa, Dr. Bradley Willcox asked the oldest Okinawans about their diet when they were younger, and the common response was "sweet potatoes for almost every meal." After completing his study, Dr. Willcox and his colleagues discovered that elderly Okinawans aged 65 and over followed a diet with a 10:1 carbohydrate-to-protein ratio. This meant that they consumed ten parts carbohydrates to one part protein each day.[12,15] This low-protein diet was predominantly made up of good carbohydrates, such as brown rice, whole grains, beans, vegetables, and sweet potatoes.

Interestingly, the 10:1 carbohydrate-to-protein ratio in the Okinawan diet has been shown to be effective in life-extending studies on laboratory animals as well.[16] Studies in both animals and humans suggest cutting protein intake by a tenth can slow down aging.

Okinawans follow the idea of "nuchi gusui," which means "food is medicine." Their healthy diet consists of purple sweet potatoes (and leaves), bitter melon, and turmeric. Their diet is low in pickles and pork. In 1950, they ate an average of only 3 g of pork daily, less than the 11-g average in mainland Japan and the 63-g average in the US in the same year.

An examination of the long-lived Okinawans' food intake revealed that out of their total daily intake (1,262 g of food), they consumed only 154 g of rice per day. Instead, they ate 849 g of purple sweet potatoes, a rich source of good carbohydrates and fiber. Okinawans also eat in moderation and stop when they are 80 percent full. Plus, these elders consumed tofu and seaweed daily and regularly drank green tea while limiting processed foods, sugar, and saturated fat.[17,18] The Okinawan diet is not only associated with increased longevity but also with improved health outcomes such as lower rates of heart disease, stroke, and cancer.

Another reason for the long, healthy lives of Okinawans is their diet. They mostly eat fresh, seasonal produce, fish, and foods made from soy. This diet has low levels of saturated fats, added sugars, and processed foods, all of which can lead to chronic diseases like heart disease, diabetes, and obesity.

Okinawa's isolation and limited food supply also forced them to rely on local plant-based food until the early 1960s. However, as they became more connected to the mainland, their traditional diet was influenced by Western and Japanese foods, leading to a shift towards a more Westernized diet. This dietary shift has also been linked to an increase in chronic diseases and a decrease in their life expectancy.

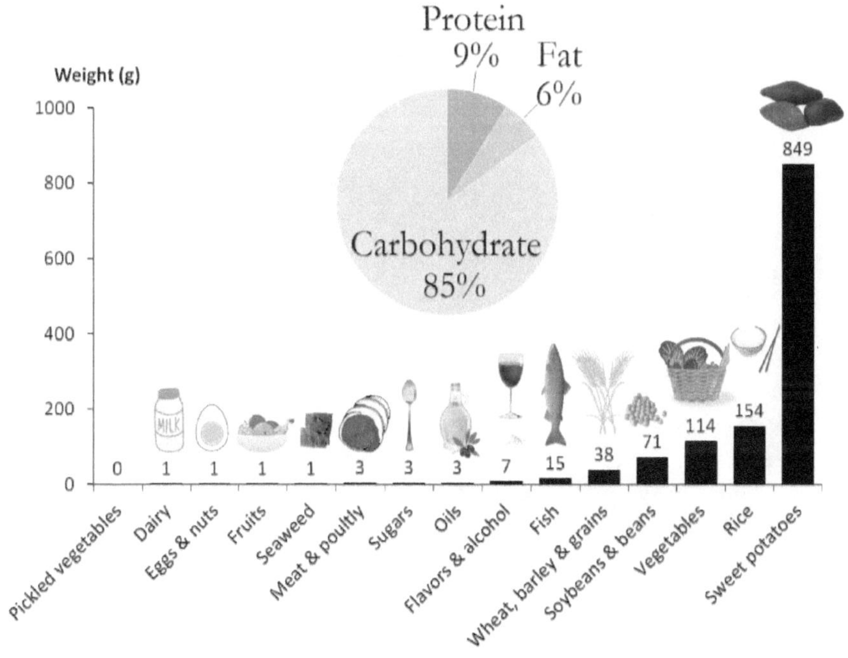

Daily food intake of long-lived Okinawans in 1950.[12]

Along with their healthy diets, Japanese people also stay active with regular activities like walking, cycling, and gardening. As mentioned earlier, being socially engaged and having community support greatly contributes to the health of older Japanese individuals. They often have strong connections with family and friends, take part in social activities, and get help from local community groups when needed.

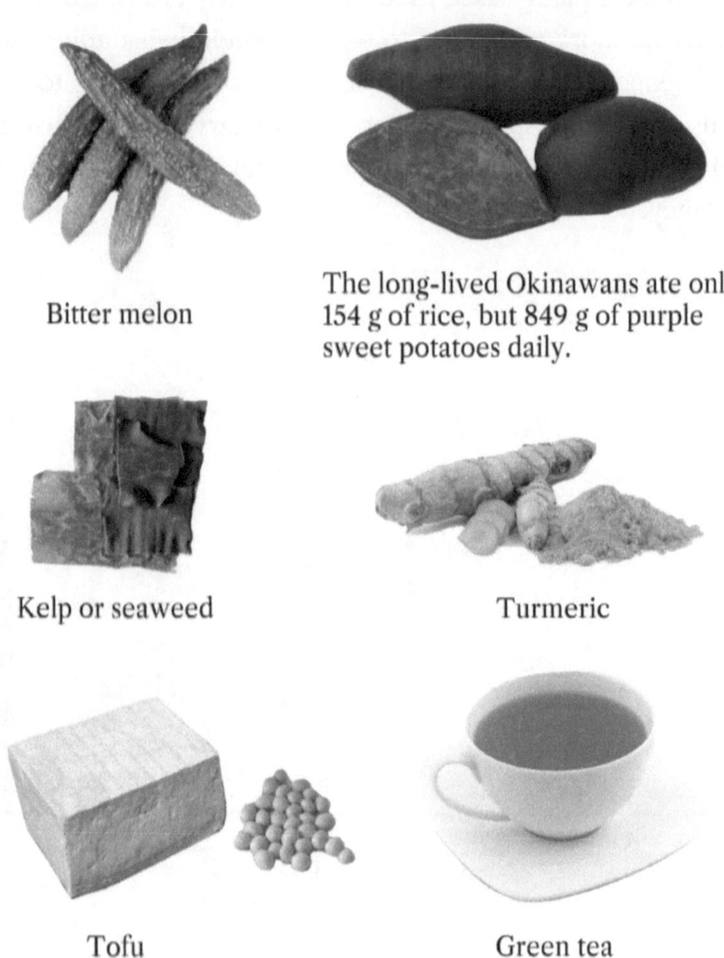

Traditional Okinawan foods eaten during the 1950s included purple sweet potatoes, bitter melon, turmeric, kelp or seaweed, tofu and green tea.

A fusion of healthy eating, active living, and a strong sense of community not only contribute the long lives of the Japanese but also offers a blueprint for global health policies. These factors can help promote healthy aging and reduce the burden of chronic diseases across the globe.

These days, Japanese people are among the healthiest people in the world. By measuring population ageing around the world based on age-related disease burden the people have, scientists know that elderly Japanese individuals experience health problems typically associated with 65-year-olds at the age of 76, which is 11 years later than people in the rest of the world.[19]

Measuring population aging also allows us to compare the level of health problems faced by different age groups across countries. For example, 76-year-olds in Japan experience the same level of health problems as 73-year-olds in Thailand, 71-year-olds in the UK, 69-year-olds in the United States, 58-year-olds in Egypt, and 46-year-olds in Papua New Guinea. This means that a 46-year-old in Papua New Guinea may face similar health problems to a 76-year-old in Japan. This research highlights the health inequality among global populations. As of 2017, the top five healthiest nations are Switzerland, Singapore, South Korea, Japan, and Italy, respectively.

Lowering daily calorie intake without causing malnutrition and consuming less protein, as seen in the Okinawan diet, has been proven to help extend one's lifespan. Conversely, eating too much protein has been linked to a shorter lifespan. Maintaining an optimal level of protein synthesis is essential for the normal function of cells. High protein intake increases the speed of protein synthesis in cells, leading to more mistakes being made in the cell.[20] This can be compared to working at a fast pace, which increases the likelihood of making errors. While your cells are normally adept at removing these abnormal proteins, as you get older, this ability decline. If an excessive amount of abnormal proteins accumulates in a cell, tissue, or organ, it can harm your health. So, it's essential to maintain accurate protein synthesis at the cellular level. For adults, the recommended protein intake is around 56 g for men and 46 g for women per day. You can obtain this amount of protein from various sources, including about 300 g of foods such as pork, chicken, fish, nuts, tofu, lentils, or Greek yogurt.

A change in energy allocation for life extension

In 1979, Kirkwood and Holiday proposed the "disposable soma theory of aging."[21] This theory suggests that living organisms have a finite amount of energy, and must choose how to allocate it—whether to use their energy resources for growth and reproduction or for maintaining their body (lifespan). From an evolutionary perspective, resources are often prioritized for growth and reproduction rather than maintenance. Once humans have successfully reproduced, we tend to age and eventually die. Therefore, increasing investment in maintaining and repairing cells, rather than growth and reproduction, could potentially lead to increased longevity.

However, it's worth noting that Kirkwood and Holiday's theory of aging only applies to females, as they are the sex responsible for reproduction. And the data supporting this theory was obtained exclusively from studies involving female subjects.

Later, this theory served as the basis for the "resource reallocation hypothesis".[22] This hypothesis focuses on the role of macronutrients, namely carbohydrates and protein. It suggests that while protein is essential for reproduction, carbohydrates are important for restoring vitality and extending lifespan. The hypothesis posits that during periods of famine, dietary carbohydrates are abundant but protein is scarce. The more you consume a diet with a higher carbohydrate-to-protein ratio, the more your body will use carbohydrates to nourish itself and potentially extend lifespan, while the amount of protein consumed may not be sufficient for reproduction.

Once conditions improve and a high-protein diet or a diet with a lower carbohydrate-to-protein ratio becomes available, the body can increase investment in reproduction. However, the amount of available carbohydrates is limited, so the body may reallocate resources towards reproduction, producing offspring rather than focusing on maintenance and repair.

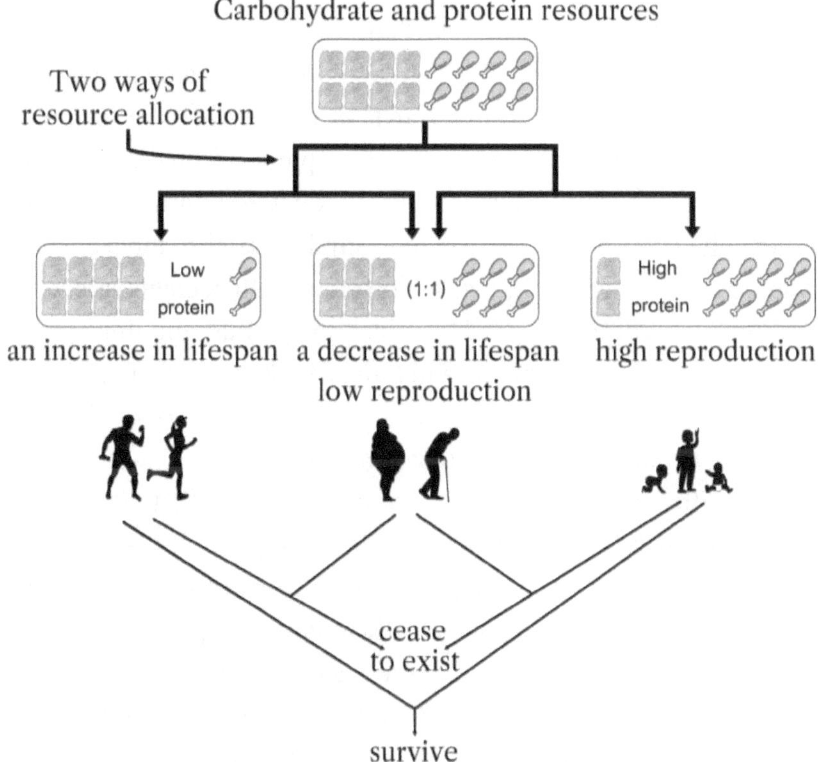

The resource reallocation hypothesis posits that during famine, the human body uses energy from carbohydrates for maintenance rather than reproduction, increasing lifespan and reducing reproduction. This helps humans survive famine, and when conditions improve, resources shift to reproduction, decreasing lifespan. The hypothesis also indicates that evenly distributed resources occur in a society with a mix of young and old. In contrast, a society with mainly middle-aged and older people may face healthcare and social service strains and challenges in maintaining workforce productivity as the working-age population declines.

So coincidentally, our bodies have a similar energy allocation mode that is consistent with the resource reallocation hypothesis.

Inside our bodies, there is a protein called mTOR that is controlled by the food we eat.[23] mTOR regulates growth and is crucial for tissue regeneration. High mTOR activity is an analog of the saying "live fast, die young." Too much mTOR activity is good for growth but bad for lifespan. Whenever food is plentiful, mTOR works to make more proteins, causing cells to divide, multiply and grow prolifically. When food is scarce, similar to the environmental conditions under which humans evolved, mTOR recognizes states of nutrient depletion and reduces its role, thus limiting protein production and cell growth. This aims to keep cell material and energy stable to combat famine. This process works for body maintenance and repair and extends lifespan.

With this knowledge, scientists think that if we can manipulate mTOR by controlling its function, it could be a strategy for slowing down the aging process. Currently, the scientific community is able to fine-tune mTOR activity using mTOR inhibitors such as rapamycin, first discovered as an antibiotic, or natural compounds like fisetin, curcumin, and resveratrol, or even through calorie restriction. Unfortunately, not only does inhibiting the mTOR pathway with rapamycin arrest aging, but it also suppresses the immune system. Compromising your body's immune system for the sake of longevity could be a risky decision.

Today, some individuals are approaching the prospect of living longer and becoming super-elders, looking younger than their actual age, including some celebrities and Instagram influencers. The elder Okinawans are among those who are considered super-elders. One of the reasons behind their longevity is their traditional diet, which has a carbohydrate to protein ratio of 10:1. A high-carbohydrate diet can trick the body into perceiving a state of famine, leading to the use of carbohydrates for restoring vitality and extending lifespan. However, the Okinawans didn't experience a period of famine; instead, they intentionally followed a high-carbohydrate diet. This provides evidence in support of the resource reallocation hypothesis in today's resource-rich world. And it has been proven that eating less protein and replacing it with healthy carbohydrates can significantly contribute to longevity.

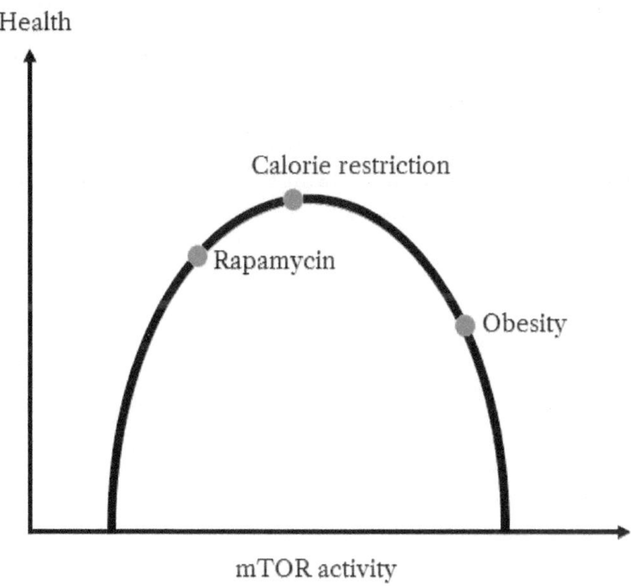

Healthspan and lifespan can be increased by inhibiting of mTOR activity.[23] Rapamycin can inhibit mTOR activity and limit protein production in cells. While calorie restriction can help regulate the level of mTOR activity, obesity accelerates it.

If inhibiting the mTOR pathway using rapamycin to slow aging also suppresses the immune system, it may not be worth the trade-off. To promote a longer and healthier life, it's better to consider combining regular exercise with a balanced approach to diet and lifestyle. Just like the long-lived Okinawans, who not only consume fewer calories but also engage in daily physical activities such as working in the fields and growing vegetables, which have been medically proven to reduce the risk of serious diseases. Relying solely on medications or supplements won't lead to a longer life without the benefits of regular physical activity.

To wrap up, it's crucial to keep in mind that the key to lasting health and longevity lies in a right blend of elements working together harmoniously. By adopting the habits of those who enjoy long, healthy lives, like the Okinawans, you can tap into your own potential for wellness and ready yourself to face the three waves of aging. Eating smart, staying active, and keeping good friends close are the secrets to a long, happy life. Remember, it's not just about living longer, it's about living better too.

CHAPTER 18

Design your own healthy plates

Charles Darwin was not the first to propose the idea of species evolution. In 1801, French biologist Jean-Baptiste Lamarck suggested that traits are inherited from parents to their offspring. To survive, species must adapt to changes in their environment, either by altering their behavior or their physical forms. Lamarck used the example of giraffes to illustrate his theory, stating that they developed long necks as a result of their ancestors stretching their necks. If a giraffe stretched its neck, a specific fluid would flow into its neck, activating certain genes and causing the neck to grow longer. Lamarck posited that giraffes passed this stretching trait to their offspring, and over time, the repeated stretching resulted in the distinct long-necked appearance that persisted through generations.[1] Importantly, the giraffe's long neck is its most valuable asset, as it allows them to access food and nutrients unavailable to other species, enabling their continued survival.

An ancient Chinese proverb states, "人生 最大 财富 是 健康," which translates to "the greatest wealth in life is health." Health is indeed more valuable than wealth, and everyone can achieve good health without necessarily being wealthy. In today's world, we find ourselves surrounded by unhealthy food options and at risk for chronic diseases. Yet, we can make conscious decisions to select healthier foods and steer clear of detrimental illnesses. To ensure our survival, it's time for us to modify our behaviors and adapt our lifestyles in order to thrive and maintain our well-being.

Feed for health and longevity

By learning from this book, you can design your own nutritious meals and use them to establish healthy eating habits that last into your golden years. The whole foods discussed in this book can be a powerful tool against chronic diseases and aging. However, even after gaining health literacy, you might still face obstacles to achieving good health. These obstacles include laziness, ingrained habits, lack of time, support, or encouragement, food-related peer pressure, and an unhealthy environment. You need to overcome these barriers to step onto a healthier lifestyle.

If you can become health literate and break through these barriers in your 30s, you may not need to work just to pay medical bills in the future. Retirement should not be synonymous with poor health. You shouldn't work hard now just to spend your savings on medical expenses during retirement.

In an era marked by global environmental shifts, consuming processed foods and leading sedentary lifestyles pose significant threats to your health. To flourish in these changing times, you have to adjust your habits and transform your body accordingly. Failing to do so may result in experiencing an array of health problems as you age, including the onset of incurable diseases that will undoubtedly lead to frustration and despair. Furthermore, you will likely be forced to confront not just one ailment, but a multitude of health issues simultaneously. Relying on medications that adversely affect cellular and organ functions will only exacerbate your problems, causing more harm than good in the long run.

Many people, especially the elderly, lack knowledge about nutrition and don't know how to use natural nutrients to repair and transform their bodies. The advantage of natural foods is that they work in harmony with the body's biochemical pathways. Although there are various anti-aging strategies available, from fasting to anti-aging foods, too few people actually utilize them. Health is a vital treasure in life, and in the end, it all boils down to who's better equipped to protect it.

As you age, your body undergoes numerous changes that can lead to various health issues and a decline in overall vitality. That is why you need to be proactive and start implementing anti-aging interventions early on, so you can better weather the storm and enjoy a healthier, more fulfilling life in your later years.

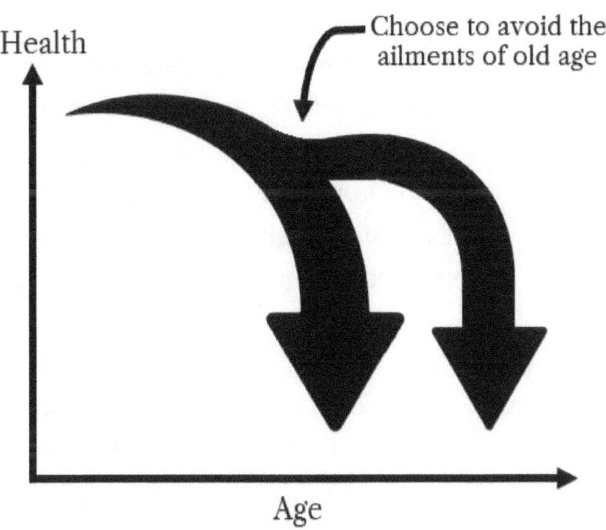

Old age descends on you like a storm. It's crucial to equip yourself with anti-aging strategies now to be well-prepared for the future.

Rather than a society filled with numerous elderly people suffering from various ailments and relying on multiple medications until they die, anti-aging foods have the potential to create a community with millions of older people who actively contribute to society until the end of their lives. Each of us has the ability to intervene in the aging process and foster a healthier body.

Similar to how a giraffe inherits its long neck from its ancestors, individuals who nourish their bodies with senolytics, stemness rejuvenators, and stemness preservers can thrive and pass on life-extending habits, health, and longevity to their offspring. In contrast, those who fail to properly nourish themselves may not be able to pass down such longevity to future generations.

***

Now design your own healthy plates

Since you consume food every day, why not make healthier choices by incorporating natural foods into your diet? Healthier natural foods include not only fruits, vegetables, whole grains, nuts, and spices, but also senolytics, stemness rejuvenators, and stemness preservers that contain phytonutrients explained in this book. These nutrients can stimulate stem cell activity, increase the body's resistance to aging, enhance the body's healing capacity, and prolong lifespan.

Many people consume insufficient amounts of vegetables or may have never even tried some of the foods mentioned in this book. As a result, it's not uncommon for individuals to experience a reaction to a specific food. However, it's essential to remember that the body's response to food varies from person to person, depending on factors such as genetics, gut microbiota, lifestyle, previous eating habits, and nutrient intake.[2]

Before starting, it's advisable to first adjust your gut environment by consuming a diet rich in fruits and vegetables for a week. Alternatively, you can eat a handful of walnuts daily to encourage the growth of good gut bacteria in the intestines and decrease the abundance of harmful gut bacteria.[3]

Next, assess if there is any chronic inflammation present in your body. To effectively restore your body's healing capacity, slow down aging, and extend your lifespan, it's important to first eliminate inflammation. If left unaddressed, inflammation can disrupt these processes and persist throughout your life. For more details on how to address this issue, refer to Chapter 10: Pain and Inflammation. In that chapter, I outline various tactics and adjustments to your lifestyle that can help you fight off chronic inflammation. It's a guide to setting you back on track towards a healthier, more extended lifespan.

In the meantime, maintain a balanced gut microbiota by filling half of your plate with vegetables and fruits, as healthy eating relies on cooperation from beneficial gut bacteria. Avoiding sugar is also vital as it can disrupt your gene activity, hinder stem cell functions, and accelerate cellular damage, potentially leading to diseases earlier in life. After these, you can proceed with the following guidelines.

Step 1 involves eradicating senescent cells with natural senolytics, such as fisetin from strawberries, curcumin from turmeric, resveratrol from Japanese Merlot grapes or mulberries, quercetin from red onions, and luteolin from celery or onion leaves (refer to Chapter 16 for more details).

After completion, move on to **Step 2**, which focuses on re-energizing your body using foods like salmon, garfish, anchovy, mackerel, bluefin tuna, red bell pepper, pistachio nuts, cashew nuts, eggs, celery leaves, and tryptophan-rich foods (as explained in Chapter 16).

Step 3 emphasizes repairing telomeres through lifestyle modifications, such as maintaining a healthy diet, exercising regularly, getting enough sleep, and fostering mental well-being. This may involve consuming American shad, Atlantic salmon, garfish, anchovy, mackerel, Bluefin tuna, Ethiopian kale leaves and sinigrin-rich vegetables like Brussels sprouts, cauliflower, cabbage, and gotu kola, as well as ensuring proper vitamin D3 intake.

Step 4 targets restoring the body's healing capacity and decelerating aging through stemness rejuvenators. Start by incorporating natural foods such as apples (remember to eat the peels as well), which are rich in fisetin and resveratrol. Additionally, intake 15-20 g of fresh turmeric roots (or 1,400 mg of turmeric powder) combined with 5-7 black peppercorns and good fats such as extra virgin oil during breakfast for a duration of 2-3 weeks, following a frequency of once or twice a week. Apples, turmeric roots, and black pepper boast both natural senolytic compounds and stemness rejuvenators, helping eliminate senescent cells and rejuvenate stem cells. Also, consider trying out these foods: tomatoes, red guavas, gac fruits, fingerroot, mango, triphala, probiotics like *Lactobacillus*, purslane, and cherries. After taking senolytics and stemness rejuvenators you might observe improvements within a few days, such as softer, firmer facial skin or feeling more energized. However, it may take up to 50 healthy days to see signs of aging reversal.

Next, in **Step 5**, consider incorporating other natural foods, rich in both stemness rejuvenators and preservers, to maintain the youthfulness or regenerative capacity of your stem cells for as long as possible.

In **Step 6**, to further enhance your body's potential for improved health and to bolster its ability to resist age-related diseases, opt for natural foods mentioned in other chapters in this book. All the anti-aging foods in this book are nature's gift for your well-being, providing nourishment for both survival and thriving. Don't forget, your lifespan depends on your body's ability to renew itself and fend off aging, both of which can be naturally strengthened by consuming anti-aging foods.

Additionally, prioritize quality sleep by setting up a consistent sleep schedule and crafting a sleep-friendly environment. Proper sleep hygiene not only rejuvenates the body and mind but also assists in hormonal balance and cellular repair, crucial for overall health and longevity. And remember, regular exercise is key. It helps keep your muscles strong, your heart healthy, and your brain sharp. Strive for a blend of strength training, aerobic exercises, and flexibility routines to address all aspects of fitness.

As we reach the end of this book, keep in mind that the journey toward longevity and optimal health starts with the choices you make every day. By embracing a diverse array of natural foods, giving importance to sleep and exercise, and adopting a mindful approach to living, you can unleash your body's full regenerative potential. Embrace foods and habits that naturally boost your body's ability to renew itself. Your lifespan, and how well you age, really depends on them. Allow this book to guide you on your path to a life brimming with vitality and happiness, as you harness the power of nature and holistic living. So go forth and start cultivating the habits that will lead you to a healthier and disease-free life.

Now design your own healthy plates.

Here are a few examples of my healthy plates

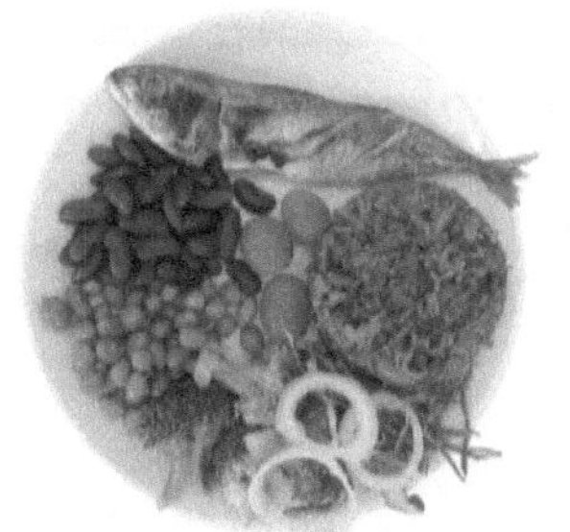 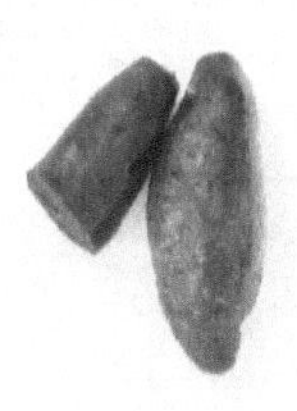 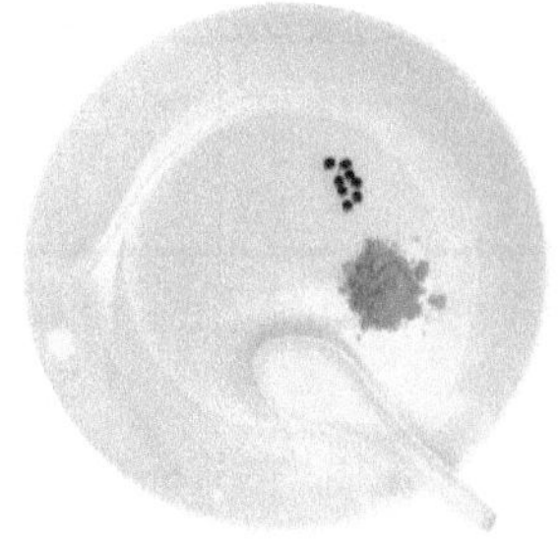

Healthy diet plan	Deageable diet plan
Vegetables, nuts and fruits ½	Sacha inchi oil or extra virgin
Fish ¼	olive oil 1 tablespoon
Riceberry rice and purple	Turmeric powder 1,400 mg
sweet potatoes ¼	5-7 black peppercorns

Now design your healthy plates

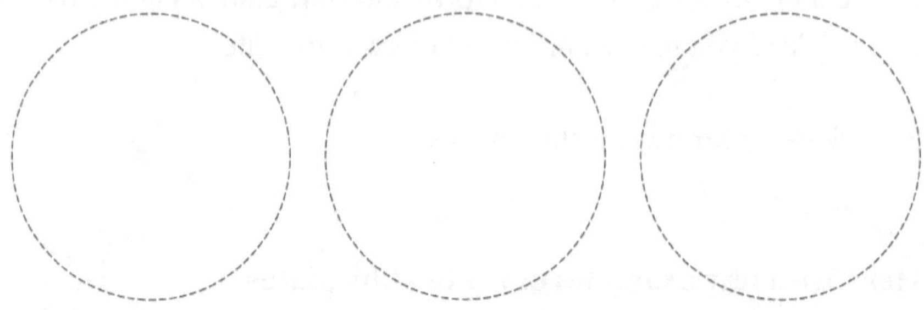

Healthy diet plan	Deageable diet plan
Vegetables, nuts and fruits ½	....
Fish, pork, chicken, etc. ¼	....
Carbohydrate ¼	....
(good carbs, beans and legumes)	....

Bibliography

CHAPTER 1: Your health is your wealth

1. TechCrunch - TechCrunch Disrupt 2019. https://en.wikipedia.org/wiki/Will_Smith

2. Crane JD, MacNeil LG, Lally JS, et al. Aging Cell. 2015;14:625–634

3. http://en.wikipedia.org/wiki/File:Jeanne-Calment-1996.jpg

4. Steven S, et al. Diabetes Care. 2016;39:808–815

5. Lean M.E.J., Leslie W.S., Barnes A.C., Brosnahan N., Thom G., McCombie L., Peters C., Zhyzhneuskaya S., Al-Mrabeh A., Hollingsworth K.G., et al. Lancet Diabetes Endocrinol. 2019.7(5): 344-355.

CHAPTER 2: Vicious cycle in the treatment of chronic disease

1. Blue Cross Blue Shield Health Index (2017). Retrieved June, 2020. www.bcbs.com/the-health-of-america/reports/the-health-of-millennials

2. Morgan TK, Williamson M, Pirotta M, Stewart K, Myers SP, Barnes J. Med J Aust. 2012;196(1):50-53

3. Qato DM, Ozenberger K, Olfson M. JAMA. 2018;319(22):2289-2298

4. Goldberg RM, Mabee J, Chan L, Wong S. Am J Emerg Med. 1996;14:447–450

5. Woodhouse KW, Wynne HA. Clin Pharmacokinet. 1988;15:287–294

6. Konrat C, Boutron I, Trinquart L, Auleley GR, Ricordeau P, Ravaud P. PLoS One. 2012;7(3):e33559

7. Dickinson J. Can Fam Physician. 2014;60(4):367-368

8. Willett W, Rockström J, Loken B, Springmann M, Lang T, Vermeulen S, et al. Lancet. 2019;393:447-92

9. https://food-guide.canada.ca/en/guidelines/ Retrieved September, 2020

CHAPTER 3: Growing old, old cells and old-cell-destroying substances

1. Genesis 5:5-27

2. Genesis 6

3. Laza I. M., Hervella M., Neira Zubieta M., de-la-Rúa C. Sci Rep. 2019.9(1):20380

4. Altekruse S.F., Kosary C.L., Krapcho M., Neyman N., Aminou R., Waldron W., Ruhl J., Howlader N., Tatalovich Z., Cho H., Mariotto A., Eisner M.P., Lewis D.R., Cronin K., Chen H.S., Feuer E.J., Stinchcomb D.G., Edwards B.K. (eds). SEER Cancer Statistics Review, 1975-2007, National Cancer Institute. Bethesda, MD, https://seer.cancer.gov/csr/1975_2007/, based on November 2009 SEER data submission, posted to the SEER web site, 2010

5. Williams, G. (1957). Evolution, 11(4), 398-411

6. Rabe T., Strowitzki T. (2007) Anti-Aging-Medizin auf dem Weg zur Wissenschaft. In: Herfarth C. (eds) Gesundheit. Heidelberger Jahrbücher, vol 50. Springer, Berlin, Heidelberg

7.   Baker DJ, Childs BG, Durik M, et al. Nature. 2016;530(7589):184–189

8.   Hickson L. J., Langhi Prata L. G. P., Bobart S. A., Evans T. K., Giorgadze N., Hashmi S. K., et al. (2019). EBioMedicine 47 446–456

9.   Miean KH, Mohamed S. J Agric Food Chem. 2001;49:3106–3112

10.   Xu M, Pirtskhalava T, Farr JN, et al. Nat Med. 2018;24(8):1246-1256

11.   FoodDB. https://foodb.ca/

12.   Muhammad F.M., Ahsm M., Abdul W. Modern Concepts & Developments in Agronomy. 2018;1

13.   Chang Q., Wong Y.S. J Agric Food Chem. 2004;22: 6694-6699

14.   Li Y., Yao J., Han C., Yang J., Chaudhry M.T., Wang S., Liu H., Yin Y. Nutrients. 2016;8:167

15.   McAnlis G.T., McEneny J., Pearce J., Young I.S. Eur J of Clin Nutr. 1999;53(2):92–96

16.   Yousefzadeh MJ, Zhu Y, McGowan SJ, Angelini L, Fuhrmann-Stroissnigg H, Xu M, Ling YY, Melos KI, Pirtskhalava T, Inman CL, McGuckian C, Wade EA, Kato JI, Grassi D, Wentworth M, Burd CE, Arriaga EA, Ladiges WL, Tchkonia T, Kirkland JL, Robbins PD, Niedernhofer LJ. EBioMedicine. 36. 2018;18–28

17.   AFFIRM: A Phase 2 Randomized, Placebo-Controlled Study of Alleviation by Fisetin of Frailty, Inflammation, and Related Measures in Older Women. https://clinicaltrials.gov/ct2/show/NCT03430037

18.   Arai Y, et al. J. Nutr. 2000;130:2243–2250

19.   Aghajanian S, Kazemi S, Esmaeili S, Aghajanian S, Moghadamnia A. International Journal of Engineering, 2020. 33; 12-17

20.   Weiskirchen S, Weiskirchen R. Adv. Nutr. 2016;7:706–18

21.   Chen T, Shen L, Yu J, et al. Aging Cell. 2011;10:908–911

22.   Lapasset L, Milhavet O, Prieur A, et al. Genes Dev. 2011;25(21):2248-2253

23.   Lee-Six H, Øbro NF, Shepherd MS, Grossmann S, Dawson K, Belmonte M, Osborne RJ, Huntly BJP, Martincorena I, Anderson E, O'Neill L, Stratton MR, Laurenti E, Green AR, Kent DG, Campbell PJ. Nature. 2018 Sep;561(7724):473-478

24.   Flindt, R. Amazing number in biology. Springer-Verlag, 2006.

25.   Suvorova II, Knyazeva AR, Petukhov AV, Aksenov ND, Pospelov VA. Cell Death Discov. 2019 Feb 4;5:61

26.   Mokhames Z, Rezaie Z, Ardeshirylajimi A, Basiri A, Taheri M, Omrani MD. In Vitro Cell Dev Biol Anim. 2020;56(4):313-321

27.   Shoba G, Joy D, Joseph T, Majeed M, Rajendran R, Srinivas PS. Planta Med. 1998;64:353–356

28.   Johnson JJ, Nihal M, Siddiqui IA, et al. Mol Nutr Food Res. 2011;55(8):1169–1176

CHAPTER 4: Sugar: the real enemy of your body

1.   Yudkin, John (2012). Pure, White and Deadly. London: Penguin Books

2.   "Diet, Nutrition and the Prevention of Chronic Diseases". WHO technical report series 916. Geneva: World Health Organization. 2003

3. Moynihan P. Adv Nutr 2016. Jan;7(1):149-156

4. Intake for Adults and Children, WHO, Geneva

5. บทความ เด็ก /คนไทยไม่กินหวาน .ไกรยง วิชกูล .สำนักงานพัฒนาระบบข้อมูลข่าวสารสุขภาพ .2544

6. Kasikorn research center

7. Kriengsinyos W, Chan P, Amarra MSV. Asia Pac J Clin Nutr. 2018;27(2):262

8. Thewjitcharoen Y, Chotwanvirat P, Jantawan A, et al. J Diabetes Res. 2018;2018:9152910

9. Zagorsky JL, Smith PK. Econ Hum Biol. 2020;38:100888

10. Burrows T, Goldman S, Olson RK, Byrne B, Coventry WL. Appetite. 2017 Sep 1;116:372-380

11. Eck KM, Dinesen A, Garcia E, et al. Nutrients. 2018;10(9):1232

12. Vij VA, Joshi AS. J Clin Diagn Res. 2013;7(9):1894-1896

13. Eweis DS, Abed F, Stiban J. Obesity Res Clin Pract 2017;11:534–43

14. Bes-Rastrollo M, Schulze MB, Ruiz-Canela M, Martinez-Gonzalez MA. PLoS Med. 2013 Dec;10(12):e1001578; dicsussion e1001578.

15. Ullah H., Akhtar M., Hussain F., Imran M. 2015;4. 354-358

16. Sanchez A, Reeser JL, Lau HS, Yahiku PY, Willard RE, McMillan PJ, Cho SY, Magie AR, Register UD (1973). Am. J. Clin. Nutr 26(11):1180–1184

17. Shodja M.M., Knutsen R., Cao J., Oda K., Beeson L.E., Fraser G.E., Knutsen S. Jacobs J Diabetes Endocrinol. 2017.8(2): 9–16

18. Thom J.A., Morris J.E., Bishop A. et al, British Journal of Urology. 1978;50:459–464

19. Khan A., Habibullah Q., Mujtaba R., Hasan A. Journal of the Liaquat University of Medical and Health Sciences. 2006.5

20. DiNicolantonio JJ, Mehta V, Zaman SB, O'Keefe JH. Mo Med. 2018;115(3):247-252

21. Douard V, Sabbagh Y, Lee J, Patel C, Kemp FW, Bogden JD, Lin S, Ferraris RP. Am J Physiol Endocrinol Metab. 2013 Jun 15;304(12):E1303-13

22. Shuto Y., Asai A., Nagao M., Sugihara H., Oikawa S. PLoS ONE. 2015;10

23. NCDs Forum in Thailand (การประชุมมหกรรมสุขภาพด้านโรคไม่ติดต่อ .(2018

24. Cheung BM, Li C. Curr Atheroscler Rep. (2012) 14:160–6

25. Softic S., Meyer J.G., Wang G.X., Gupta M.K., Batista T.M., Lauritzen H., Fujisaka S., Serra D., Herrero L., Willoughby J., et al. Cell Metab. 2019;30:735–753

26. Stanhope KL, Schwarz JM, Keim NL, et al. J Clin Invest. 2009;119(5):1322-1334

27. Lecoultre V, Egli L, Carrel G, Theytaz F, Kreis R, Schneiter P, Boss A, Zwygart K, Lê KA, Bortolotti M, Boesch C, Tappy L. Obesity (Silver Spring). 2013 Apr;21(4):782-5

28. Whitlock G, Lewington S, Sherliker P, Clarke R, Emberson J, Halsey J, et al. Lancet. 2009;373(9669):1083–1096

29. Apovian CM. JAMA. 2004;292:978–9

30. Goran MI, Ulijaszek SJ, Ventura EE. Glob Public Health. 2013;8(1):55-64

31. WHO. 2015. Guideline: sugars intake for adults and children

32. Bouchard C, et al. N. Engl. J. Med. 1990;322:1477–1482

33. Moore J.B., Horti A., Fielding B.A. BMJ Open. 2018;8:1–11

34. Sheiham A, James WP. J Dent Res. 2015;94:1341–1347

35. Irigoyen ME, Mejía-González A, Zepeda-Zepeda MA, Betancourt-Linares A, Lezana-Fernández MÁ, Álvarez-Lucas CH. Med Oral Patol Oral Cir Bucal. 2012;17(5):e825-e832

36. Trakoon-osot W, Sotanaphun U, Phanachet P, Porasuphatana S, Udomsubpayakul U, Komindr S. J Pharm Res 2013;6:859-64

37. Fuangchan A, Sonthisombat P, Seubnukarn T, et al. J Ethnopharmacol. 2011;134(2):422-428

38. Shimizu K., Ozeki M., Tanaka K., Itoh K., Nakajyo S., Urakawa N., Atsuchi M. J. Vet. Med. Sci. 1997;59:753–757

39. Li Y., Zheng M., Zhai X., Huang Y., Khalid A., Malik A., et al. (2015). Acta Pol. Pharm. 72, 981–985

40. Shanmugasundaram E., Gopinath K., Shanmugasundaram K., Rajendran V. (1990. a). J. Ethnopharmacol. 30 (3), 265–279

41. Ahmed ABA, Rao AS, Rao MV. Phytomedicine. 2010;17(13):1033–1039

42. Tiwari P., Mishra B.N., Sangwan N.S. Biomed. Res. Int. 2014;2014:830285

43. Sugihara Y, Nojima H, Matsuda H, Murakami T, Yoshikawa M, Kimura I. Journal of Asian Natural Products Research. 2000;2(4):321–327

44. Wang J, Zhang X, Lan H, Wang W. Food Nutr Res. 2017;61(1):1377571

45. Chuengsamarn S., Rattanamongkolgul S., Luechapudiporn R., Phisalaphong C., Jirawatnotai S. Diabetes Care. 2012. 35:2121-2127

46. Den Hartogh DJ, Gabriel A, Tsiani E. Nutrients. 2019;12(1):58

47. Na L.-X., Li Y., Pan H.-Z., Zhou X.-L., Sun D.-J., Meng M., Li X.-X., Sun C.-H. Mol. Nutr. Food Res. 2013;57:1569–1577

48. Na L.X., Yan B.L., Jiang S., Cui H.L., Li Y., Sun C.H. Environ. Sci. 2014;27:902–906

49. Arcaro CA, Gutierres VO, Assis RP, et al. PLoS One. 2014;9(12):e113993

50. Shoba G, Joy D, Joseph T, Majeed M, Rajendran R, Srinivas PS. Planta Med. 1998;64:353–356

51. Chacko E. Scientifica (Cairo). 2016;2016:4045717

CHAPTER 5: Karma of eating

1. Domingo JL, Nadal M. Food Chem Toxicol. 2017;105:256–261

2. Cancer Research UK, WHO

3. Ward M.H., Cross A.J., Abnet C.C., Sinha R., Markin R.S., Weisenburger D.D. Eur. J. Cancer Prev. 2012;21:134-138

4. Kopp T, Vogel U, Tionneland A, Anderson V. Am J Clin Nutr. 2018;107:465–479

5. Benarba B. EXCLI J. 2018;17:792–797

6. Zhong VW, Van Horn L, Greenland P, Carnethon MR, Ning H, Wilkins JT, Lloyd-Jones DM, Allen NB. JAMA Intern Med. 2020 Apr 1;180(4):503-512

7. Cho, C. E. et al. Mol. Nutr. Food Res. 2017.61, 1600324

8. Velasquez M.T., Ramezani A., Manal A., Raj D.S., Vanholder R. Toxins. 2016;8:326

9. Boini KM, Hussain T, Li P-L, et al. Cell Physiol Biochem 2017;44:152-162

10. Zhu W, Gregory JC, Org E, et al. Cell. 2016;1165:111-124

11. Blausen 0012 AdiposeTissue. By BruceBlaus. Blausen.com staff (2014). "Medical gallery of Blausen Medical 2014". WikiJournal of Medicine 1 (2). DOI:10.15347/wjm/2014.010. ISSN 2002-4436.

12. FAO/WHO Consultation on the Health Implications of Acrylamide in Food; Geneva, 25–27 June 2002, Summary Report. (PDF). Retrieved June, 2020

13. United States Food and Drug Administration [FDA]. (2004). Acrylamide in foods. Washington, DC: United States Food and Drug Administration

14. United States Food and Drug Administration Center for Food Safety and Applied Nutrition [FDA/CFSAN]. (2002). Exploratory date on acrylamide in foods. Washington, DC: United States Food and Drug Administration

15. Ritz E, Hahn K, Ketteler M, Kuhlmann MK, Mann J. Dtsch Arztebl Int. 2012;109:49–55

16. Merve Yanar G, Barry A F. Nutri Food Sci Int J. 2020. 9(5): 555775

17. León JB, Sullivan CM, Sehgal AR. J. Ren. Nutr. 2013;23:265–270

18. https://www.pepsicobeveragefacts.com/home/phosphorus. Retrieved September, 2020

19. Dhingra R, Sullivan L, Fox C, Wang T, D'Agostino R, Gaziano M, Vasan RS. Arch Intern Med 2007;167:879–85

20. Kendrick J., Ix J.H., Targher G., Smits G., Chonchol M. Am. J. Cardiol. 2010;106:564–568

21. Dhingra R., Gona P., Benjamin E. J., Wang T. J., Aragam J., D'Agostino R. B., Sr., et al. . Eur. J. Heart Fail.2010; 12, 812–818

22. Chang AR, Lazo M, Appel LJ, et al.. Am J Clin Nutr. 2014;99:320–327

23. Chetty R, Stepner M, Abraham S, et al. JAMA. 2016;315(16):1750-1766

24. Stephen AM, Champ MM, Cloran SJ et al. Nutrition Research Reviews. 2017. 30: 149–90

25. Reynolds A, Mann J, Cummings J, Winter N, Mete E, Te Morenga L. Lancet 2019; 393(10170)434– 445

26. Katagiri R., Goto A., Sawada N., Yamaji T., Iwasaki M., Noda M., Iso H., Tsugane S. Am J Clin Nutr. 2020. 28 Jan. pii: nqaa002

27. Mori B, Nakaji S, Sugawara K, Ohta M, Iwane S, Munakata A, Yoshida Y, Ohi G. Nutr Res.1996.16;53-60

28. Ma W, Nguyen LH, Song M, et al. Am J Gastroenterol. 2019;114(9):1531-1538

29. https://en.wikipedia.org/wiki/Diverticulosis. Retrieved August, 2020

30. Reynolds A, Mann J, Cummings J, Winter N, Mete E, Te Morenga L. Lancet. 2019 Feb 2;393(10170):434-445

31. Heart disease facts. https://www.cdc.gov/heartdisease/facts.htm. Retrieved August, 2020

32. U.S. Department of Agriculture, Agricultural Research Service. FoodData Central, 2019. fdc.nal.usda.gov

33. Chen PY., Li S., Koh YC., Wu JC., Yang MJ., Ho CT., Pan MH. J Agric Food Chem. 2019; 67 (28): 7869-7879

34. Wang Z, Roberts AB, Buffa JA, et al. Cell 2015;163:1585–95

35. Wu W.K., Panyod S., Ho C.T., Kuo C.H., Wu M.S., Sheen L.Y. J Funct Foods.2015.15: 408-417

36. Barabási A., Menichetti G. & Loscalzo J. Nat Food (2019) doi:10.1038/s43016-019-0005-1

37. FoodDB. https://foodb.ca/

38. Shi X, Lv Y, Mao C, et al. Nutrients. 2019;11(7):1504

39. Wang J, Zhang X, Lan H, Wang W.Food Nutr Res. 2017;61(1):1377571

40. Blausen.com staff (2014), "Medical gallery of Blausen Medical 2014", WikiJournal of Medicine, 1 (2), doi:10.15347/WJM/2014.010, ISSN 2002-4436, Wikidata Q44276831

CHAPTER 6: Reversible type 2 diabetes

1. Dietary Guidelines for Indians-A Manual. Hyderabad: National Institute of Nutrition (2011)

2. Dasgupta R, Pillai R, Kumar R, Arora NK. Indian J Community Med. 2015;40(2):71–4

3. Statista (2019) Sugar consumption worldwide in 2018/2019, by leading country in million metric tons. accessed May 18, 2020. https://www.statista.com/statistics/496002/sugar-consumption-worldwide/

4. บทความ เด็ก /คนไทยไม่กินหวาน .ไกรยง วิชฎล .สำนักงานพัฒนาระบบข้อมูลข่าวสารสุขภาพ .2544

5. International Diabetes Federation IDF Diabetes Atlas: Top 10 countries or territories for number of adults (20-79 years) with diabetes, 9th ed. (2019). Available online at: https://www.diabetesatlas.org/en/sections/demographic-and-geographic-outline.html (accessed May 17, 2020)

6. Institute for Health Metrics and Evaluation-IHME. https://ourworldindata.org. Retrieved June, 2020

7. Balachandra H. Reports of Health Visits to Outer Atolls to Ministry of Health and Environment. Majuro: Marshall Islands. Unpublished Ministry of Health Documents; (2002)

8. Davis B.C., Jamshed H., Peterson C.M., et al. Front Nutr. 2019;6:79

9. Danaei, G. The Lancet. 378 (9785): 31–40

10. Jakob Suckale, Michele Solimena - Solimena Lab and Review Suckale Solimena 2008 Frontiers in Bioscience , preprint PDF from Nature Proceedings, original data: Daly et al. 1998 PMID:18508724

11. Nichols GA, Hillier TA, Brown JB. Am J Med. 2008;121:519-524

12. Malmström H, Walldius G, Carlsson S, Grill V, Jungner I, Gudbjörnsdottir S, et al. Diabetes Obes Metab. 2018. 6:1419-1426

13. Di Nicolantonio J.J., O'Keefe J.H., Wilson W.L. Br. J. Sports Med. 2018;52:910–913

14. Singh GM, Micha R, Khatibzadeh S, et al. Circulation. 2015;132(8):639–666

15. Taylor R. Calorie restriction for long-term remission of type 2 diabetes. Clin Med (Lond). 2019;19(1):37–42

16. Taylor R, Holman RR. Clin Sci (Lond) 2015;128:405–410

17. Adam Heller, Karalee Jarvis, and Sheryl S. Coffman. Chemical Research in Toxicology 2018. 6: 506-509

18. Knowler WC, Barrett-Connor E, Fowler SE, et al. N Engl J Med. February 7 2002;346(6):393–403

19. Tuomilehto J, Lindström J, Eriksson JG, et al. N Engl J Med. 2001;344:1343–50

20. Astbury N. M., Aveyard P., Nickless A., et al. BMJ. 2018;362, article k3760

21. Lean MEJ, Leslie WS, Barnes AC, et al. Lancet Diabetes Endocrinol. 2019;7(5):344-355

22. Ge L., et.el. BMJ. 2020.1;369:m696

23. Nichols GA, Hillier TA, Brown JB. Am J Med. 2008;121:519-524

24. Malmström H, Walldius G, Carlsson S, Grill V, Jungner I, Gudbjörnsdottir S, et al. Diabetes Obes Metab. 2018. 6:1419-1426

25. Diabetes Prevention Program (DPP) Research Group Reduction in the incidence of type 2 diabetes with lifestyle intervention or metformin. N Engl J Med. 2002;346:393–403

26. Lindstrom J., Louheranta A., Mannelin M., Rastas M., Salminen V., Eriksson J., Uusitupa M., Tuomilehto J. Diabetes Care. 2003;26(12):3230–3236

27. Taylor R. Calorie restriction for long-term remission of type 2 diabetes. Clin Med (Lond). 2019;19(1):37–42

28. Xu J., Stanislaus S., Chinookoswong N., Lau Y.Y., Hager T., Patel J., Ge H., Weiszmann J., Lu S.C., Graham M., et al. Am J Physiol Endocrinol Metab. 2009;297:E1105–E1114

29. Coskun T, Bina HA, Schneider MA, Dunbar JD, Hu CC, Chen Y, et al. Endocrinology. 2008;149:6018–6027

30. MacDonald TL, Pattamaprapanont P, Pathak P, et al. Nat Metab. 2020;10.1038/s42255-020-0240-7

31. Chuengsamarn S., Rattanamongkolgul S., Luechapudiporn R., Phisalaphong C., Jirawatnotai S. Diabetes Care. 2012. 35:2121-2127

32. Pothitirat W., Gritsanapan W. Current Science. 2006. 91

33. Shoba G, Joy D, Joseph T, Majeed M, Rajendran R, Srinivas PS. Planta Med. 1998;64:353–356

34. Cheng CW, Villani V, Buono R, Wei M, Kumar S, Yilmaz OH, Cohen P, Sneddon JB, Perin L, Longo VD. Cell. 2017.23;168(5):775-788

35. Jones EC, Rylands JC, Jardet CL. Case Rep Endocrinol. 2018;2018:6147349

36. Cancer Research UK - Original email from CRUK. https://en.wikipedia.org/wiki/Pancreatic_cancer

37. Wang P, Alvarez-Perez JC, Felsenfeld DP, et al. Nat Med. 2015;21(4):383–388

38. Harrington N. Journal of Student Research. 2012.1(1): 23–32

39. Jun H.J., Lee J.H., Jia Y., Hoang M.H., Byun H., Kim K.H., Lee S.J. J. Nutr. 2012;142:432–440

40. Kang J.H., Jeong I.S., Kim M.Y. Evid Based Complement Alternat Med. 2018:4381205

41. Lee J., Chae K., Ha J., et al. Journal of Ethnopharmacology. 2008;115(2):263–270

42. Javid A.Z., Haybar H., Dehghan P. Asia Pac J Clin Nutr. 2018;27(4):785-791

43. Kim IH, Kisseleva T, Brenner DA. Curr Opin Gastroenterol 2015;31:184-191

44. Ito Y, Sørensen KK, Bethea NW, et al. Exp Gerontol. 2007;42(8):789-797

45. Jin YR, Jin JL, Li CH, Piao XX, Jin NG. Pharm Biol. 2012;50(4):523–528

46. FoodDB. https://foodb.ca/

CHAPTER 7: Cut out the junk food and maintain healthy weight

1. Clarke R.E., Dordevic A.L., Tan S.M., Ryan L., Coughlan M.T. Nutrients. 2016;8:125

2. Schulte EM, Avena NM, Gearhardt AN. PLoS One. 2015 Feb 18;10(2):e0117959

3. Alonso-Pedrero L, Ojeda-Rodríguez A, Martínez-González MA, Zalba G, Bes-Rastrollo M, Marti A. Am J Clin Nutr. 2020;111(6):1259-1266

4. Hall K. D., Ayuketah A., Brychta R., Cai H., Cassimatis T., Chen K. Y., et al. Cell Metab. 2019.30 66.e3–77.e3

5. Romaguera D., Ängquist L., Du H., Jakobsen M.U., Forouhi N.G., Halkjær J., et al. PLoS One. 2011;6:e23384

6. Pounis G, Castelnuovo AD, Costanzo S, et al. Nutr Diabetes. 2016;6(7):e218

7. Blausen.com staff (2014), "Medical gallery of Blausen Medical 2014", WikiJournal of Medicine, 1 (2), doi:10.15347/WJM/2014.010, ISSN 2002-4436, Wikidata Q44276831

8. Chen L.W., Aris I.M., Bernard J.Y., Tint M.T., Colega M., Gluckman P.D., Tan K.H., Shek L.P.C., Chong Y.S., Yap F., et al. Am. J. Clin. Nutr. 2017;105:705–713

9. Hall KD, Butte NF, Swinburn BA, & Chow CC (2013). Lancet Diabetes Endocrinol, 1(2), 97–105

10. World food consumption patterns – trends and drivers. EU Agricultural Markets Briefs. No 6. June 2015

11. Bouchard C, Tremblay A, Després JP, et al. N Engl J Med. 1990;322(21):1477-1482

12. https://en.wikipedia.org/wiki/Brown_adipose_tissue. Hg6996 - Own work

13. Vague J. Am J Clin Nutr. 1956.4: 20–34.

14. Nutrition and Biotechnology in Heart Disease and Cancer. John B. Longenecker, David Kritchevsky, and Marc K. Drezner, Eds. Plenum, New York, 1995. 267 pp

15. Lebel A, Kestens Y, Pampalon R, et alJ Obes 2012;2012:1–9

16. Courtemanche CJ, Pinkston JC, Ruhm CJ, Wehby GL. Southern Econ J.2016;82:1266–1310

17. Sturm R, An R. CA Cancer J Clin. 2014 Sep-Oct;64(5):337-50

18. Boucher, J. G., Boudreau, A., Ahmed, S., & Atlas, E. (2015). Environmental Health Perspectives, 123,1287–1293

19. Liu B, Lehmler HJ, Sun Y, Xu G, Liu Y, Zong G, et al. Lancet Planet Health 2017;1:e114-22

20. Elliot J.G., Donovan G.M., Wang K.C.W., Green F.H.Y., James A..L, Noble P.B. Eur Respir J. 2019;54(6). pii: 1900857

21. World food consumption patterns – trends and drivers. EU Agricultural Markets Briefs. No 6. June 2015

22. Sørensen TB, Matsuzaki M, Gregson J, Kinra S, Kadiyala S, Shankar B, Dangour AD. PLoS One. 2020 Mar 31;15(3):e0230744

23. https://ourworldindata.org/

24. Ministry of Health of Brazil. Dietary Guidelines for the Brazilian Population 2nd edn. http://www.fao.org/nutrition/education/food-based-dietary-guidelines/regions/countries/brazil/en/. Published 2014

25. Romaguera D., Ängquist L., Du H., Jakobsen M.U., Forouhi N.G., Halkjær J., et al. PLoS One. 2011;6:e23384

26. Gomes P, Fleming Outeiro T, Cavadas C. Trends Pharmacol Sci. (2015) 36:756–68

27. Wilkinson MJ, Manoogian ENC, Zadourian A, Lo H, Fakhouri S, Shoghi A, Wang X, Fleischer JG, Navlakha S, Panda S, Taub PR. Cell Metab. 2020 Jan 7;31(1):92-104.e5

28. Guan D, Xiong Y, Trinh TM, et al. Science. 2020;eaba8984

29. Iwayama K, Kurihara R, Nabekura Y, Kawabuchi R, Park I, Kobayashi M, et al. EBioMedicine. (2015) 2:2003–9

30. Murray B, Rosenbloom C. Nutr Rev. 2018;76(4):243-259

31. Masood W, Annamaraju P, Uppaluri RK. Ketogenic Diet. https://www.ncbi.nlm.nih.gov/books/NBK499830/. Retrieved August, 2020

32. Zemel MB, Shi H, Greer B, Dirienzo D, Zemel PC. FASEB J. 2000 Jun;14(9):1132-8

33. Zemel MB, Thompson W, Milstead A, Morris K, Campbell P. Obes Res. 2004 Apr;12(4):582-90

34. Rodríguez-Rodríguez E, Perea JM, López-Sobaler AM, Ortega RM; Research Group: 920030. Ann Nutr Metab. 2010;57(2):95-102

35. Ge L., et.el. BMJ. 2020.1;369:m696

36. Rinott E, Youngster I, Meir AY, et al. Gastroenterology. 2020;S0016-5085(20)35111-8

37. Kahleova H, Fleeman R, Hlozkova A, Holubkov R, Barnard ND. Nutr Diabetes. 2018;8(1):58

38. Wang S, Liang X, Yang Q, Fu X, Rogers CJ, Zhu M, Rodgers BD, Jiang Q, Dodson MV, Du M. Int J Obes (Lond). 2015 Jun;39(6):967-76

39. Grahame HD. Acta Pharm Sin B. 2016;6(1):1–19

40. Winder W.W., Hardie D.G. Am. J. Physiol. Metab. 1996;270:E299–E304

41. Carpéné C, Les F, Cásedas G, et al. Antioxidants (Basel). 2019;8(3):74

42. The US Burden of Disease Collaborators. JAMA. 2018;319(14):1444–72

43. OECD OBESITY UPDATE 2017. Retrieved from https://www.oecd.org/health/obesity-update.htm

44. Nankervis SA, Mitchell JM, Charchar FJ, McGlynn MA, Lewandowski PA. Longev Healthspan. 2013;2:4

45. Reynolds A, Mann J, Cummings J, Winter N, Mete E, Te Morenga L. Lancet 2019; 393(10170)434– 445

46. Yashin AI, Arbeev KG, Akushevich I, Ukraintseva SV, Kulminski A, Arbeeva LS, Culminskaya I. Biogerontology. 2010 Jun;11(3):257-65

47. Rauber F, da Costa Louzada ML, Steele EM, Millett C, Monteiro CA, Levy RB. Nutrients. 2018;10(5):587

48. Unwin J.D., Haslam D., Livesey G. J. Insul. Resist. 2016;1:1–9

49. Korem T, Zeevi D, Zmora N, Weissbrod O, Bar N, Lotan-Pompan M, Avnit-Sagi T, Kosower N, Malka G, Rein M, Suez J, Goldberg BZ, Weinberger A, Levy AA, Elinav E, Segal E. Cell Metab. 2017.25(6):1243-1253.e5

50. Mohan V, Spiegelman D, Sudha V, et al. Diabetes Technol Ther. 2014;16(5):317-325

51. Tsai CH, Chen EC, Tsay HS, Huang CJ. Nutr J. 2012;11:4

CHAPTER 8: Real atherosclerosis begins in childhood

1. Zech LA, Hoeg JM. Lipids Health Dis. 2008;7

2. Agouridis AP, Elisaf MS, Nair DR, Mikhailidis DP. Arch Med Sci. 2015;11(6):1145-55

3. Afrodriguezg/Wikimedia Commons/CC BY 4.0

4. Med Chaos/Wikimedia Commons/CC BY 4.0

5. Centers for Disease Control and Prevention (US); National Center for Chronic Disease Prevention and Health Promotion (US); Office on Smoking and Health (US). How Tobacco Smoke Causes Disease: The Biology and Behavioral Basis for Smoking-Attributable Disease: A Report of the Surgeon General. Atlanta (GA): Centers for Disease Control and Prevention (US); 2010. 6, Cardiovascular Diseases. Available from: https://www.ncbi.nlm.nih.gov/books/NBK53012/

6. Tobacco kills up to half of its users – Accelerated efforts needed to tackle Afghanistan's tobacco crisis. WHO. 2017

7. Willcox BJ, Tranah GJ, Chen R, Morris BJ, Masaki KH, He Q, Willcox DC, Allsopp RC, Moisyadi S, Poon LW, Rodriguez B, Newman AB, Harris TB, Cummings SR, Liu Y, Parimi N, Evans DS, Davy P, Gerschenson M, Donlon TA. Aging Cell. 2016 Aug;15(4):617-24

8. Davy PMC, Willcox DC, Shimabukuro M, Donlon TA, Torigoe T, Suzuki M, Higa M, Masuzaki H, Sata M, Chen R, Murkofsky RL, Morris BJ, Lim E, Allsopp RC, Willcox BJ. J Gerontol A Biol Sci Med Sci. 2018 Oct 8;73(11):1448-1452

9. Thorin E, Hamilton C, Dominiczak AF, Dominiczak MH, Reid JL. Atherosclerosis. 1995;114(2):185–195

10. Alexopoulos N, McLean DS, Janik M, Arepalli CD, Stillman AE, Raggi P. Atherosclerosis. 2010 May;210(1):150-4

11. Blausen.com staff (2014), "Medical gallery of Blausen Medical 2014", WikiJournal of Medicine, 1 (2), doi:10.15347/WJM/2014.010, ISSN 2002-4436, Wikidata Q44276831

12. Merghani A, Maestrini V, Rosmini S, Cox AT, Dhutia H, Bastiaenan R, David S, Yeo TJ, Narain R, Malhotra A, et al. Circulation. 2017;136:126–137

13. Currens JH, White PD. N Engl J Med. 1961;265:988–993

14. Antero-Jacquemin J, Pohar-Perme M, Rey G, Toussaint JF, Latouche A. Eur J Epidemiol. 2018;33(6):531–43

15. Hong Y.M. Korean Circ. J. 2010;40:1–9

16. Akoumianakis I, Sanna F, Margaritis M, et al. Sci Transl Med. 2019;11(510):eaav5055

17. Nephron - Own work. https://en.wikipedia.org/wiki/Atherosclerosis. Retrieved August, 2020

18. Ed Uthman. https://en.wikipedia.org/wiki/Atheroma. Retrieved August, 2020

19. Brunner FJ, Waldeyer C, Ojeda F, et al. Lancet. 2019.394(10215):2173-2183

20. Nehra A, Alterowitz R, Culkin DJ, et al. J Urol. 2015;194(3):745-753

21. Stuntz M, Perlaky A, des Vignes F, Kyriakides T, Glass D. PLoS One. 2016;11(2):e0150157

22. Chilton CP, Castle WM, Westwood CA, Pryor JP. Br J Urol. 1982;54(6):748-750

23. Hempel A, Maasch C, Heintze U, Lindschau C, Dietz R, Luft FC & Haller H (1997) Circ Res 81, 363–371

24. Funk SD, Yurdagul A, Orr AW. Int J Vasc Med 2012;2012:1–19

25. Hall H, Perelman D, Breschi A, Limcaoco P, Kellogg R, McLaughlin T, Snyder M. PLOS Biology 2018. 16 e2005143

26. Shuto Y., Asai A., Nagao M., Sugihara H., Oikawa S. PLoS ONE. 2015;10

27. DiNicolantonio J.J., Lucan S.C., O'Keefe J.H. Prog. Cardiovasc. Dis. 2016;58:464–472

28. Kearns CE, Schmidt LA, Glantz SA. JAMA Intern Med 2016;176:1680-5

29. Bai W, Li J, Liu J. Clin Chim Acta 2016;461:76–82

30. Gutierrez OM, Isakova T, Enfield G, Wolf M. J Ren Nutr. 2011 Mar;21(2):140–148

31. Ritz E., Hahn K., Ketteler M., Kuhlmann M.K., Mann J. Dtsch. Arztebl. Int. 2012;109:49–55.

32. Ogola B.O., Zimmerman M.A., Clark G.L., Abshire C.M., Gentry K.M., Miller K.S., Lindsey S.H. Am. J. Physiol. Heart Circ. Physiol. 2018;315:H1073–H1087

33. Li D. Y., and Tang W. H. W. 2017. Curr. Atheroscler. Rep. 19: 39

34. Wikoff WR, Anfora AT, Liu J, Schultz PG, Lesley SA, Peters EC and Siuzdak G (2009).Proc Natl Acad Sci U S A 106(10): 3698–3703

35. Menni C, et al. Eur. Heart J. 2018;39:2390–2397

36. Randrianarisoa E., Lehn-Stefan A., Wang X., Hoene M., Peter A., Heinzmann S.S., Zhao X., Konigsrainer I., Konigsrainer A., Balletshofer B., et al. Sci. Rep. 2016;6:26745

37. Bogiatzi C., Gloor G., Allen-Vercoe E., Reid G., Wong R.G., Urquhart B.L. et al. . (2018) Atherosclerosis 273, 91–97

38. Domínguez F, Fuster V, Fernández-Alvira JM, Fernández-Friera L, López-Melgar B, Blanco-Rojo R, Fernández-Ortiz A, García-Pavía P, Sanz J, Mendiguren JM, Ibañez B, Bueno H, Lara-Pezzi E, Ordovás JM. J Am Coll Cardiol. 2019 Jan 22;73(2):134-144

39. Vallat R, Shah VD, Redline S, Attia P, Walker MP. PLoS Biol. 2020 Jun 4;18(6):e3000726

40. McAlpine CS, Kiss MG, Rattik S, et al. Nature. 2019;566(7744):383-387

41. Vallat R, Shah VD, Redline S, Attia P, Walker MP. PLoS Biol. 2020 Jun 4;18(6):e3000726

42. Mostafa MN, Osama M. Exp Biol Med (Maywood). 2020 Sep;245(15):1376-1384.

43. Esselstyn CB, Jr, Ellis SG, Medendorp SV, Crowe TD. J Fam Pract. 1995 Dec;41(6):560–8

44. Esselstyn CB., Jr. Prev Cardiol. 2001 Autumn;4(4):171–7

45. Amengual J, Coronel J, Marques C, Aradillas-García C, Morales JMV, Andrade FCD, Erdman JW, Teran-Garcia M. J Nutr. 2020 Aug 1;150(8):2023-2030

46. Jenkins DJ, Kendall CW, Marchie A, Faulkner DA, Wong JM, de Souza R, Emam A, Parker TL, Vidgen E, Trautwein EA, Lapsley KG, Josse RG, Leiter LA, Singer W, Connelly PW. Am J Clin Nutr. 2005 Feb;81(2):380-7

47. Lin X, Racette SB, Lefevre M, et al. Eur J Clin Nutr. 2010;64(12):1481-1487

48. FoodDB. https://foodb.ca/

49. Ornish D, Scherwitz LW, Billings JH, et al. JAMA. 1998;280(23):2001-2007

50. BruceBlaus - Own work, https://en.wikipedia.org/wiki/Coronary_catheterization

51. Khalil A. Can J Physiol Pharmacol. 2002 Jul;80(7):662-9

52. Paulis G, Brancato T, D'Ascenzo R, et al. Andrology. 2013;1(1):120-128

53. Varshney R, Budoff MJ. J Nutr. 2016 Feb;146(2):416S-421S

54. Elosta A, Slevin M, Rahman K, Ahmed N. Sci Rep. 2017;7:39613

55. Budoff MJ, Takasu J, Flores FR, Niihara Y, Lu B, Lau BH, Rosen RT, Amagase H. Prev Med. 2004 Nov;39(5):985-91.

56. Lawson, L. D. (1993). Bioactive organosulphur compounds of garlic and garlic products: role in reducing blood lipids. In Kinghorn, A. D. & Balandrin, M. F. (Ed), Human medicinal agents from plants (pp. 176-179). Whashington: American Chemical Society (ACS Symposium Series, n. 534)

57. Schurgers LJ, Spronk HM, Soute BA, Schiffers PM, DeMey JG, Vermeer C. Blood. 2007 Apr 1;109(7):2823-31

58. Knapen MH, Braam LA, Drummen NE, Bekers O, Hoeks AP, Vermeer C. Thromb Haemost. 2015 May;113(5):1135-44

59. Gast GC, de Roos NM, Sluijs I, Bots ML, Beulens JW, Geleijnse JM, Witteman JC, Grobbee DE, Peeters PH, van der Schouw YT. Nutr Metab Cardiovasc Dis. 2009 Sep;19(7):504-10

60. Geleijnse JM, Vermeer C, Grobbee DE, et al. J Nutr. 2004;134(11):3100-3105

61. Imamura Haruki, Yamaguchi Takashi, Nagayama Daiji, Saiki Atsuhito, Shirai Kohji, Tatsuno Ichiro. International Heart Journal. 2017;58(4):577–583

62. Nagata C., Wada K., Tamura T., Konishi K., Goto Y., Koda S. Am. J. Clin. Nutr. 2017;105(2):426–431

63. Tokede OA, Onabanjo TA, Yansane A, Gaziano JM, Djoussé L. Br J Nutr. 2015;114(6):831-843

64. Willcox BJ, Willcox DC, Todoriki H et al. Ann N Y Acad Sci 2007; 1114: 434–55

65. Kinoshita H, Ogata Y. Evid Based Complement Alternat Med. 2018 Nov 8;2018:4915784

66. Roager HM, Licht TR. Nat Commun. 2018;9(1):3294

67. Kohara K., Tabara Y., Ochi M., et al. Scientific Reports. 2018;8(1)

68. Chung R.W.S., Leanderson P., Lundberg A.K., Jonasson L. Atherosclerosis. 2017;262:87–93

69. Gruber M., Chappell R., Millen A., LaRowe T., Moeller S.M., Iannaccone A., Kritchevsky S.B., Mares J. J. Nutr. 2004;134:2387–2394

70. Moran R, Nolan JM, Stack J, et al. J Nutr Health Aging. 2016. pp. 1–8

71. Bovier ER, Lewis RD, Hammond BR., Jr. Nutrients. 2013;5:750–757

72. Jalal F, Nesheim MC, Agus Z, Sanjur D, Habicht JP. Am J Clin Nutr. 1998 Sep;68(3):623-9

73. Prysyazhna O., Wolhuter K., Switzer C., Santos C., Yang X., Lynham S., Shah A.M., Eaton P., Burgoyne J.R. Circulation. 2019;140:126–137

74. Tome-Carneiro J., Gonzalvez M., Larrosa M., Yanez-Gascon M.J., Garcia-Almagro F.J., Ruiz-Ros J.A., Garcia-Conesa M.T., Tomas-Barberan F.A., Espin J.C. Am. J. Cardiol. 2012;110:356–363

75. Iwabu M., Okada-Iwabu M., Yamauchi T., Kadowaki T. NPJ Aging Mech. Dis. 2015;1:15013

76. Tomé-Carneiro J, Gonzálvez M, Larrosa M, et al. Cardiovasc Drugs Ther. 2013;27(1):37-48

77. Wasilewski GB, Vervloet MG, Schurgers LJ. Front Cardiovasc Med. 2019;6:6

CHAPTER 9: Repairable heart

1. Lazar E, Sadek HA, Bergmann O. Eur Heart J. 2017;38(30): 2333–2342

2. Wencker D., Chandra M., Nguyen K., Miao W., Garantziotis S., Factor S.M. et al. J Clin Invest 2003; 111: 1497–1504

3. Robert E. et. al. Proceedings of the National Academy of Sciences Oct 2019, 116 (40) 19905-19910

4. Piano M.R. Alcohol Res. 2017;38:219–241

5. Zaitsu, M., Takeuchi, T., Kobayashi, Y. and Kawachi, I. Cancer.2020. 126: 1031-1040

6. https://ourworldindata.org/

7. Stockdale W. T., Lemieux M. E., Killen A. C., Zhao J., Hu Z., Riepsaame J., Hamilton N., Kudoh T., Riley P. R., Van Aerle R. et al. (2018). Cell Rep. 25, 1997-2007

8. Cho W. J., Chow A. K., Schulz R., Daniel E. E. Canadian Journal of Physiology and Pharmacology. 2010;88(1):73–76

9. Jasmin JF, Rengo G, Lymperopoulos A, Gupta R, Eaton GJ, Quann K, et al. (2011). Am J Physiol Heart Circ Physiol, 300: H1274-81

10. Uray IP, Connelly JH, Frazier OH, et al. Cardiovasc Res. 2003;59:57–66

11. Lee YJ, Hsu JD, Lin WL, Kao SH, Wang CJ. Food Funct. 2017;8:397–405.

12. Hada Y, Uchida HA, Otaka N, et al. Int J Mol Sci. 2020;21(12):4527. Published 2020 Jun 25. doi:10.3390/ijms21124527

13. Tian L, Su CP, Wang Q, et al. J Cell Mol Med. 2019;23(7):4666-4678

14. Zhao Y, Wang J, Ballevre O, Luo H, Zhang W. Hypertens Res. 2012;35(4):370-374

15. Raish M. International Journal of Biological Macromolecules. 2017;97:544–551

16. Tan HF, & Gan CY. International Journal of Biological Macromolecules.2016. 85; 487–496

17. Deng Y., Tang Q., Zhang Y., Zhang R., Wei Z. Food & Nutrition Research. 2017;61(1):1–12

18. Douthit MK, Fain ME, Nguyen JT, et al. J Nutr. 2017;147(10):1960–1967

19. Rhéaume-Bleue K (2012). Vitamin K2 and the Calcium Paradox. John Wiley & Sons, Canada

20. Magyar K., Halmosi R., Palfi A., Feher G., Czopf L., Fulop A., Battyany I., Sumegi B., Toth K., Szabados E. Clin. Hemorheol. Microcirc. 2012;50:179–187

21. Olson ER, Naugle JE, Zhang X, Bomser JA, Meszaros JG. Am J Physiol Heart Circ Physiol. 2005 Mar;288(3):H1131-8

22. Shrikanta A, Kumar A, Govindaswamy V. J Food Sci Technol. 2015;52(1):383-390

CHAPTER 10: Pain and inflammation

1. Bertolini, A., Ferrari, A., Ottani, A., Guerzoni, S., Tacchi, R., and Leone, S. CNS Drug Rev. 2006.12; 250–275

2. https://abcnews.go.com/Health/wireStory/california-list-common-pain-killer-carcinogen-68424692: date 21Jan 2020

3. Furman D. et al. Nat Med. 2019: 25(12): 1822-1832

4. Wang X, Liang T, Qiu J, et al. Stem Cells Int. 2019;2019:6568394

5. Chung S, Lapoint K, Martinez K, Kennedy A, Boysen Sandberg M, McIntosh MK. Endocrinology. 2006;147:5340–51

6. Ruan Y, Tang J, Guo X, Li K, Li D. Curr Alzheimer Res. 2018;15(9):869-876

7. Chowdhury R, Warnakula S, Kunutsor S, et al. Ann Intern Med. 2014;160(6):398-406

8. Simopoulos AP. Biomed Pharmacother. 2006;60(9):502–507

9. Simopoulos AP. Nutrients. 2016;8:128

10. Simopoulos A.P. Exp. Biol. Med. 2008;233:674–688.

11. Rizzo AM, Montorfano G, Negroni M, et al. Lipids Health Dis. 2010;9:7

12. https://en.wikipedia.org/wiki/Fatty_acid_ratio_in_food. Retrieved August, 2020

13. Kodahl N. Planta. 2020;251(4):80

14. Zatonski W, Campos H, Willett W. Eur J Epidemiol. 2008;23(1):3–10

15. Zatonski WA, McMichael AJ, Powles JW. BMJ1998;316:1047-51

16. Kesteloot H, Sans S, Kromhout D. Eur Heart J. 2006; 27(1): 107–113

17. Denk F, Crow M, Didangelos A, Lopes DM, McMahon SB. Cell Rep. 2016 May 24;15(8):1771-81

18. Simpson RJ, Lowder TW, Spielmann G, Bigley AB, LaVoy EC, Kunz H. Ageing Res Rev. 2012;11(3):404-420

19. Spielmann G, McFarlin BK, O'Connor DP, Smith PJ, Pircher H, Simpson RJ. Brain Behav Immun. 2011;25(8):1521-1529

20. Youm Y-H, Nguyen KY, Grant RW, et al. Nat Med 2015;21:263–9

21. Newman JC, Verdin E. Annu Rev Nutr. 2017;37:51-76

22. Koeslag JH, Noakes TD, Sloan AW. J Physiol. 1980 Apr;301:79-90

23. Jordan S, Tung N, Casanova-Acebes M, Chang C, Cantoni C, Zhang D, Wirtz TH, Naik S, Rose SA, Brocker CN, Gainullina A, Hornburg D, Horng S, Maier BB, Cravedi P, LeRoith D, Gonzalez FJ, Meissner F, Ochando J, Rahman A, Chipuk JE, Artyomov MN, Frenette PS, Piccio L, Berres ML, Gallagher EJ, Merad M. Cell. 2019 Aug 22;178(5):1102-1114

24. Collins N., Han S. J., Enamorado M., Link V. M., Huang B., Moseman E. A. Cell.2019. 178(1088);e15–1101.e15

25. Traba J, Kwarteng-Siaw M, Okoli TC, et al. J Clin Invest. 2015;125(12):4592-4600

26. Vargas-Ortiz K, Pérez-Vázquez V, Figueroa A, Díaz FJ, Montaño-Ascencio PG, Macías-Cervantes MH. Eur J Sport Sci. 2018 Mar;18(2):226-234

27. Nerurkar PV, Johns LM, Buesa LM, Kipyakwai G, Volper E, Sato R, Shah P, Feher D, Williams PG, Nerurkar VR. J Neuroinflammation. 2011 Jun 3;8:64

28. Traba J, Geiger SS, Kwarteng-Siaw M, et al. J Biol Chem. 2017;292(29):12153-12164

29. Farnaghi S., Prasadam I., Cai G., Friis T., Du Z., Crawford R., et al. . (2017). J. 31, 356–367

30. Rayati F, Hajmanouchehri F, Najafi E. Dent Res J (Isfahan) 2017 Jan-Feb;14(1):1–7

31. Kuptniratsaikul V, Dajpratham P, Taechaarpornkul W, et al. Clin Interv Aging 2014; 9: 451–458

32. Daily J.W., Yang M., Park S. J. Med. Food. 2016;19:717–729

33. Shoba, G. , Joy, D. , Joseph, T. , Majeed, M. , Rajendran, R. , & Srinivas, P. S. Planta Medica.1998. 64(4); 353–356

34. https://en.wikipedia.org/wiki/Intestinal_villus. WikipedianProlific

35. Beauchamp GK, Keast RS, Morel D, Lin J, Pika J, Han Q, Lee CH, Smith AB, Breslin PA. Nature. 2005 Sep 1;437(7055):45-6

36. Al-Waeli H., Nicolau B., et al. Sci Rep. 2020.10(1):468

CHAPTER 11: You have to have the right bacteria to live a longer life

1. Tamburini S, Shen N, Wu HC, Clemente JC. Nat. Med. 2016;22:713–722

2. Robertson RC, Manges AR, Finlay BB, Prendergast AJ. Trends Microbiol. (2019) 27:131–47

3. Hehemann JH, Correc G, Barbeyron T, Helbert W, Czjzek M, Michel G. Nature. (2010) 464:908–12

4. David L. A., Maurice C. F., Carmody R. N., Gootenberg D. B., Button J. E., Wolfe B. E., et al. . (2014). Nature 505, 559–563

5. Bamberger C., Rossmeier A., Lechner K., Wu L., Waldmann E., Fischer S., Stark R.G., Altenhofer J., Henze K., Parhofer K.G. Nutrients. 2018;10:244

6. Roager HM, Vogt JK, Kristensen M, et al Gut. 2019.68(1):83-93.

7. Hunter P. EMBO Rep. 2012;13(11):968-970

8. Yano JM, et al. Cell. 2015;161:264–276

9. Jovanovic-Malinovska R, Kuzmanova S, Winkelhausen E. Int J Food Prop 2014;17:949–65

10. Caetano B.F., de Moura N.A., Almeida A.P., Dias M.C., Sivieri K., Barbisan L.F. Nutrients. 2016;8

11. Roager HM, Vogt JK, Kristensen M, et al. Gut. 2019.68(1):83-93.

12. Wassermann B., Müller H., Berg G. An Apple a Day: Front Microbiol. 2019.24;10:1629

13. Cooley, M. B., Chao, D., and Mandrell, R. E. J. Food Prot. 2006.69; 2329–2335

14. Wan S.Z., Liu C., Huang C.K., Luo .FY., Zhu X. Front Pharmacol. 2019;10:1321

15. Wan S, Huang C, Wang A, Zhu X. PeerJ. 2020 Apr 24;8:e9050

CHAPTER 12: Bone loss is a significant global health concern

1. Barrere F, van Blitterswijk CA, de Groot K. Int J Nanomedicine. 2006; 1: 317–332

2. Unni J., Garg R., Pawar R. J Midlife Health. 2010;1:19–22

3. Chen P, Li Z, Hu Y. BMC Public Health. 2016;16(1):1039–1049

4.   Handa R, Kalla AA, Maalouf G. Best Practice and Research Clinical Rheumatology. 2008;22(4):693-708

5.   Kotlarz H, Gunnarsson CL, Fang H, Rizzo JA. Arthritis Rheum. 2009 Dec;60(12):3546-53

6.   Asomaning K., Bertone-Johnson E.R., Nasca P.C., Hooven F., Pekow P.S. J. Womens Health. 2006;15:1028–1034

7.   Shamsul A. Khan, Habibullah Qureshi, Mujtaba Farooq Rana, Khemomal Asudo Karira, Hasan Ali.2006.Jan-Apr.JLUMHS.

8.   Thom JA, Morris JE, Bishop A, Blacklock NJ. Br J Urol. 1978;50(7):459-464

9.   Ochs-Balcom H.M. et al. J Bone Miner Res. 2019. doi: 10.1002/jbmr.3879

10.   Iqbal J., Sun L., Cao J., Yuen T., Lu P., Bab I., Leu N.A., Srinivasan S., Wagage S., Hunter C.A., et al. Proc. Natl. Acad. Sci. USA. 2013;110:11115–11120

11.   Naganathan V, et al. Arch Intern Med. 2000;160:2917–2922

12.   Weaver CM, Gordon CM, Janz KF, Kalkwarf HJ, Lappe JM, Lewis R, et al. Osteoporos Int. (2016) 27:1281–386

13.   Malmgren L, McGuigan F, Christensson A, Akesson KE. Osteoporos Int. 2017;28(12):3463-3473

14.   Messa P. Nephrol Dial Transplant 2013; 28:3–7

15.   Wallace T, Jun S, Zou P, Weaver C, Bailey RL. Curr Dev Nutr. 2020;4(Suppl 2):1500

16.   Weaver CM, Gordon CM, Janz KF, Kalkwarf HJ, Lappe JM, Lewis R, et al. Osteoporos Int. (2016) 27:1281–386

17.   Illingworth CM. J Pediatr Surg. 1974 Dec;9(6):853-58

18.   Hsueh M.F, Önnerfjord P, Bolognesi M.P, Easley M.E, Kraus V.B. Sci Adv. 2019;5(10):eaax3203

19.   Jeon O.H., Kim C., Laberge R.M., Demaria M., Rathod S., Vasserot A.P., Chung J.W., Kim D.H., Poon Y., David N., et al. Nat. Med. 2017;23:775–781

20.   Institute of Medicine (US) Committee to Review Dietary Reference Intakes for Vitamin D and Calcium; Ross AC, Taylor CL, Yaktine AL, et al., editors. Dietary Reference Intakes for Calcium and Vitamin D. Washington (DC): National Academies Press (US); 2011. 6, Tolerable Upper Intake Levels: Calcium and Vitamin D. Available from: https://www.ncbi.nlm.nih.gov/books/NBK56058/

21.   L'Abbé M.R.Calcium Physiology. Encyclopedia of Food Sciences and Nutrition (2nd Ed). 2003; 771-779

22.   Blausen.com staff (2014), "Medical gallery of Blausen Medical 2014", WikiJournal of Medicine, 1 (2), doi:10.15347/WJM/2014.010, ISSN 2002-4436, Wikidata Q44276831

23.   Clark S, Horton R. Lancet. 2018;391(10137):2302

24.   Shiri R, Karppinen J, Leino-Arjas P, Solovieva S, Viikari-Juntura E. Am J Epidemiol. 2010;171:135–154

25.   Dieleman JL, Baral R, Birger M, Bui AL, Bulchis A, Chapin A, Hamavid H, Horst C, Johnson EK, Joseph J, et al. JAMA. 2016;316(24):2627–2646

26.   Shipton, E.A. Pain Ther. 2018. 7:127–137

27.   Zhang J., Valverde P., Zhu X., Murray D., Wu Y., Yu L., Jiang H., Dard M.M., Huang J., Xu Z., Tu Q., Chen J. Bone Research.2017. 5;16056

28. Colaianni G, Sanesi L, Storlino G, Brunetti G, Colucci S, Grano M. Cells. 2019;8(5):451

29. Zhang J., Valverde P., Zhu X., Murray D., Wu Y., Yu L., Jiang H., Dard M.M., Huang J., Xu Z., Tu Q., Chen J. Bone Research.2017. 5;16056

30. Colaianni G, Sanesi L, Storlino G, Brunetti G, Colucci S, Grano M. Cells. 2019;8(5):451

31. Ahmed M.F., El-Sayed A.K., Chen H., Zhao R., Yusuf M.S., Zuo Q., Zhang Y., Li B. Exp. Ther. Med. 2019;17:4154–4166

32. Ozaki K, Kawata Y, Amano S, Hanazawa S. Biochem Pharmacol. (2000) 59:1577–81

33. Riva A, Togni S, Giacomelli L, et al. Eur Rev Med Pharmacol Sci. 2017;21:1684–1689

34. Kim JY, Cheon YH, Kwak SC, et al. J Bone Miner Res. 2014;29:1541-1553

35. Yang F, Yuan PW, Hao YQ, Lu ZM. BMC Complement Altern Med. 2014;14:74.24565373

36. Lee S.-U., Shin H.K., Min Y.K., Kim S.H. Int. Immunopharmacol. 208;8:741-747

37. Jang, Hae Won et al. Conference Proceedings. 2018

38. Lin L., Ni B., Lin H., et al. J Ethnopharmacol. 2015;159:158-183

39. Di X., Wang X., Di X., Liu Y. J. Pharm. Biomed. Anal. 2015;115:144-149

40. Huh J.E., Koh P.S., Seo B.K., Park Y.C., Baek Y.H., Lee J.D., Park D.S. Int. J. Mol. Sci. 2014;15:16025–16042

41. Bai Y, et al. 2018. FASEB J. 32(8):4573-4584

42. Li Y, Wu Y, Jiang K, et al. Oxid Med Cell Longev. 2019;2019:8783197

43. Lucas A. Edralin, Perkins-Veazie Penelope, Smith J. Brenda, Clarke Stephen, Kuvibidila Solo, Lightfoo A. Stanley. Effects of mango on bone parameters in mice fed high fat diet.2010

44. DiNicolantonio JJ, Mehta V, Zaman SB, O'Keefe JH. Mo Med. 2018;115(3):247-252

45. Fam VW, Holt RR, Keen CL, Sivamani RK, Hackman RM. Nutrients. 2020 Nov 4;12(11):E3381

46. L'Abbé M.R.Calcium Physiology. Encyclopedia of Food Sciences and Nutrition (2nd Ed). 2003; 771-779

47. Wortsman J, Matsuoka LY, Chen TC, Lu Z, Holick MF. Am J Clin Nutr. 2000;72(3):690-693

48. Marantes I, Achenbach SJ, Atkinson EJ, Khosla S, Melton LJ 3rd, Amin S. J Bone Miner Res. 2011;26(12):2860-2871

49. Hassan-Smith ZK, Jenkinson C, Smith DJ, et al. PLoS One. 2017;12(2):e0170665

50. Amrein K, Scherkl M, Hoffmann M, et al. Eur J Clin Nutr. 2020;1-16

51. Heaney RP. Am J Clin Nutr. 2004;80(6 Suppl):1706S-9S

52. Turner Biomechanics Laboratory - http://www.osseon.com/osteoporosis-overview/

53. Holick MF. N Engl J Med. 2007;357(3):266-281

54. Bügel S. Proc Nutr Soc. 2003 Nov;62(4):839-43

55. Misra D, Booth SL, Tolstykh I, et al. Am J Med 2013;126:243–8

56. Knapen M.H., Schurgers L.J., Vermeer C. Osteoporosis Int. 2007;18:963–972

57. Maresz K. Integr Med (Encinitas). 2015;14:34-39

58. van den Heuvel EG, Muys T, van Dokkum W, Schaafsma G. Am J Clin Nutr. 1999 Mar;69(3):544-8

59. Abrams SA, Griffin IJ, Hawthorne KM, Liang L, Gunn SK, Darlington G, Ellis KJ. Am J Clin Nutr. 2005 Aug;82(2):471-6.

60. Holloway L, Moynihan S, Abrams SA, Kent K, Hsu AR, Friedlander AL. Br J Nutr. 2007 Feb;97(2):365-72

61. Wetli HA, Brenneisen R, Tschudi I, Langos M, Bigler P, Sprang T, Schürch S, Mühlbauer RC. J Agric Food Chem. 2005 May 4;53(9):3408-14

CHAPTER 13: The very big problem of the aged: muscle loss

1. Kim KM, Jang HC, Lim S. Korean J Intern Med. 2016;31:643–650

2. Williams D, Kuipers A, Mukai C, Thirsk R. CMAJ. 2009;180:1317–1323

3. Fernández-Garrido J., Ruiz-Ros V., Buigues C., Navarro-Martinez R., Cauli O. Arch. Gerontol. Geriatr. 2014;59:7–17

4. Wilson D, Jackson T, Sapey E, Lord JM. Ageing Res Rev. 2017 Jul;36:1-10

5. Kenny AM, Dawson L, Kleppinger A, Iannuzzi-Sucich M, Judge JO. J Gerontol A Biol Sci Med Sci. 2003 May;58(5):M436-40

6. Xia MF, Chen LY, Wu L, Ma H, Li XM, Li Q, Aleteng Q, Hu Y, He WY, Gao J, Lin HD, Gao X. Clin Nutr. 2020 Jun 13:S0261-5614(20)30293-4

7. Gruther W, Benesch T, Zorn C, et al. J Rehabil Med. 2008;40(3):185-189

8. https://en.wikipedia.org/wiki/Muscle_atrophy. OpenStax - https://cnx.org/contents/FPtK1zmh@8.25:fEI3C8Ot@10/Preface.

9. Dridi H, Kushnir A, Zalk R, Yuan Q, Melville Z, Marks AR. Nat Rev Cardiol. 2020 Nov;17(11):732-747

10. Andreux PA, van Diemen MPJ, Heezen MR, Auwerx J, Rinsch C, Groeneveld GJ, and Singh A (2018). Sci. Rep. 8, 8548

11. Marzetti E, Csiszar A, Dutta D, Balagopal G, Calvani R, Leeuwenburgh C. Am J Physiol Heart Circ Physiol. 2013;305(4):H459–H476

12. van Dronkelaar C, van Velzen A, Abdelrazek M, van der Steen A, Weijs PJM, Tieland M. J Am Med Dir Assoc. 2018 Jan;19(1):6-11.e3

13. Schoenfeld B. J. Acta Physiol. 2018; 222: e12990

14. Wang J., Leung K.-S., Chow S.K.-H., Cheung W.-H. J. Orthop. Translat. 2017;10:94–101

15. Golomb BA, Evans MA. Am J Cardiovasc Drugs. 2008;8(6):373–418

16. Andreux PA, Blanco-Bose W, Ryu, D. et al. Nat Metab 2019. 1, 595–603

17. Cortés-Martín, A. , García-Villalba, R. , González-Sarrías, A. , Romo-Vaquero, M. , Loria-Kohen, V. , Ramírez-de-Molina, A. , … Espín, J. C. (2018). Food & Function, 9(8), 4100–4106

18. García-Villalba R., Espín J.C., Tomás-Barberán F.A. J. Chromatogr. A. 2015;1428:162–175

19. FoodDB. https://foodb.ca/

20. Kunkel S.D., Suneja M., Ebert S.M., Bongers K.S., Fox D.K., Malmberg S.E. Cell Metab. 2011;13:627–638

21. Cho Y. H., Lee S. Y., Kim C. M., et al. Evidence-Based Complementary and Alternative Medicine. 2016;2016:9

22. Lahiri S, Kim H, Garcia-Perez I, et al. Sci Transl Med. 2019;11(502):eaan5662

23. Buigues C., Fernandez-Garrido J., Pruimboom L., Hoogland A.J., Navarro-Martinez R., Martinez-Martinez M., Verdejo Y., Mascaros M.C., Peris C., Cauli O. Int. J. Mol. Sci. 2016;17:932

24. Jovanovic-Malinovska R, Kuzmanova S, Winkelhausen E. Int J Food Prop 2014;17:949–65

CHAPTER 14: Exercise is the key to a healthier and longer life

1. Schumacher L.M., Thomas J.G., Raynor H.A., Rhodes R.E., O'Leary K.C., Wing R.R., Bond D.S. Obesity (Silver Spring). 2019;27(8):1285-1291

2. Vigelsø A, Gram M, Wiuff C, Andersen JL, Helge JW, Dela F. J Rehabil Med. 2015;47(6):552-560

3. Contrepois K., Wu S., Moneghetti K.J., et al. Cell. 2020;181(5):1112-1130

4. Nedeltcheva AV, Kilkus JM, Imperial J, Schoeller DA, Penev PD. Ann Intern Med. 2010 Oct 5;153(7):435-41

5. Charles J. Weschler. Environmental Science & Technology, 1978; 12 (8): 923

6. Crane J., MacNeil L., Lally J., Ford R., Bujak A., Brar I., Kemp B., Raha S., Steinberg G., Tarnopolsky M. Aging Cell. 2015;14:625–634

7. Pollock RD, O'Brien KA, Daniels LJ, Nielsen KB, Rowlerson A, Duggal NA, Lazarus NR, Lord JM, Philp A, Harridge SDR. Aging Cell. 2018 Apr;17(2):e12735

8. Tanimura Y, Aoi W, Takanami Y, et al. Physiol Rep. 2016;4(12):e12828

9. Kharitonenkov A, DiMarchi R. Trends Endocrinol Metab. 2015 Nov;26(11):608-617

10. Zhang Y, et al. eLife. 2012;1:e00065.

11. Kim KH, Kim SH, Min YK, Yang HM, Lee JB, Lee MS. PLoS One. 2013;8(5):e63517

12. Ekelund U, Tarp J, Fagerland MW, Johannessen JS, Hansen BH, Jefferis BJ, Whincup PH, Diaz KM, Hooker S, Howard VJ, Chernofsky A, Larson MG, Spartano N, Vasan RS, Dohrn IM, Hagströmer M, Edwardson C, Yates T, Shiroma EJ, Dempsey P, Wijndaele K, Anderssen SA, Lee IM. Br J Sports Med. 2020 Dec;54(24):1499-1506

13. Wen CP, Wai JP, Tsai MK, Yang YC, Cheng TY, Lee MC, Chan HT, Tsao CK, Tsai SP, Wu X. Lancet. 2011 Oct 1;378(9798):1244-53

CHAPTER 15: Under stress, depression and lack of sleep

1. Greer SM, Goldstein AN, Walker MP. Nat Commun. 2013;4:2259

2. DiFeliceantonio AG, Coppin G, Rigoux L, Edwin Thanarajah S, Dagher A, Tittgemeyer M, Small DM. Cell Metab. 2018 Jul 3;28(1):33-44.e3

3. Altena E, Chen IY, Daviaux Y, Ivers H, Philip P, Morin CM. Brain Sci. 2017 Apr 14;7(4):41

4. Chao A.M., Jastreboff A.M., White M.A., Grilo C.M., Sinha R. Obesity. 2017;25:713–720

5. Kain ZN, Zimolo Z, Heninger G. J Clin Endocrinol Metab. 1999;84:2438–2442

6. Spiegel K, Tasali E, Penev P, et al. Ann Intern Med 2004;141:846–50

7. Bahrami-Nejad Z, Zhao ML, Tholen S, et al. Cell Metab. 2018;27(4):854-868.e8

8. Chen Y, Lyga J. Inflamm Allergy Drug Targets. 2014;13:117–190

9. Institute of Medicine (US) Committee on Sleep Medicine and Research; Colten HR, Altevogt BM, editors. Sleep Disorders and Sleep Deprivation: An Unmet Public Health Problem. Washington (DC): National Academies Press (US); 2006. 2, Sleep Physiology. Available from: https://www.ncbi.nlm.nih.gov/books/NBK19956/

10. Mouland J.W., Martial F., Watson A., Lucas R.J., Brown T.M. Curr. Biol. 2019;29:4260–4267

11. Chang AM, Aeschbach D, Duffy JF, Czeisler CA. Proc Natl Acad Sci USA. 2015;1232:(4)112–1237

12. Patel D, Steinberg J, Patel P. J Clin Sleep Med. 2018;14(6):1017-1024

13. Hublin C, Partinen M, Koskenvuo M, Kaprio J. Sleep. 2007;30(10):1245-1253

14. Long sleep and mortality: rationale for sleep restriction. Sleep Med Rev. 2004;8(3):159-174

15. Everson C.A., Bergmann B.M., Rechtschaffen A. Sleep.1989. 12: 13–21

16. Gabriel BM, Zierath JR. Nat. Rev. Endocrinol. 2019;15:197–206

17. Tordjman S., Chokron S., Delorme R., Charrier A., Bellissant E., Jaafari N., Fougerou C. 2017. Curr Neuropharmacol 15:434–443

18. Vallat R., Shah V.D., Redline S., Attia P., Walker M.P. PLoS Biol. 2020;18(6):e3000726

19. Shokri-Kojori Ehsan, Wang Gene-Jack, Wiers Corinde E., Demiral Sukru B., Guo Min, Kim Sung Won, Lindgren Elsa, Ramirez Veronica, Zehra Amna, Freeman Clara, Miller Gregg, Manza Peter, Srivastava Tansha, De Santi Susan, Tomasi Dardo, Benveniste Helene, Volkow Nora D. Proc Natl Acad Sci USA. 2018;115(17):4483–4488

20. Lucey BP, Hicks TJ, McLeland JS, et al. Ann Neurol. 2018;83(1):197-204

21. Greer SM, Goldstein AN, Walker MP. Nat Commun. 2013;4:2259

22. Nedeltcheva AV, Kilkus JM, Imperial J, Schoeller DA, Penev PD. Ann Intern Med. 2010 Oct 5;153(7):435-41

23. Chaput JP, Després JP, Bouchard C, Tremblay A. Sleep. 2008;31(4):517-523

24. Vallat R., Shah V.D., Redline S., Attia P., Walker M.P. PLoS Biol. 2020;18(6):e3000726

25. Everson C.A., Bergmann B.M., Rechtschaffen A. Sleep.1989. 12: 13-21

26. https://www.bbc.com/future/article/20180118-the-boy-who-stayed-awake-for-11-days. Retrieved November, 2020

27. https://www.telegraph.co.uk/sport/football/competitions/euro-2012/9348993/Chinese-man-dies-after-Euro-2012-viewing-marathon.html. Retrieved November, 2020

28. Zimmermann RC, McDougle CJ, Schumacher M, et al. J Clin Endocrinol Metab. 1993;76(5):1160-1164

29. Gabriel BM, Zierath JR. Nat. Rev. Endocrinol. 2019;15:197–206

30. Fuller PM, Lu J, Saper CB. Science. 2008 May 23;320(5879):1074-7

31. Wehrens SMT, Christou S, Isherwood C, et al. Curr Biol. 2017;27(12):1768-1775.e3

32. Ju D., Zhang W., Yan J., Zhao H., Li W., Wang J., Liao M., Xu Z., Wang Z. et al. Sci Transl Med. 2020.12(542). pii: eaba0769

33. Huang, L., Q. Li, Y. Chen, X. Wang and X. Zhou. African Journal of Microbiology Research.2009. 3(12): 957-961

34. Wada K, Yata S, Akimitsu O, et al. J Circadian Rhythms. 2013;11:4

35. Wang XS, Armstrong ME, Cairns BJ, Key TJ, Travis RC. Occup Med (Lond). 2011;61(2):78-89

36. Esmaily H, Sahebkar A, Iranshahi M, Ganjali S, Mohammadi A, Ferns G, et alChin J Integr Med. 2015;21:332–8

37. Ng Q.X., Koh S.S.H., Chan H.W., Ho C.Y.X. J. Am. Med. Dir. Assoc. 2017;18:503–508

38. Kanchanatawan B, Tangwongchai S, Sughondhabhirom A, Suppapitiporn S, Hemrunrojn S, Carvalho AF, Maes M. Neurotox Res. 2018 Apr;33(3):621-633

39. Sanmukhani J, Satodia V, Trivedi J, Patel T, Tiwari D, Panchal B, Goel A, Tripathi CB. Phytother Res. 2014 Apr;28(4):579-85

40. Shoba, G. , Joy, D. , Joseph, T. , Majeed, M. , Rajendran, R. , & Srinivas, P. S. Planta Medica.1998. 64(4); 353–356

41. Ngamsuttha N. 2012. Turmeric, varieties Trang 1 and 84-2. Kasikorn Hospital, Year 85, Issue 4.July - August. Department of Agriculture, Bangkok: 108-111

42. Furuyashiki A., Tabuchi K., Norikosh K., Kobayashi T., & Oriyama S. (2019). Environmental Health and Preventive Medicine, 24(46), 1–11

43. Antonelli M., Barbieri G., Donelli D Int. J. Biometeorol. 2019;63:1117–1134

44. Murtagh EM, Murphy MH, Boone-Heinonen J. Curr Opin Cardiol. 2010;25(5):490-496

45. https://blog.23andme.com/health-traits/what-patients-say-works-for-depression. Retrieved August, 2020

46. Heinzel S, Lawrence JB, Kallies G, Rap M A, Heissel A. GeroPsych: The Journal of Gerontopsychology and Geriatric Psychiatry.2015. 28(4), 149–162

47. Childs E, de Wit H. Front Physiol. 2014;5:161

48. Qato DM, Ozenberger K, Olfson M. JAMA. 2018;319(22):2289-2298

49. https://www.who.int/news-room/fact-sheets/detail/depression. Retrieved December, 2020

50. Noonan S, Zaveri M, Macaninch E, et al. BMJ Nutrition, Prevention & Health 2020;bmjnph-2019-000053

51. Mohammadi AA, Jazayeri S, Khosravi-Darani K, Solati Z, Mohammadpour N, Asemi Z, Adab Z, Djalali M, Tehrani-Doost M, Hosseini M, Eghtesadi S. Nutr Neurosci. 2016 Nov;19(9):387-395

52. Yong SJ, Tong T, Chew J, Lim WL. Front Neurosci. 2020 Jan 14;13:1361

53. Tamarkin L, Danforth D, Lichter A et al. Science. 1982. 216:1003–1005

54. Karasek M. Exp Gerontol. 2004;39(11-12):1723-1729

55. Hikichi T, Tateda N, Miura T. Clin Ophthalmol. 2011;5:655-660

56. Bubenik GA. J Physiol Pharmacol. 2008;59 Suppl 2:33-51

57. Zimmermann RC, McDougle CJ, Schumacher M, et al. J Clin Endocrinol Metab. 1993;76(5):1160-1164

58. Wada K, Yata S, Akimitsu O, et al. J Circadian Rhythms. 2013;11:4

59. Fukushige H, Fukuda Y, Tanaka M, et al. J Physiol Anthropol. 2014;33(1):33

60. Nagashima S, Yamashita M, Tojo C, Kondo M, Morita T, Wakamura T. J Physiol Anthropol. 2017;36(1):20

61. Karasek M. Exp Gerontol. 2004;39(11-12):1723-1729

62.   Hikichi T, Tateda N, Miura T. Clin Ophthalmol. 2011;5:655-660

63.   Hunter CM, Figueiro MG. Biol Res Nurs. 2017;19(4):365-374

64.   Youngstedt SD, Kripke DFSleep Med Rev. 2004;8(3):159-174

65.   Suhner A, Schlagenhauf P, Johnson R, Tschopp A, Steffen RChronobiol Int. 1998;15(6):655–666

66.   Burkhardt S, Tan DX, Manchester LC, Hardeland R, Reiter RJ. J Agric Food Chem. 2001;49:4898–4902

67.   Howatson G, Bell PG, Tallent J, Middleton B, McHugh MP, Ellis J. Eur J Nutr. 2012 Dec;51(8):909-16

68.   Bubenik GA. J Physiol Pharmacol. 2008;59 Suppl 2:33-51

CHAPTER 16: Biohacking your body to rejuvenate old cells and slow down aging

1.   Baker DJ, Childs BG, Durik M, Wijers ME, Sieben CJ, Zhong J, et al. Flindt, R. Amazing number in biology. Springer-Verlag, 2006.

2.   Okuda T, Yokotsuka K. Am J Enol Vitic 1996;67:93–9

3.   Shrikanta A, Kumar A, Govindaswamy V. J Food Sci Technol. 2015;52(1):383-390

4.   Ling L., Gu S., Cheng Y. Mol. Med. Rep. 2017.15; 1188–1194

5.   Covarrubias, A.J., Kale, A., Perrone, R. et al. Nat Metab. 2020: 2; 1265–1283

6.   Chini C, Hogan KA, Warner GM, Tarragó MG, Peclat TR, Tchkonia T, Kirkland JL, Chini E. Biochem Biophys Res Commun. 2019 May 28;513(2):486-493

7.   Connell NJ, Houtkooper RH, Schrauwen P. Diabetologia. 2019;62(6):888-899

8.   Camacho-Pereira J, Tarragó MG, Chini CCS, et al. Cell Metab. 2016;23(6):1127-1139

9.   Escande C, Nin V, Price NL, Capellini V, Gomes AP, Barbosa MT, O'Neil L, White TA, Sinclair DA, Chini EN. Diabetes. 2013 Apr;62(4):1084-93

10.   Balan E, Decottignies A, Deldicque L. Nutrients. 2018;10(12):1942

11.   Ornish D, Lin J, Chan JM, Epel E, et al. Lancet Oncol. 2013;14:1112–1120

12.   Tran HTT., Schreiner M., Schlotz N., Lamy E. Nutrients. 2019;11(4). pii: E786

13.   Horbowicz M. Vegetable Crops Research Bulletin.2003.58;23-40

14.   Tsoukalas D, Fragkiadaki P, Docea AO, et al. Mol Med Rep. 2019;20(4):3701-3708

15.   Tsoukalas D, Fragkiadaki P, Docea AO, et al. Mol Med Rep. 2019;20(4):3701-3708

16.   Zhu H, Guo D, Li K, et al. Int J Obes (Lond). 2012;36(6):805-809

17.   Qi H, Pei D. Cell Res. 2007 Jul;17(7):578-80

18.   Hou P, Li Y, Zhang X, Liu C, Guan J, Li H, Zhao T, Ye J, Yang W, Liu K, Ge J, Xu J, Zhang Q, Zhao Y, Deng H. Science. 2013 Aug 9;341(6146):651-4

19.   Suvorova II, Knyazeva AR, Petukhov AV, Aksenov ND, Pospelov VA. Cell Death Discov. 2019;5:61

20.   Spehar K, Pan A, Beerman I. Stem Cells. 2020 Sep;38(9):1060-1077

21.   Ding DF, Li XF, Xu H, Wang Z, Liang QQ, Li CG, Wang YJ. J Integr Med. 2013 Nov;11(6):389-96

22.   Banaszewski K, Park E, Edirisinghe I, Cappozzo JC, Burton-Freeman BM. J. Berry Res. 3 (2), 113-126

23.   Huang W, Li ML, Xia MY, Shao JY. Int J Mol Med. 2018;42(1):208-218

24. Suvorova II, Knyazeva AR, Petukhov AV, Aksenov ND, Pospelov VA. Cell Death Discov. 2019;5:61

25. Ling L., Gu S., Cheng Y. Mol. Med. Rep. 2017.15; 1188–1194

26. Tripathi V, Chhabria S, Jadhav V, Bhartiya D, Tripathi A. Stem Cell Rev Rep. 2018 Apr;14(2):213-222

27. Johnson J.J., Nihal M., Siddiqui I.A., Scarlett C.O., Bailey H.H., Mukhtar H., Ahmad N. Mol. Nutr. Food Res. 2011;55:1169–1176

28. La Porte C, Voduc N, Zhang G, Seguin I, Tardiff D, Singhal N, et al. Clin Pharmacokinet. (2010) 49:449–54

29. Smoliga JM, Blanchard O. Molecules. 2014;19:17154–72

30. Wightman EL, Reay JL, Haskell CF, Williamson G, Dew TP, Kennedy DO. Br J Nutr. 2014;112(2):203–213

31. Gehm BD, McAndrews JM, Chien PY, Jameson JL. Proc Natl Acad Sci U S A. 1997;94(25):14138-14143

32. Bayele H. K. Sci Rep. 2020.10(1):5338

33. Bo S, Togliatto G, Gambino R, et al. Acta Diabetol. 2018;55(4):331-340

34. Walle T., Hsieh F., DeLegge M.H., Oatis J.E., Jr., Walle U.K. Drug Metab. Dispos. 2004;32:1377–1382

35. Wightman EL, Reay JL, Haskell CF, Williamson G, Dew TP, Kennedy DO. Br J Nutr. 2014;112(2):203–213

36. Peltz L., Gomez J., Marquez M., Alencastro F., Atashpanjeh N., Quang T. et al. PLoS One. 2012;7:e37162

37. Smoliga JM, Blanchard O. Molecules. 2014;19:17154–72

38. Walle T., Hsieh F., DeLegge M.H., Oatis J.E., Jr., Walle U.K. Drug Metab. Dispos. 2004;32:1377–1382

39. Ortuño J., Covas M.-I., Farre M., Pujadas M., Fito M., Khymenets O., Andres-Lacueva C., Roset P., Joglar J., Lamuela-Raventós M., Torre R. Food Chem, 2010.120;1123-1130

40. Okuda T, Yokotsuka K. Am J Enol Vitic 1996;67:93–9

41. Shrikanta A, Kumar A, Govindaswamy V. J Food Sci Technol. 2015;52(1):383-390

42. Ramírez-Garza S.L., Laveriano-Santos E.P., Marhuenda-Muñoz M. Nutrients. 2018.10(12): 1892

43. Gehm BD, McAndrews JM, Chien PY, Jameson JL. Proc Natl Acad Sci U S A. 1997;94(25):14138-14143

44. Heinrich U., Tronnier H., Stahl W., Béjot M., Maurette J.-M. Skin Pharmacol. Physiol. 2006;19:224–231

45. Darvin M, Patzelt A, Gehse S, et al. Eur J Pharm Biopharm. 2008;69(3):943–947

46. Meinke M.C., Nowbary C.K., Schanzer S., Vollert H., Lademann J., Darvin M.E. Nutrients. 2017;9:775

47. Yanti Y, Rukayadi KH, Lee JK, et al. J Oral Sci. 2009;51(1):87–95

48. Shim J.-S., Kwon Y.-Y., Hwang J.-K. Planta Medica. 2008;74(3):239–244

49. Shim JS, Choi EJ, Lee CW, Kim HS, Hwang JK. Journal of Medicinal Food. 2009;12(3):601–607

50. Woo SW, Rhim DB, Kim C, Hwang JK. Prev Nutr Food Sci. 2015;20(1):15–21

51. Fam VW, Holt RR, Keen CL, Sivamani RK, Hackman RM. Nutrients. 2020 Nov 4;12(11):E3381

52. https://en.wikipedia.org/wiki/Ataulfo_(mango). asitkghosh@yahoo.com Thaumaturgist - Own work. Retrieved June, 2020

53. Esquirol Y., Ferrieres J.,Marquie JC., Huo Yung Kai S., Niezborala ., Berard E., Bongard V., Ruidavets JB. Congress of the European Society of Cardiology, Munich, 26 August, 2018

54. Westfall S, Lomis N, Prakash S. Scientific Reports. 2018;8:8362

55. Liao N., Shi Y., Zhang C., Zheng Y., Wang Y., Zhao B., Zeng Y., Liu X., Liu J. Stem Cell Res. Ther. 2019;10:306

56. Scholtens RM, van Munster BC, van Kempen MF, de Rooij SE. J Psychosom Res. 2016 Jul;86:20-7

57. Fanelli S, Francioso A, Cavallaro RA, d'Erme M, Mosca L, et al. (2018) Int J Clin Nutr Diet 4: 134

58. Richie JP Jr, Nichenametla S, Neidig W, Calcagnotto A, Haley JS, Schell TD, Muscat JE. Eur J Nutr. 2015 Mar;54(2):251-63

59. Ornish D, Lin J, Chan JM, Epel E, et al. Lancet Oncol. 2013;14:1112–1120

60. Valcavi R, Dieguez C, Azzarito C, Edwards CA, Dotti C, Page MD, Portioli I, Scanlon MF. Clin Endocrinol (Oxf). 1987 Apr;26(4):453-8

61. Wright J, Aldhous M, Franey C, English J, Arendt J. Clin Endocrinol (Oxf). 1986;24(4):375-382

62. Meeking DR, Wallace JD, Cuneo RC, Forsling M, Russell-Jones DL. Eur J Endocrinol. 1999;141(1):22-26

63. Nassar E, Mulligan C, Taylor L, et al. J Int Soc Sports Nutr. 2007;4:14

64. Redman LM, Veldhuis JD, Rood J, et al. Aging Cell. 2010;9(1):32-39

65. Sources: https://en.wikipedia.org, https://gerontology.wikia.org and https://enacademic.com

66. Lenton KJ, Sané AT, Therriault H, Cantin AM, Payette H, Wagner JR. Am J Clin Nutr. 2003 Jan;77(1):189-95

CHAPTER 17: Eat less and live longer

1.   Lehallier B., Gate D., Schaum N. et al. Nat Med. 2019.25; 1843–1850

2.   Yu BP, Masoro EJ, Murata I, Bertrand HA, Lynd FT. Journals Gerontol. 1982;37(2):130–41

3.   Kagawa Y. Preventive medicine. 1978;7:205–217

4.   Bureau of Agricultural Economics, U.S. Supplement for 1949 to Consumption of food in the United States, 1909–48. In: U.S. Dept. of Agriculture, B.o.A.E., editor. Miscellaneous publication (United States. Dept. of Agriculture) Washington, D.C.: 1950. p. 52

5.   Kalm LM, Semba RD. The Journal of nutrition. 2005;135:1347–1352

6.   Cangemi R, Friedmann AJ, Holloszy JO, Fontana L. Aging Cell. 2010 Apr;9(2):236-42

7. Rayner JJ, Abdesselam I, Peterzan MA, Akoumianakis I, Akawi N, Antoniades C, Tomlinson JW, Neubauer S, Rider OJ. Int J Obes (Lond) 2019;43:2536–2544

8. https://www.pbrc.edu/research-and-faculty/calculators/weight-loss-predictor/

9. Racette SB, Weiss EP, Villareal DT, Arif H, Steger-May K, Schechtman KB, Fontana L, Klein S, Holloszy JO. Journals of Gerontology Series A: Biological Sciences and Medical Sciences. 2006b;61:943–950

10. Civitarese AE, Carling S, Heilbronn LK, et al. PLoS Med. 2007;4(3):e76

11. Redman L. M., Smith S. R., Burton J. H., Martin C. K., Il'yasova D., Ravussin E., Cell Metab. 2018.27;805–815.e4

12. Willcox BJ, Willcox DC, Todoriki H et al. Ann N Y Acad Sci 2007; 1114: 434–55

13. Cangemi R, Friedmann AJ, Holloszy JO, Fontana L. Aging Cell. 2010 Apr;9(2):236-42

14. Fontana L, Klein S, Holloszy JO, Premachandra BN. J Clin Endocrinol Metab. 2006 Aug;91(8):3232-5

15. Le Couteur DG, et al. Age and Ageing. 2016;45:443–447

16. Le Couteur DG, Solon-Biet S, Cogger VC et al. Cell Mol Life Sci 2016; 73: 1237–52

17. Willcox D.C., Scapagnini G., Willcox B.J. Mech. Ageing Dev. 2014;136–137:148–162

18. Sho H. Asia Pac. J. Clin. Nutr. 2001;10:159–164

19. Chang A.Y., Skirbekk V.F., Tyrovolas S., Kassebaum N.J., Dieleman J.L. Lancet Public Health. 2019;4:e159–e167

20. Xie J, de Souza Alves V, von der Haar T, O'Keefe L, Lenchine RV, Jensen KB, Liu R, Coldwell MJ, Wang X, Proud CG. Curr Biol. 2019 Mar 4;29(5):737-749.e5

21. Kirkwood T. B. L. and Holliday Robin. Proc. R. Soc. Lond. B. 1979. 205531–546

22. Moatt JP, Savola E, Regan JC, Nussey DH, Walling CA. Bioessays. 2020;e1900241

23. Sabatini D.M. Proc. Natl. Acad. Sci. USA. 2017;114:11818–11825

24. Escobar KA, Visconti LM, Wallace AW, VanDusseldorp TA. Adv Geriatr Med Res. 2020;2(1):e200002

CHAPTER 18: Design your own healthy plates

1. https://evolution.berkeley.edu/evolibrary/article/history_09 (accessed June 20,2020)

2. Berry S, Valdes A, Davies R, et al. Curr Dev Nutr. 2019;3(Suppl 1):nzz037.OR31-01-19

3. Bamberger C., Rossmeier A., Lechner K., Wu L., Waldmann E., Fischer S., Stark R.G., Altenhofer J., Henze K., Parhofer K.G. Nutrients. 2018;10:244

4. Wang Y, Chang J, Liu X, et al. Aging (Albany NY). 2016;8(11):2915-2926